Infertility Management Series

Basic Laboratory
Procedure in ART

Infertility Management Series
Basic Laboratory
Procedure in ART

Series Editors

Juan A Garcia-Velasco MD PhD
Director IVI Madrid
Madrid, Spain
IVI Director
Nova IVI Fertility, India and
GCC, Abu Dhabi, UAE
Professor
Obstetrics and Gynecology
Rey Juan Carlos University
Madrid, Spain

Manish Banker MD DGO
Director
Nova IVI Fertility and Pulse Women's Hospital
Ahmedabad, Gujarat, India
Past President
Indian Society for Assisted Reproduction (ISAR)

Editors

Irene Rubio Palacios PhD
Co-Head, IVF Department, NIF India
Medical Affairs, IVI-RMA Global, Spain

Javier Herrero Zapata PhD
Co-Head, IVF Department, NIF India
Medical Affairs, IVI-RMA Global, Spain

Foreword

Nicolás Prados Dodd PhD
Laboratory Coordinator IVI-RMA Global
Associate Professor
Pablo Olavide University
Sevilla, Spain

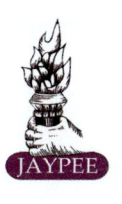

The Health Sciences Publisher
New Delhi | London | Panama

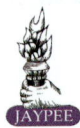 **Jaypee Brothers Medical Publishers (P) Ltd**

Headquarters
Jaypee Brothers Medical Publishers (P) Ltd.
4838/24, Ansari Road, Daryaganj
New Delhi 110 002, India
Phone: +91-11-43574357
Fax: +91-11-43574314
E-mail: jaypee@jaypeebrothers.com

Overseas Offices
JP Medical Ltd.
83 Victoria Street, London
SW1H 0HW (UK)
Phone: +44-20 3170 8910
Fax: +44(0)20 3008 6180
E-mail: info@jpmedpub.com

Jaypee-Highlights Medical Publishers Inc.
City of Knowledge, Bld. 235, 2nd Floor, Clayton
Panama City, Panama
Phone: +1 507-301-0496
Fax: +1 507-301-0499
E-mail: cservice@jphmedical.com

Jaypee Brothers Medical Publishers (P) Ltd.
17/1-B, Babar Road, Block-B, Shyamoli
Mohammadpur, Dhaka-1207
Bangladesh
Mobile: +08801912003485
E-mail: jaypeedhaka@gmail.com

Jaypee Brothers Medical Publishers (P) Ltd.
Bhotahity, Kathmandu, Nepal
Phone: +977-9741283608
E-mail: kathmandu@jaypeebrothers.com

Website: www.jaypeebrothers.com
Website: www.jaypeedigital.com

Inquiries for bulk sales may be solicited at: jaypee@jaypeebrothers.com

Infertility Management Series: Basic Laboratory Procedure in ART
First Edition: **2018**

ISBN: 978-93-5270-061-5

Printed at: Samrat Offset Pvt. Ltd.

Contributors

Aila Coello MSc
Embryologist
IVI Valencia
Valencia, Spain

Alberto Pacheco PhD
Director
Andrology Laboratory
IVI Madrid, Spain
Associate Professor
Alfonso X "El Sabio" University
Madrid, Spain

Alberto Tejera PhD
Embryologist
IVI Valencia
Valencia, Spain

Ana Cobo PhD
Director
Cryopreservation Laboratory
IVI Valencia, Valencia
Associate Professor
Rey Juan Carlos University
Madrid, Spain

Carlos Simón PhD
IVI-INCLIVA Foundation
Valencia
Associate Professor
Valencia University
Valencia, Spain

Carmela Albert PhD
IVF Laboratory Supervisor
IVI Valencia
Valencia, Spain

Cristina González-Ravina PhD
Director
Andrology Laboratory
IVI Sevilla, Sevilla
Associate Professor
Pablo Olavide University
Sevilla, Spain

Irene Rubio Palacios PhD
Co-Head, IVF Department
NIF India
Medical Affairs
IVI-RMA Global, Spain

Javier Herrero Zapata PhD
Co-Head, IVF Department
NIF, India
Medical Affairs
IVI-RMA Global, Spain

José V Medrano PhD
Health Research Institute La Fe
Valencia, Spain

Marcos Meseguer PhD
IVF Scientific Supervisor
IVI Valencia, Valencia
Associate Professor
Valencia University
Valencia, Spain

Mª José de los Santos PhD
Director
IVF Laboratory
IVI Valencia, Valencia
IVI-INCLIVA Foundation
Valencia, Spain

Pilar Gámiz PhD
IVF Laboratory Supervisor
IVI Valencia
Valencia, Spain

Deven Patel MSc
Clinical Embryologist and
Regional Manager
NIF Ahmedabad
Ahmedabad, Gujarat, India

Hetal Shukla MSc
Chief Andrologist
NIF Ahmedabad
Ahmedabad, Gujarat, India

Preeti Shah MSc
Clinical Embryologist and
Regional Manager
NIF Ahmedabad
Ahmedabad, Gujarat, India

Pallavi Menon MSc
Clinical Embryologist and
Lab Manager
NIF Sadashivanagar
Bengaluru, Karnataka, India

Carol Rubina D'Souza MSc
Clinical Embryologist
NIF Sadashivanagar
Bengaluru, Karnataka, India

Belén Aparicio MSc
Embryologist
IVI Valencia
Valencia, Spain

Aditi Kotdawala MSc
Clinical Embryologist and
Lab Manager
NIF Ahmedabad
Ahmedabad, Gujarat, India

Anisha Uberoi MSc
Clinical Embryologist and
Lab Manager
NIF Delhi West
New Delhi, India

Himani Agnihotri MSc
Clinical Embryologist
NIF Delhi West
New Delhi, India

Rishina Bansal MSc
Clinical Embryologist and
Lab Manager
NIF Andheri
Mumbai, Maharashtra, India

Shridutt Gaitonde BSc
Clinical Embryologist
NIF Andheri
Mumbai, Maharashtra, India

Navin Desai MSc
Clinical Embryologist
NIF Andheri
Mumbai, Maharashtra, India

Natalia Basile PhD
Clinical Embryologist
IVI Madrid
Madrid, Spain

Foreword

In this edition of the series about infertility management, we wanted to include one of the fundamental aspects of any treatment of assisted reproduction: all the procedures performed in the laboratories of in vitro fertilization (IVF) and andrology. Each couple that needs to undergo a fertility cycle deserves the widest range of treatments available, from the simplest to the most complex, to find the most convenient solution for their specific problem.

The purpose of this book is to provide a reliable and updated version of the techniques performed in an IVF unit and to give an idea of the state-of-the art technologies. Another important point to consider is the design, set-up and staff that form the IVF unit, as ultimately it will impact also in the consecution of the clinical objectives.

I am sure that this book will be a reference for the professionals of the field, as well as, for the students that want to increase their knowledge about the current trends from a clinical perspective. At the same time, the publication of this book continues the formative work of Nova IVI Fertility, in its spirit to contribute to the maximum in the formation and enrichment of the professionals of Human Assisted Reproduction.

Nicolás Prados Dodd PhD
Laboratory Coordinator IVI RMA Global
Associate Professor
Pablo Olavide University
Sevilla, Spain

Preface

The progress in assisted reproductive technique (ART) has involved putting a new technology in constant evolution at the service of the population. This implies the idea of being able to recover it when desired, not being necessarily, so much less when it is directly linked to age. For these reasons, it seems that the tendency is not to decrease, but quite the opposite. This implies an enormous effort at the clinical level, due to the difficulties involved in the diagnosis and the treatment of the reproductive disorders of each member of the couple; and at the technological level, in the search for progress that provides solutions for the majority of infertile couples. From the most basic techniques, as the conventional in vitro fertilization or the embryo transfer, to the most complex as the genetic diagnosis, the magnetic cell sorting of sperm cells or the use of stem cells to develop into gametes, all have the same importance for the couple whose problem needs solution. This book aims to provide an overview of all the procedures being offered in ART and help to improve the practice of the professionals of the field.

Irene Rubio Palacios PhD
Javier Herrero Zapata PhD

Acknowledgments

The editors thank all the authors for their great contribution, professional commitment and enthusiasm displayed.

We also like to express our gratitude to Mr Jitendar P Vij (Group Chairman), Mr Ankit Vij (Group President), Ms Chetna Malhotra Vohra (Associate Director—Content Strategy), and Ms Angima Shree (Senior Development Editor) of Jaypee Brothers Medical Publishers, New Delhi, India, for shaping up of the book.

Contents

Chapter 1

Semen Analysis and Sperm Preparation

Hetal Shukla, Deven Patel, Preeti Shah

INTRODUCTION

Semen analysis though being imperfect is an important tool in the diagnosis of male infertility.[1] Cellular and chemical components of human semen can provide information on the functional properties of the organs producing this fluid, i.e. the testis, epididymis, and accessory glands.[2]

In Table 1.1, we can see the historic evolution from the first semen observations to the latest guidelines published about the topic.

While semen analysis is an important tool in diagnosing male infertility, it is to be remembered that reference ranges given by the World Health Organization (WHO) manual are not diagnostic cutoff values but only results obtained out of an observation of a fertile population. Male fertility cannot be determined solely on the result of a semen analysis, as there is no evidence stating the exact number and quality of sperm required for a man to be considered fertile. As Christopher De Jonge has rightly said, semen analysis is still the subject of both commendation and condemnation.[3]

SEMEN ANALYSIS

Semen analysis involves different steps to be followed:
- Semen sample collection
- Examining the physical characteristics of the seminal fluid
- Enumerating and classifying the morphological aspects of sperms and other cells
- Evaluating the functional status of the sperm
- Detecting perceptible immunological effects in semen
- Estimating concentrations of the various biochemical substances present in the seminal plasma to understand functional properties of the organs producing this fluid, i.e. the testis, epididymis, and accessory glands.

Semen Sample Collection and Handling

Semen ejaculate of the patient must be collected in a sterile container preferably by masturbation in a special private room provided. Hands and genitals

Table 1.1: History and milestones on the semen sample analysis.		
1677	Anton van Leeuwenhoek	First observed human spermatozoa from an ejaculate, along with his student, Johan Ham. The microscope used was created by him and saw millions of small motile "animals" which he called animalcules[4] and he was the first to observe the serpentine motion of the animalcules and different shapes of spermatozoa across different species[5]
1771	Lazzaro Spallanzani	After extensive work on artificial insemination, observed spermatic animalcules in various species and documented the fertilizing capacity of the sperm.[6]
1837	Rudolf Wagner	Documented his observations on spermatozoa of more than 400 species, including humans. He concluded "the motility of the sperm was greatest at the point of ejaculation and was less in sperm taken from vas deferens and even lesser or nonexistent in sperm taken from testis"[7]
1866	J Marion Sims	He made an important observation after postcoital cervical mucus test that the presence of spermatozoa indicates that the male is not barren[8]
1929	Macomber and Sanders	Quantitatively assessed spermatozoa. From the study which involved 294 males, it was deduced that a "normal" reference value of above 60 million/mL significantly increases the chances of pregnancy. They also tried to establish a method for counting spermatozoa with the help of a blood counting chamber[9]
1951	John Macleod	After his remarkable study on 1800 men comparing sperm characteristics between fertile and infertile populations—normal reference value was brought down to 20 million/mL[10]
1980	World Health Organization (WHO)	Published first manual on semen analysis to help establish uniformity in methods of evaluating spermatozoa worldwide. It has been updated periodically with the fifth edition currently being in use[11]
1981	Rune Eliasson	Stated that it was not justified to discriminate a semen sample with 5 million/mL sperm concentration as infertile[2]
1990s	CellSoft, Hamilton-Thorne and SQM	Introduction of computer-assisted semen analysis (CASA)

must be washed and dried using soap and dry tissues before collection. Before sample collection, the WHO manual recommends a maximum interval of abstinence between 2 days and 7 days, but recommends that the interval should be "as constant as possible". Therefore, standardization of, "abstinence time" to 3–4 days is strongly advised.[12] As the initial portion of the semen is rich in sperm quantity, spillage if any either initial or later must be recorded.

Some men may have difficulties in producing a semen sample at the laboratory. In these cases, the man may collect a first sample at home and deliver it to the laboratory within 60 minutes.[12,13] During the transport sample container must be tightly closed and kept in polystyrene box to protect from the temperature variation. Rarely, for the man unable to ejaculate through masturbation may use a special, nonspermicidal condom to collect a sample at intercourse.

Semen sample collection container must be properly labeled with patient's name, the clinical history number if any, date of collection and task to be performed. The sample submission must be registered with the patient at the laboratory and acknowledgment signature with relevant consent must be taken duly signed.

As semen sample can show variations, semen samples with compromised semen parameters should be checked a minimum of two properly collected samples, ideally collected over two spermatogenic cycles, examined at 37°C is a good recommendation.

Safety Considerations while Performing Semen Analysis

Semen samples are potentially hazardous due to possible presence of bacteria, protozoan related to sexually transmitted diseases and infectious virus. In the andrology laboratory technicians handling, the semen sample must take utmost care to protect oneself and the semen sample and the laboratory environment.

Following precautions must be taken:
- Routine disinfection of the platform and the surfaces of the andrology laboratory
- Carry out all the procedures under the laminar air flow unit (LAFU)
- Use disposable gloves, laboratory coat and protective face mask
- Avoid sample spillage in the work area
- Disinfect all the laboratory equipment before and after the work
- Wash hands and disinfect the hands at the end of the analysis
- Careful disposal of all the waste material, segregated in different bins, i.e. biohazardous material, for sharp material and decomposable material
- Do not consume food or drinks in the work area.

Physical Examination of Semen

Coagulation and Liquefaction

Normally, semen is ejaculated in a liquid state, which gels shortly thereafter. Absence of coagulation of the sample indicates ejaculatory duct obstruction or congenital absence of vas deferens and seminal vesicles.[14]

Occasionally, samples may not liquefy, making semen evaluation difficult. In these cases, additional treatment, mechanical mixing or enzymatic digestion may be necessary. There are different approaches in those cases:

- Some samples can be induced to liquefy by the addition of an equal volume of physiological medium (e.g. Dulbecco's phosphate-buffered saline; followed by repeated pipetting).[12]
- Inhomogeneity can be reduced by repeated (6–10 times) gentle passage through a blunt gauge 18 (internal diameter 0.84 mm) or gauge 19 (internal diameter 0.69 mm) needle attached to a syringe.[12]
- Digestion by bromelain/physiological medium, a broad specificity proteolytic enzyme, may help to promote liquefaction: prepare 10 IU/mL bromelain in Dulbecco's phosphate-buffered saline; it is difficult to dissolve but, with mixing, most should dissolve within 15–20 minutes. Dilute semen 1 + 1 (1:2) with the 10 IU/mL bromelain, stir with a pipette tip, and incubate at 37°C for 10 minutes. Mix the sample well before further analysis.[12]

Comment: These treatments may affect seminal plasma biochemistry, sperm motility and sperm morphology, and their use must be recorded. The 1 + 1 (1 : 2) dilution of semen with bromelain must be accounted for when calculating sperm concentration.

Viscosity measures the seminal fluid's resistance to flow. High viscosity may interfere with determination of sperm motility, concentration, and antibody coating of spermatozoa. Normally, semen coagulates upon ejaculation and usually liquefies within 15–20 minutes. Semen that remains a coagulum is termed nonliquefied, whereas that which pours in thick strands instead of drops is termed hyperviscous. The clinical significance of abnormalities in liquefaction remains controversial.[15] Exact liquefaction time is of no diagnostic importance unless more than 2 hours elapse without any change. Failure to liquefy is usually a sign that there is inadequate secretion by the prostate of the proteolytic enzymes fibrinolysin, fibrinogenase, and aminopeptidase.[16] Importantly, liquefaction should be differentiated from viscosity, as abnormalities in viscosity can be the result of abnormal prostate function and/or the use of an unsuitable type of plastic container.

Color

Greyish, white, milky white with opacity is the normal color. Pathologically, seminal discoloration may be due to fresh blood, drugs, jaundice, or contamination of semen with urine (e.g. bladder neck dysfunction).

Physiologic yellowish tinge in samples with prolonged abstinence is due to carotene pigment.

Odor

Normal sample may be unpleasant to some but normally it smells spicy or musky. Abnormal semen sample with possible infection or high sperm oxidation may cause malodorous, and pungent smell. Abnormal prostate function may be the reason of odorless semen sample.

pH

Normal semen pH is in the range of 7.2–7.8 and it tends to increase with time after ejaculation as natural buffering decreases. Changes are usually due to inflammation of the prostate or seminal vesicles. In cases of acute prostatitis, vasculitis or bilateral epididymitis the pH will be more than 8 and in cases of chronic infection of these organs or in cases where only prostatic fluids are present the pH will invariably less than 7.2.

Osmolality

Osmolality can be measured by freezing point or vapor pressure osmometer. This is to be determined in the seminal plasma separating it by low speed centrifugation. Normal range of semen osmolality is 340–380 mOsmol/kg. Low osmolality is usually associated with morphologically abnormal sperms.[17]

Volume

Measuring volume should be as precise as possible to the nearest 0.1 mL in graduated centrifuge tube. Lower reference value of semen volume as per WHO manual is 1.5 mL. Volume more than 6 mL may be due to prolonged abstinence or excessive secretion from the accessory sex glands. If a laboratory weighs the semen to find the volume, semen density to be considered varies between 1.043 g/mL and 1.102 g/mL.[18,19]

Aspermia

No sperm seen in ejaculate after orgasm.

Hypospermia

Less than 1.5 mL of semen (Table 1.2).

Hyperspermia

More than 6 mL of semen ejaculated (Table 1.2).
Comment: Improper collection, hypogonadism, retrograde ejaculation, and obstruction of lower urinary tract may yield low volume.

Table 1.2: Summary of the main semen characteristics and its reference values.

Characteristics	Normal (fertile)	Abnormal (subfertile)
Coagulation	Present	Absent
Liquefaction	15–30 minutes	>60 minutes
Odor	Musky or spicy	Malodorous
Color	Greyish or white	Reddish/brown/yellow
Volume	1.5–4.5 mL	<1.5 mL, >6 mL
pH	7.2–7.8	Variable
Osmolality	340–380 mOsmol/kg	Variable

Microscopic Evaluation of Semen

Ideally, microscopic evaluation of semen should be carried out using phase contrast microscope with 20X, 40X, and 100X objective lenses.

Motility

The first aspect of sperm function to assess is sperm motility. This assessment should begin immediately to avoid temperature drop or dehydration of the preparation. As per WHO guidelines 2010,[12] the motility score is represented in percentage progressive motile sperms, percentage of nonprogressively motile sperms and percentage of nonmotile sperms. Rapid and slow progressive motility is calculated by the speed at which sperm moves with flagellar movement in a given volume as a percentage (range 0–100%) by counting 200 sperms.

The efficient passage of spermatozoa through cervical mucus is dependent on rapid progressive motility,[20,21] that is, spermatozoa with a forward progression of at least 25 μm/s. Reduced sperm motility can be a symptom of disorders related to male accessory sex gland secretion and the sequential emptying of these glands.

According to previous editions of the WHO manual motility was scored in following four grades:

1. Rapid progressive motility (i.e. >25 μm/s at 37°C and >20 μm/s at 20°C; note: 25 μm is approximately equal to five head lengths or half a tail length)
2. Slow or sluggish progressive motility
3. Nonprogressive motility (<5 μm/s)
4. Immobility.

A normal semen analysis must contain at least 50% grade A and B, progressively motile spermatozoa. If greater than 50% sperms are immotile then the sperms should be checked for viability. Persistent poor motility is a good predictor of failure in fertilization, an outcome that is actually more important when making decisions regarding a couple's treatment options.[22]

Sperm Concentration

A phase contrast microscope using volumetric dilution and hemocytometry is recommended for all examinations of unstained preparations of fresh or washed semen and is reported as millions of sperm per milliliters.

Improved Neubauer hemocytometer, Makler chamber, Cell-Vu chamber and computer-assisted semen analysis (CASA) can be used to measure sperm count. Hu Ya et al. in their comparative study of accuracy and precision of four methods including hemocytometer, Makler chamber, Cell-Vu chamber, and computer-aided semen analysis for determining sperm concentration concluded that there was not any significant difference between Cell-Vu chamber and CASA.[23] In another study by Sukcharoen et al.[24] a comparison of Makler counting chamber and improved Neubauer hemocytometer was carried out and the sperm concentration obtained with Makler counting chamber was not statistically different from those determined by improved Neubauer hemocytometer in semen samples with concentrations over 40×10^6/mL. But using Makler counting chambers caused a shift in concentration, which were overestimated significantly (p-value < 0.0001) in semen samples with concentrations less than 40×10^6/mL. Overall, Makler chamber counts were 11.2% higher. Although less complicated than the improved Neubauer hemocytometer method, measurement of sperm concentration by Makler counting chamber is an inaccurate method, especially in semen samples with concentrations less than 40×10^6/mL.

Anyway, each laboratory can select its own proper method for manual or computer-aided analysis. Although use of—Makler chamber is showing subjective variations the ease of use with acceptable accuracy, it is commonly used in semen analysis to determine the sperm concentration.

Aggregation of Spermatozoa

The adherence of immotile spermatozoa to each other or of motile spermatozoa to mucus strands, either nonsperm cells or debris is considered to be nonspecific aggregation and should be recorded as such.

Agglutination of Spermatozoa

The tight junctions of sertoli cells forming the blood-testis barrier provide immunologic protection to sperm antigens. The spermatozoon evokes an immune response when exposed to the systemic immune defense system in conditions in which this barrier is disrupted, leading to the formation of antisperm antibodies (ASAs). Certain ASAs have a cytotoxic effect on the spermatozoa and can cause cell death and immobilization of sperm cells. Other effects of ASAs include creating agglutinated clumps of moving sperm in the semen sample, hampering passage of sperm through the cervical mucus, and zonal binding and passage.[25]

Agglutination specifically refers to motile spermatozoa sticking to each other, head-to-head, tail-to-tail or in a mixed way. The motility is often vigorous with a frantic shaking motion, but sometimes the spermatozoa are so agglutinated that their motion is limited. Any motile spermatozoa that stick to each other by their heads, tails or mid pieces should be noted.

Two current methods of detecting antibodies bound to the surface of motile sperm are the mixed agglutination reaction assay [MAR test; only for immunoglobulins G (IgGs)] and the immunobead-binding assay (for IgA, IgG, and IgMs).[26] A positive finding of more than 50% of motile sperm with attached beads is considered to be clinically significant, but with the advent of assisted reproductive technology (ART), ASAs testing has lost its relevance.

The major type of agglutination [reflecting the degree (grades 1–4) and the site of attachment (grades A–E)] should be recorded (Rose et al., 1976):[27]

- *Grade 1:* Isolated, less than 10 spermatozoa per agglutinate, many free spermatozoa
- *Grade 2:* Moderate, 10–50 spermatozoa per agglutinate, free spermatozoa
- *Grade 3:* Large, agglutinates of more than 50 spermatozoa, some spermatozoa still free
- *Grade 4:* Gross, all spermatozoa agglutinated and agglutinates interconnected.

Note:

- *Motile spermatozoa stuck to cells or debris or immotile spermatozoa stuck to each other (aggregation) should not be scored as agglutination*
- *The presence of agglutination is not sufficient evidence to deduce an immunological cause of infertility, but is suggestive of the presence of ASAs; further testing is required*
- *Severe agglutination can affect the assessment of sperm motility and concentration.*

Cellular Elements Other than Spermatozoa

The ejaculate contains cells other than spermatozoa, some of which may be clinically relevant (infection of the male reproductive tract can directly or indirectly cause infertility[28]). These include epithelial cells from the genitourinary tract, as well as leukocytes and immature germ cells, the latter two collectively referred to as "round cells".[29] They can be identified by examining a stained smear at 1000X magnification. These cells can be more precisely

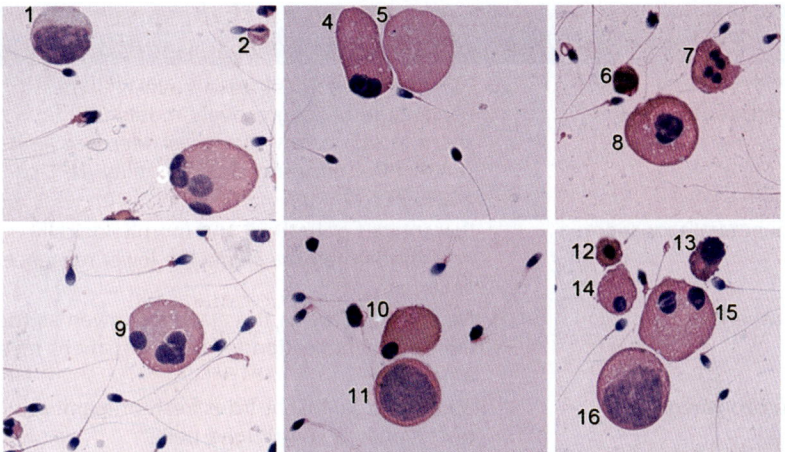

Fig. 1.1: Cellular elements other than spermatozoa. (1-11-16 macrophage, 2 abnormal sperm, 3 and 4 dividing spermatid, 5 cytoplasm, 6 unknown, and 7-8-9-10-12-13-14-15 degenerating spermatid).

identified and quantified by detecting peroxidase activity or the antigen CD45. Their concentration can be estimated as for spermatozoa, from wet preparations or from the ratio of these cells to the number of spermatozoa on the stained smear and the sperm concentration.

Pyospermia is a laboratory finding categorized as the abnormal presence of leukocytes in human ejaculate and may indicate genital tract inflammation.[30] To differentiate round cells from polymorphonuclear (PMN) leukocytes, which are primary sources of reactive oxygen species (ROS) generation, peroxidase staining is used. Neutrophils, polynuclear leukocytes, and macrophages are peroxidase-positive granulocytes (PMN should be 1×10^6/mL), whereas degranulated PMNs, lymphocytes, and immature germ cells are peroxidase-negative (Fig. 1.1 and Table 1.3).[31-33]

SPERM MORPHOLOGY

Historical Evolution of Sperm Morphology

Up to 1970s, only the head of the spermatozoa was considered while assessing morphology. In 1971, Rune Eliasson emphasized the importance of evaluation of the whole spermatozoon including the mid-piece and tail. Eliasson was one of the first to standardize this parameter through a classification system containing three groups—head, mid-piece and tail.[34] Evaluation of sperm morphology has seen two approaches—liberal and strict. The liberal approach as followed by MacLeod, considered all forms to be normal except those that were highly distorted, therefore no criteria was put forth for normal spermatozoa.[35] But in the strict criteria, as described by

Table 1.3: Nomenclature related to semen quality [World Health Organization (WHO) manual, fifth edition].

Aspermia	No semen (no or retrograde ejaculation)
Asthenozoospermia	Percentage of progressively motile (PR) spermatozoa below the lower reference limit [≥40% PR + nonprogressive motility (NP), or ≥32% PR]
Asthenoteratozoospermia	Percentages of both PR and morphologically normal spermatozoa below the lower reference limits
Azoospermia	No spermatozoa in the ejaculate (given as the limit of quantification for the assessment method employed)
Cryptozoospermia	Spermatozoa absent from fresh preparations but observed in a centrifuged pellet
Hemospermia (hematospermia)	Presence of erythrocytes in the ejaculate
Leukospermia (leukocytospermia, pyospermia)	Presence of leukocytes in the ejaculate above the threshold value
Necrozoospermia	Low percentage of live, and high percentage of immotile, spermatozoa in the ejaculate
Normozoospermia	Total number (or concentration, depending on outcome reported)* of spermatozoa, and percentages of PR and morphologically normal spermatozoa, equal to or above the lower reference limits
Oligoasthenozoospermia	Total number (or concentration lower reference value ≥15 million/mL or ≥39 million total sperm count, depending on outcome reported)* of spermatozoa, and PR spermatozoa, below the lower reference limits
Oligoasthenoteratozoospermia	Total number (or concentration lower reference value ≥15 million/mL or ≥39 million total sperm count, depending on outcome reported)* of spermatozoa, and percentages of both PR and morphologically normal spermatozoa, below the lower reference limits
Oligoteratozoospermia	Total number (or concentration lower reference value ≥15 million/mL or ≥39 million total sperm count, depending on outcome reported)* of spermatozoa, and percentage of morphologically normal spermatozoa, below the lower reference limits
Oligozoospermia	Total number (or concentration lower reference value ≥15 million/mL or ≥39 million total sperm count, depending on outcome reported)* of spermatozoa below the lower reference limit
Teratozoospermia	Percentage of morphologically normal spermatozoa below the lower reference limit

*Preference should always be given to total number, as this parameter takes precedence over concentration.

Menkveld and Kruger, even borderline forms are to be considered abnormal.[36] A normal spermatozoa was defined on the basis of spermatozoa obtained from the internal cervical os (after coitus) and from those tightly bound to zona pellucid,[36] thereby providing guidelines which were adopted by the WHO manual. The WHO manual in its first two editions followed the liberal approach after which it implemented the stricter criteria;[34] this would explain the dramatic reduction in the normal morphology reference value from 80% (1st edition)[11] to 4% (5th edition).[12]

The clinical implications of poor morphology scores remain highly controversial. The initial studies using rigid criteria reported that patients undergoing *in vitro* fertilization (IVF) who had greater than 14% normal forms had better fertilization rates.[37] Later studies reported that most impairment in fertilization rates occurred with morphology scores of less than 4% (Fig. 1.2).[38]

The staining of a seminal smear (Papanicolaou, Giemsa, Shorr, and Diff-Quik) allows the quantitative evaluation of normal and abnormal sperm morphological forms in an ejaculate. Smears can be scored for morphology using the WHO classification, or by Kruger's strict criteria classification.[38] WHO method classifies abnormally shaped sperm into specific categories based on specific head, tail, and midpiece abnormalities, which is based on the appearance of sperm recovered from postcoital cervical mucus or from the surface of zona pellucida (>30% normal forms). In contrast, Kruger's strict criteria classifies sperm as normal only if the sperm shape falls within strictly defined parameters of shape and all borderline forms are considered abnormal (>14% normal forms).

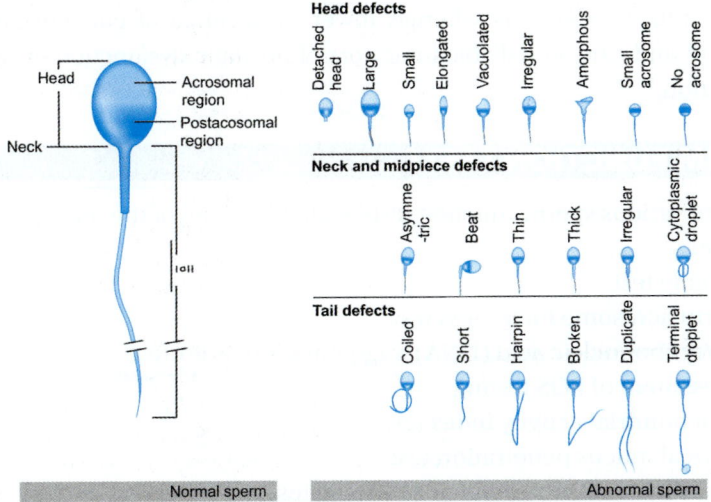

Fig. 1.2: There is a sperm with normal shape and on the right side the multiple defects the sperms can have; these can affect the head, neck or tail region.

- *Head defects:* Large, small, tapered, pyriform, round, amorphous, vacuolated (>20% of the head area occupied by unstained vacuolar areas) heads with small acrosomal area (<40% of head area), double heads, any combination of these
- *Neck and midpiece defects:* Bent neck, asymmetrical insertion of midpiece into head, thick, irregular midpiece, abnormally thin midpiece, any combination of these
- *Tail defects:* Short, multiple, hairpin, broken, bent, kinked, coiled tails, or any combination of these
- *Cytoplasmic droplets:* Greater than one-third of the area of a normal sperm head.

Morphology should be used along with other parameters, and not as an isolated parameter, when determining clinical implications. It is important to realize that, in general, pregnancy is possible with low morphology scores and that both motility and morphology have also demonstrated prognostic value, as do combinations of parameters.[39,40]

BIOCHEMICAL ANALYSIS OF SEMINAL PLASMA

Biochemical analysis of seminal plasma is an important exercise to assess the impairment of epididymal, vesicular, and prostatic function and which may be clinically relevant in patients with hyperviscous semen and to understand genital fluid interactions during the semen coagulation-liquefaction process.

Fructose reflects secretory function of seminal vesicles and in cases of azoospermia absence of fructose points the congenital absence of seminal vesicles and vas deferens whereas lower or absence of concentrations of citric acid and zinc are reliable indicators of prostatic dysfunction or prostatic obstruction.[41-43]

SPERM FUNCTION TESTS

There are various sperm-function tests available; some of the most commonly used are:
- Viability test
- Sperm acrosome intactness test
- Deoxyribonucleic acid (DNA) fragmentation index test
- Assessment of ROS testing
- Mitochondrial activity index test
- Cervical mucus penetration test
- Hemizona and zona pellucida binding test
- Sperm penetration assay (SPA)/zona-free hamster oocyte penetration test/sperm capacitation test.

Viability Test

If the semen sample shows significantly low or no motility it is difficult to judge the percentage of viable sperms. Sperm viability testing is used to determine if nonmotile sperm are alive or dead and are indicated when sperm motility is less than 5–10%. It is useful in primary ciliary dyskinesia where ultrastructural defects in sperm flagella result in absent or extremely low motility but with high viability. Also used to select sperm for intracytoplasmic sperm injection (ICSI), in surgically retrieved testicular tissue, sperms are alive but generally nonmotile, because of lack of epididymal transit.[44,45]

A functional membrane is requisite for the fertilizing ability of spermatozoa, as it plays an integral role in sperm capacitation, acrosome reaction (AR), and binding of the spermatozoon to the egg surface. Viability testing is based on the membrane permeability and it can be done by dye exclusion assays or hypo-osmotic swelling (HOS) test.

- *Dye exclusion assays:* This test relies on the ability of live sperm to resist absorption of certain dyes, whereas these dyes (Eosin Y and Nigrosin or Eosin Y and Trypan blue) penetrate and stain nonviable sperm. Trypan blue and Eosin Y stains, which do not stain live sperm, are the most commonly employed. However, as the technique requires air drying after staining, sperms are killed and not practically useful (Fig. 1.3).[46]
- *Hypo-osmotic swelling test:* The HOS test evaluates the functional integrity of the sperm's plasma membrane and serves as a useful indicator of fertility potential of sperm. When live cells are placed in hypo-osmotic media, water enters the cytoplasm causing the cell to swell, particularly the

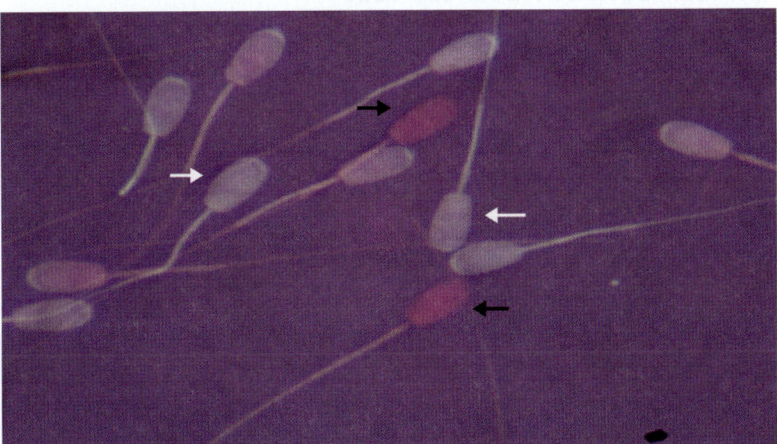

Fig. 1.3: Image of sperm viability test evaluated under a light microscope (1000x) following Eosin-Nigrosin staining. Sperm with an unstained head (white arrows) were regarded as the live sperm. Sperm having red head (black arrows) were deemed as dead sperm.

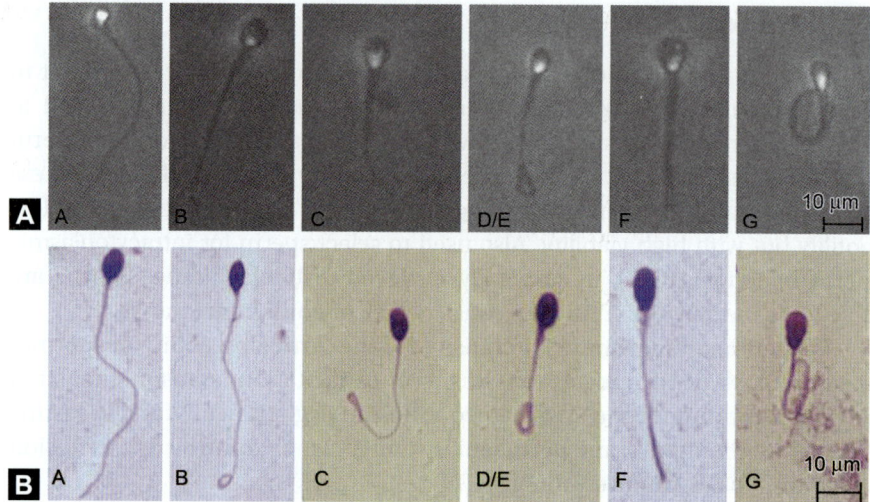

Figs. 1.4A and B: Microscopic observation of different grades of sperm swelling. The different sperm swelling grades (A–G) as observed using (A) Phase-contrast microscopy (1000x magnification) of fresh samples; and (B) Fixed and stained samples using normal light microscopy.

tail, which is calculated as a percentage. This assay does not damage or kill the sperm and is very useful for identifying viable, and nonmotile sperm for ICSI. HOS has a limited ability to predict male fertility, but an HOS result less than 50% is associated with increased miscarriage rates (Figs. 1.4A and B).

Sperm Acrosome Intactness Test

With the use of the ICSI the role of AR in fertilization is minimal, but the percentage value of acrosome intactness can still be of an important tool to predict the male factor, especially when it is idiopathic and repeated failures in natural conception or intrauterine insemination (IUI) with most semen parameters being normal.

Deoxyribonucleic Acid Fragmentation Index Test

Mammalian fertilization involves the direct interaction of the sperm and the oocyte, fusion of the cell membranes, and union of male and female gamete genomes. Although a small percentage of spermatozoa from fertile men also possess detectable levels of DNA damage, (which is repaired by oocyte cytoplasm), there is evidence to show that the spermatozoa of infertile men possess substantially more DNA damage and that this damage may adversely affect reproductive outcomes.[47,48] There appears to be a threshold of sperm DNA damage, which can be repaired by oocyte cytoplasm (i.e. abnormal chromatin packaging, protamine deficiency) beyond which embryo development and pregnancy are impaired.[49,50] We have different tests to assess the DNA fragmentation grade:

Deoxyribonucleic Acid Damage—Direct Tests

- Terminal deoxynucleotidyl transferase-mediated deoxyuridine triphosphate (dUTP) nick end-labeling (TUNEL) assay
- Deoxyribonucleic acid oxidation measurement.

Deoxyribonucleic Acid Damage—Indirect Tests

- Sperm chromatin structure assay (SCSA)
- Sperm chromatin dispersion assay
- Sperm fluorescence in situ hybridization (FISH) analysis.

Assessment of Reactive Oxygen Species Testing

Reactive oxygen species, also referred to as free radicals, are formed as a byproduct of oxygen metabolism. Contaminating leukocytes are the predominant source of ROS in these suspensions.[51] They can be eradicated by enzymes (e.g. catalase or glutathione peroxidase) or by nonenzymatic antioxidants, such as albumin, glutathione, and hypotaurine, as well as by vitamins C and E. Small amounts of ROS may be necessary for the initiation of critical sperm functions, including capacitation and the AR. On the other hand, a high ROS level produces a state known as oxidative stress that can lead to biochemical or physiologic abnormalities with subsequent cellular dysfunction or cell death. Significant levels of ROS can be detected in the semen of 25% of infertile men, whereas fertile men do not have a detectable level of semen ROS.[52–54]

Sperm ROS can also be measured by using cellular probes coupled with flow cytometry by detection of chemiluminescence.[55] Briefly, this is done by incubating fresh semen or sperm suspensions with a redox-sensitive, light-emitting probe (e.g. luminol) and by measuring the light emission over time with a light meter (luminometer).

The clinical value of semen ROS determination in predicting IVF outcome remains unproved but identifying oxidative stress as an underlying cause of sperm dysfunction has the advantage that it suggests possible therapies. Administration of antioxidants has been attempted in several trials with mixed results. But at this point there are no established semen ROS cutoff values that can be used to predict reproductive outcomes.[56,57]

Hemizona and Zona Pellucida Binding Test

The interaction between spermatozoa and the zona pellucida is a critical event leading to fertilization and reflects multiple sperm functions (i.e. completion of capacitation as manifested by the ability to bind to the zona pellucida and to undergo ligand-induced AR).[58-60]

The two most common sperm-zona pellucida binding tests currently utilized are the hemizona assay (HzA)[61] and a competitive intact-zona binding assay.[57] The HzA, which uses nonfertilized oocytes is useful in couples who have failed to fertilize during regular IVF, to determine the cause of the failure. Because the binding is species-specific,[62,63] human zona must be used, thus limiting the utility of these assays.

The induced-AR assays appear to be equally predictive of fertilization outcome and are simpler in their methodologies. The use of a calcium ionophore to induce AR is at the present time the most widely used methodology.[64,65]

Sperm Penetration Assay/Zona-Free Hamster Oocyte Penetration Test/Sperm Capacitation Test

The concept of the SPA was introduced by Yanagamachi.[66] It yields information regarding the fertilizing capacity of human spermatozoa by testing capacitation, AR, sperm or oolemma fusion, sperm incorporation into the ooplasm, and the decondensation of the sperm chromatin during the process. However, penetration of the zona pellucida and normal embryonic development are not tested. The SPA utilizes the golden hamster egg, which is unusual in that removal of its zona pellucida results in loss of all species specificity to egg penetration. Thus, a positive SPA does not guarantee fertilization of intact human eggs nor their embryonic development, whereas a negative SPA has not been found to correlate with poor fertilization in human IVF.[67]

The acrosin assay an indirect measure of sperm penetrating capability measures acrosin, which may be responsible for penetration of the zona pellucida and also triggering the AR.[68] Measurement of acrosin is thought to correlate with sperm binding and penetration of the zona pellucida.[63,69]

Sperm Mitochondrial Activity Index Test

The lack of mitochondrial enzymes impairs sperm motility and may lead to subfertility. This test estimates the incidence of spermatozoa having full complement of mitochondria containing respiratory enzymes which provides energy to sperm for motility. In this test sperms are scored on the basis of the amount of nitroblue tetrazolium (NBT) precipitate. NBT precipitation is classified as standard, substandard, low, residual or nil. Sperm mitochondrial activity index (SMAI) more than 50% is characteristics of fertile semen sample.[70]

Cervical Mucus Penetration Test

The ejaculated spermatozoa must traverse the cervical mucus—a barrier to sperms attempting entry into uterus. It is important to determine the ability of sperms to traverse the natural barrier—mucus. The cervical mucus penetration test is an *in vitro* test wherein the distance traveled by sperms in a mucus filled capillary tube placed in the reservoir containing semen. The capillary is examined under microscope at different intervals of 10 minutes, 30 minutes, and 3 hours to determine linear progression, density of penetration and motility.

SPERM PREPARATION

Isolation of a sperm fraction that contains highly motile, mostly morpho-logically normal sperm free of other cells and debris. The importance of separa-ting the spermatozoa from the seminal plasma is to remove decapacitating factors, reduce the concentration of ROS and to remove contaminating round cells as (leukocytes and immature sperm) responsible for the release of cytotoxic and cytostatic factors.

There are different methods to prepare a semen sample:

Pellet—Swim-up

- Liquefied semen is mixed well in a 6 mL/14 mL round-bottom tube (or in the collection jar) with fresh sperm wash medium up to 1:1 dilution, according to the initial sperm count
- Centrifuge at 600 g for 10 minutes with cap tightly closed. Remove the supernatant and layer with approximately 0.7 mL fresh sperm wash media without disturbing the pellet
- Place the tube in the conventional incubator with tight cap in a slanting position for a period of 20–45 minutes, or until a cloudy middle layer forms
- Collect the upper 0.5 mL cloudy layer and load a drop on the Makler chamber for assessing the final count.

Density Gradient

- In a 15 mL conical tube, make gradients with 1.0 mL of 90% density gradient medium, gently over-laid with 1.0 mL of 45% density gradient medium. Layer up to 2 mL of semen sample on top of the upper gradient layer*
- Spin at 300 g for 20 minutes. Cells, debris and immotile or abnormal sperm accumulate at the interfaces, and the pellet would contain functionally normal sperm
- Carefully collect the pellet, suspend in approximately 0.7 mL sperm wash medium and centrifuge in a second round at 600 g for 5 minutes to remove the remaining gradients
- Resuspend the pellet with 0.5 mL sperm wash medium
- Assess count and motility by loading on the Makler chamber.

---

*Volume of gradient layers can be changed according to the sperm count and debris (Fig. 1.5).

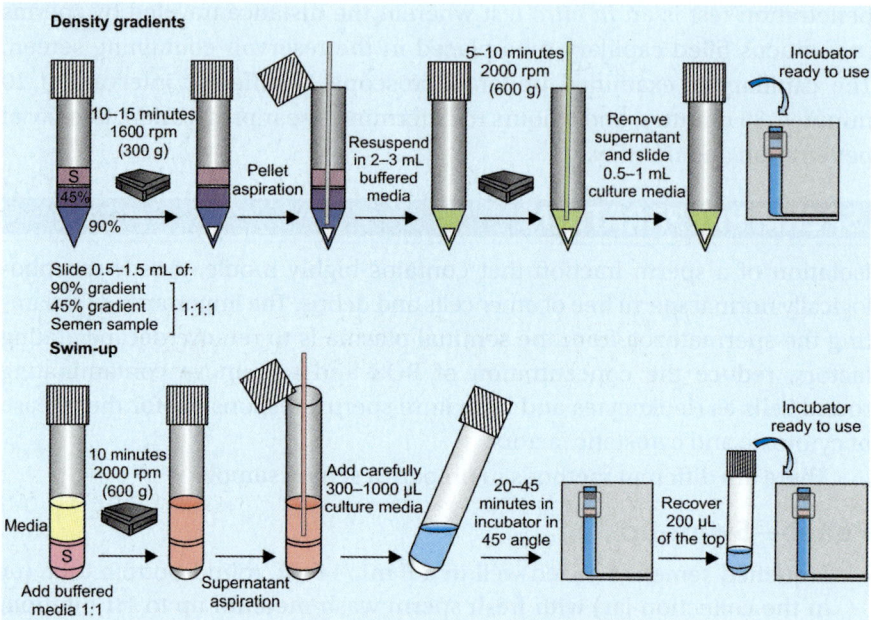

Fig. 1.5: Scheme of the density gradient and swim-up techniques.

Layering (Underlay and Overlay)

- 2 mL of culture medium is pipetted into a 6 mL/14 mL round-bottom tube. Approximately 1.0 mL neat semen is then gently pipetted underneath (underlay) the medium (being very careful not to disturb the interface formed between the semen and the medium) (Fig. 1.6).
- Alternatively 2 mL of medium is gently layered over 1.5–2 mL semen already taken in a 6 mL tube (overlay) (Fig. 1.6).
- Tightly cap the tube and keep it in the conventional incubator or heating block in a standing position for up to 45–60 minutes or until a cloudy middle layer forms
- Pipette 0.5 mL cloudy middle layer in a 6 mL round bottom tube and use it for the IUI/IVF/ICSI, etc.

MAGNETIC-ACTIVATED CELL SORTING

This is a novel technique that enables the immune magnetic separation of healthy spermatozoa by maintaining the structure, viability and functionality of the sperm. This technique is aimed to be used in IUI, IVF or IVF-ICSI cycles as the sperm thus obtained can be used in real time.

Currently, selection of sperm during ICSI is mainly based on motility and morphology. In spite of correlation between sperm motility and morphology with the aforementioned sperm functional markers, invisible anomalies

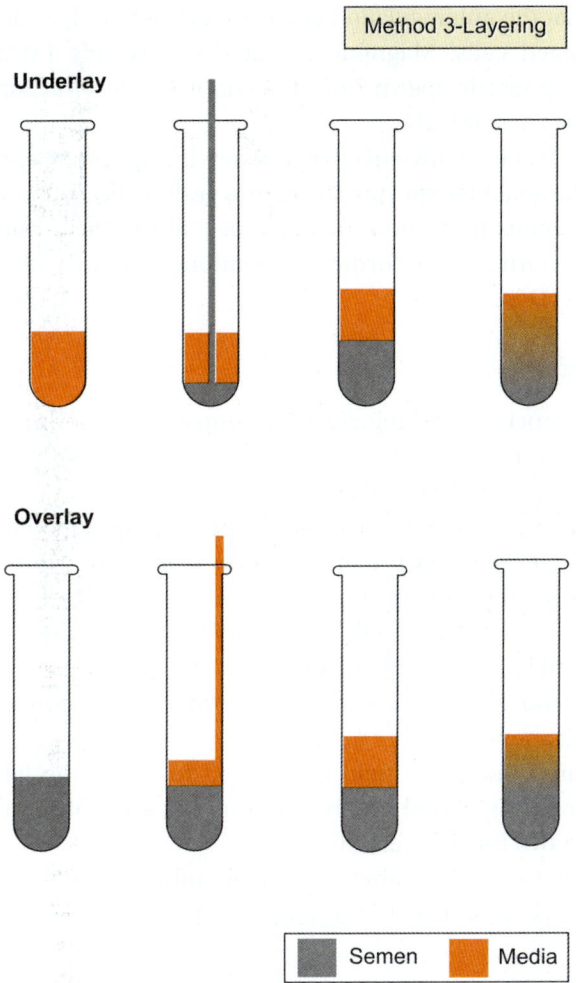

Fig. 1.6: Scheme of the layering technique.

such as programmed cell death (apoptosis), disruption of mitochondrial membrane potential (MMP), caspase-3 activity and damaged chromatin are relatively ignored. This novel sperm selection technique has recently been implemented to ensure that the selected sperms have intact chromatin.

The DNA sperm fragmentation due to apoptosis (programmed cell death), is a regulation process of the cell cycle. This may be due to either inherent (spermatogenesis) or external factors like addiction. DNA damage represented by fragmentation and subsequent sperm apoptosis may be a cause of male infertility that standard methods of semen evaluation, sperm concentration, morphology assessment and motility analysis cannot detect. Several case studies on infertile patients show that there is a high level of apoptotic spermatozoa found in an ejaculate in comparison to a fertile male.

This means that the autoregulation process has failed or that there was a high level of damaged cells. Magnetic-activated cell sorting (MACS) helps to remove such apoptotic sperm from the cohort for fertilization which have less possibilities of survival.

Despite MACS is highly effective at removing apoptotic sperm cells, it is not able to eliminate leukocytes, immature germ cells, seminal plasma and other contaminants from the semen sample. This is the reason why MACS separation is normally performed in conjunction with density gradient centrifugation (DGC).

Mode of Action

- In the presence of physiological Ca^+, phosphatidylserine (PS) has high affinity for annexin-V, which is phospholipid-binding protein showing highly selective binding to PS
- Annexin-V beads, binds to disturbed integrity of sperm membrane but do not have ability to pass the intact sperm membrane. These microbeads are biodegradable superparamagnetic beads conjugated to proteins or antibodies to label target cells (annexin V)
- Externalized PS is early sign of apoptosis
- Efficient removal of caspase in spermatozoa, which represents the main pathway of apoptosis
- High-gradient magnetic field is required to retain the labeled cells in specific columns. Based on annexin binding and subsequent magnetic separation two fractions are obtained:
  - *Annexin negative:* Unlabeled, intact membrane and nonapoptotic
  - *Annexin positive:* Labeled, altered membrane and apoptotic (Fig. 1.7).

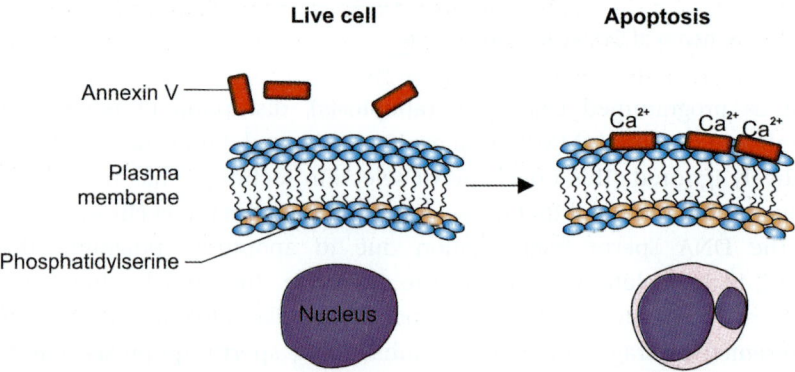

Fig. 1.7: Binding of annexin V beads with externalized phosphatidylserine (PS) on the plasma membrane of the apoptotic cell in the presence of Ca^{2+} in binding buffer solution whereas annexin V does not bind live cell with intact plasma membrane without PS externalization.

PROTOCOL

- Prepare 1X binding buffer using sterile distilled water from the 10X stock binding buffer supplied in the kit and warm it to 37°C. It will act as working binding buffer
- Prepare 200 μL of capacitated sperms in a 6 mL tube (the capacitation method can be either density gradient or swim up).
- Add 300 μL working binding buffer to the 200 μL capacitated sperm to complete a total volume of 500 μL. Mix well.
- Add 100 μL of annexin-V beads (the volume of annexin V beads may be reduced to 50 μL in case of poor samples)
- Tightly close the tube, cover it with aluminum foil and incubate for 25 minutes (it can be used an autoshaker or can be shaked manually each 5 minutes)
- 5 minutes before the incubation ends, place the MS column in the magnetic block
- Equilibrate the MS column by washing it whith 1 mL binding buffer, twice
- Pour the annexin-V beads processed sample from the MS column
- Collect the eluted sperms in a clean 6 mL round-bottom tube and add 100 μL of culture medium
- Centrifuge the filtrate at 250 g for 3 minutes, remove the supernatant
- Add 0.4 mL of culture media and mix the sperm pellet. Check the sperm count and motility
- Incubate for at least 15 minutes before use.

Notes:
1. The semen samples that will be used for ICSI should have a total count post-capacitation of at least 3×10^6 sperms
2. The kit has to be put back in the refrigerator immediately after use
3. Annexin-V is light sensitive, so it is recommended to avoid the prolonged exposure of the beads to light (Fig. 1.8).

MACS might be indicated for:
- Previous ART failure (more than 2 cycles without achieving pregnancy)
- Repeated miscarriages
- Patients who have poor embryo quality which is not attributable to the oocytes
- Infertile patients who have a high level of DNA fragmentation in their spermatozoa
- Frozen semen samples
- Addiction like smoking, tobacco chewing and alcohol
- Extensive exposure to external heat (e.g. laptop), hazardous chemicals and pollutants.

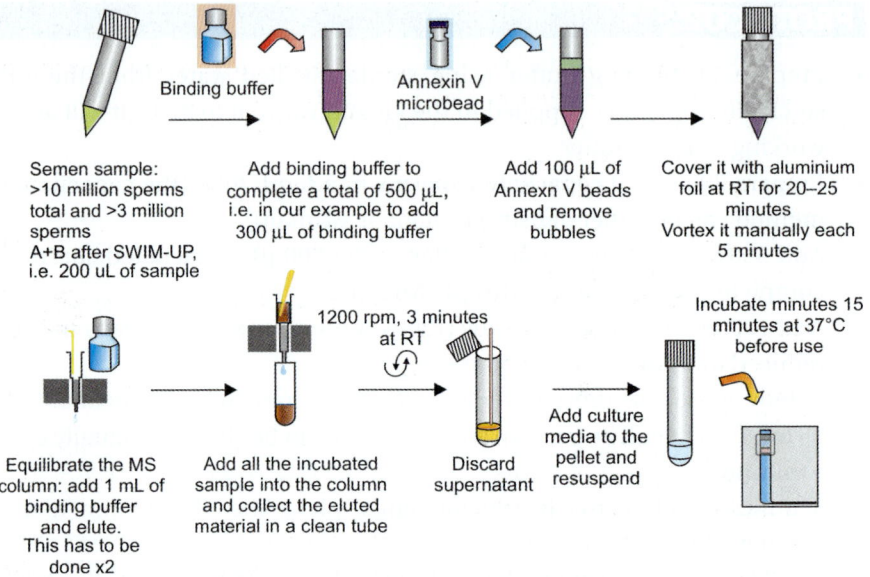

Semen sample: >10 million sperms total and >3 million sperms A+B after SWIM-UP, i.e. 200 uL of sample

Add binding buffer to complete a total of 500 µL, i.e. in our example to add 300 µL of binding buffer

Add 100 µL of Annexn V beads and remove bubbles

Cover it with aluminium foil at RT for 20–25 minutes
Vortex it manually each 5 minutes

Equilibrate the MS column: add 1 mL of binding buffer and elute. This has to be done x2

Add all the incubated sample into the column and collect the eluted material in a clean tube

1200 rpm, 3 minutes at RT

Discard supernatant

Add culture media to the pellet and resuspend

Incubate minutes 15 minutes at 37°C before use

Fig. 1.8: Scheme of the magnetic-activated cell sorting (MACS) protocol.

CONCLUSION

The larger point of concern with the andrology laboratories is to obtain objective and reproducible results of semen parameters like sperm count, morphology and motility. A sperm preparation is always critical in andrology laboratories. Nowadays, MACS sperm preparation technique is remedy to sperm DNA damage and the details to it in this chapter will be useful to the laboratories performing semen analysis and preparing sperm for the assisted reproduction. MACS demand more research to adopt them as a routine tool of sperm preparation for ICSI.

Computer-assisted semen analysis, microfluidic sperm sorting techniques and flow cytometry may become integral tools of objective semen analysis in near future.

ACKNOWLEDGMENTS

To Dr SS Vasan, Director, Ankur, (Bangalore, India), for his valuable contribution through the "Semen analysis and sperm function tests: How much to test?" publication in the Indian Journal of Urology, 2011. E-mail: moc.liamg@nasavrd.

Also to Daniel R Franken, PhD (Free State University, South Africa) and his contribution to "WHO, normal abnormal sperm images and images of cellular components of semen".

REFERENCES

1. Prathima T, Ranjani S, Pandiyan N. From the pages of history: history of semen analysis. Chettinad Health City Med J. 2015;4(1):63-4.
2. Eliasson R. Analysis of semen. In: Burger H, de Kretser DM (Eds). The Testis. New York: Raven Press; 1981 pp. 381-99.
3. De Jonge C. Semen analysis: looking for an upgrade in class. Fertil Steril. 2012; 97(2):260-6.
4. Van Leeuwenhoek A. De natis è semine genital animalculis. R Soc (Lond) Philos Trans. 1678;12:1040-3.
5. Karamanou M, Poulakou-Rebelakou E, Tzetis M, et al. Anton van Leeuwenhoek (1632-1723): father of micromorphology and discoverer of spermatozoa. Rev Argent Microbiol. 2010;42(4):311-4.
6. Capanna E. Lazzaro Spallanzani: At the roots of modern biology. J Exp Zool. 1999;285(3):178-96.
7. Birkhead TR, Montgomerie R. Three centuries of sperm research. In: Birkhead TR, Hosken DJ, Pitnick SS (Eds). Sperm Biology: An Evolutionary Perspective, 1st edition. USA: Elsevier; 2008.
8. Sims JM. Clinical Notes on Uterine Surgery: With Special Reference to the Management of the Sterile Condition. New York: William Wood; 1866. p. 430.
9. Macomber D, Sanders MB. The spermatozoa count: its value in the diagnosis, prognosis and treatment of sterility. N Engl J Med. 1929;200:981-4.
10. MacLeod J. Semen quality in 1000 men of known fertility and in 800 cases of infertile marriage. Fertil Steril. 1951;2(2):115-39.
11. World Health Organization (WHO). WHO Laboratory Manual for the Examination of Human Semen and Sperm-Cervical Mucus Interaction, 1st edition. UK: Cambridge University Press; 1980.
12. World Health Organization (WHO). WHO Laboratory Manual for the Examination and Processing of Human Semen, 5th edition. Geneva: WHO press; 2010.
13. The Nordic Association for Andrology (NAFA), European Society of Human Reproduction and Embryology (ESHRE) (2002). Manual on Basic Semen Analysis. [online] Available from www.slideshare.net/netopenscienart/manual-on-basic-semen-analysis. [Accessed February, 2017].
14. Gopalkrishnan K, Anand Kumar TC. Simple method to evaluate semen viscosity: model to test male contraception. Adv Cont Deliv Syst. 1990;5:355-60.
15. Keel BA. The semen analysis. In: Keel BA, Webster BW (Eds). Handbook of the Laboratory Diagnosis and Treatment of Infertility. Boca Raton: CRC Press; 1990. pp. 27-69.
16. Amelar RD. Coagulation, liquefaction and viscosity of human semen. J Urol. 1962;87:187-90.
17. Gopalkrishnan K, Hinduja IN, Anand Kumar TC. Determining the osmolality of seminal fluid aids in the rapid diagnosis of the fertilizing potential of spermatozoa. J IVF-ET. 1989;6:119-21.
18. Huggins C, Scott WW, Heinen JH, et al. Chemical composition of human semen and of the secretions of the prostate and seminal vesicles. Am J Physiol. 1942;136:467-73.
19. Cooper TG, Brazil C, Swan SH, et al. Ejaculate volume is seriously underestimated when semen is pipetted or decanted into cylinders from the collection vessel. J Androl. 2007;28:1-4.

20. Björndahl L. The usefulness and significance of assessing rapidly progressive spermatozoa. Asian J Androl. 2010;12(1):33-5.
21. Lindholmer C. The importance of seminal plasma for human sperm motility. Biol Reprod. 1974;10(5):533-42.
22. Aitken RJ, Sutton M, Warner P, et al. Relationship between the movement characteristics of human spermatozoa and their ability to penetrate cervical mucus and zona-free hamster oocytes. J Reprod Fertil. 1985;73(2):441-9.
23. Hu YA, Lu JC, Lu NQ, et al. Comparison of four methods for sperm counting. Zhonghua Nan Ke Xue. 2006;12(3):222-4.
24. Sukcharoen N, Ngeamjirawat J, Chanprasit Y, et al. A comparison of Makler counting chamber and improved Neubauer hemocytometer in sperm concentration measurement. J Med Assoc Thai. 1994;77(9):471-6.
25. Mortimer D. Antisperm antibodies. In: Mortimer D (Ed). Practical Laboratory Andrology. Oxford: Oxford University Press; 1994. pp. 111-25.
26. Jarow JP, Sanzone JJ. Risk factors for male partner antisperm antibodies. J Urol. 1992;148(6):1805-7.
27. Rose NR, Hjort T, Rümke P, et al. Techniques for detection of iso- and auto-antibodies to human spermatozoa. Clin Exp Immunol. 1976;23(2):175-99.
28. Mortimer D. Semen microbiology and virology. In: Mortimer D (Ed). Practical Laboratory Andrology. Oxford: Oxford University Press; 1994. pp. 127-33.
29. Johanisson E, Campana A, Luthi R, et al. Evaluation of 'round cells' in semen analysis: a comparative study. Hum Reprod Update. 2000;6(4):404-12.
30. Anderson DJ. Should male infertility patients be tested for leukocytospermia? Fertil Steril. 1995;63(2):246-8.
31. Punab M, Lõivukene K, Kermes K, et al. The limit of leucocytospermia from the microbiological viewpoint. Andrologia. 2003;35(5):271-8.
32. Politch JA, Wolff H, Hill JA, et al. Comparison of methods to enumerate white blood cells in semen. Fertil Steril. 1993;60(2):372-5.
33. Wolff H, Panhans A, Zebhauser M, et al. Comparison of three methods to detect white blood cells in semen: leukocyte esterase dipstick test, granulocyte elastase enzymeimmunoassay, and peroxidase cytochemistry. Fertil Steril. 1992;58(6):1260-2.
34. Coetzee K, Kruge TF, Lombard CJ. Predictive value of normal sperm morphology: a structured literature review. Hum Reprod Update. 1998;4(1):73-82.
35. MacLeod J, Gold RZ. The male factor in fertility and infertility. IV. Sperm morphology in fertile and infertile marriage. Fertil Steril. 1951;2(5):394-414.
36. Menkveld R, Stander FS, Kotze TJ, et al. The evaluation of morphological characteristics of human spermatozoa according to stricter criteria. Hum Reprod. 1990;5(5):586-92.
37. Menkveld R, Holleboom CA, Rhemrev JP. Measurement and significance of sperm morphology. Asian J Androl. 2011;13(1):59-68.
38. Menkveld R, Stander FS, Kotze TJ, et al. The evaluation of morphological characteristics of human spermatozoa according to stricter criteria. Hum Reprod. 1990;5:586-92.
39. Van Waart J, Kruger TF, Lombard CJ, et al. Predictive value of normal sperm morphology in intrauterine insemination (IUI): a structured literature review. Hum Reprod Update. 2001;7(5):495-500.
40. Keegan BR, Barton S, Sanchez X, et al. Isolated teratozoospermia does not affect in vitro fertilization outcome and is not an indication for intracytoplasmic sperm injection. Fertil Steril. 2007;88(6):1583-8.

41. Johnsen O, Eliasson R. Evaluation of a commercially available kit for the colorimetric determination of zinc in human seminal plasma. Int J Androl. 1987; 10(2):435-40.
42. Cooper TG, Yeung CH, Nashan D, et al. Improvement in the assessment of human epididymal function by the use of inhibitors in the assay of alphaglucosidase in seminal plasma. Int J Androl. 1990;13(4):297-305.
43. Mortimer D. Biochemistry of spermatozoa and seminal plasma. In: Mortimer D (Ed). Practical Laboratory Andrology. Oxford: Oxford University Press; 1994. pp. 89-109.
44. Bachtell NE, Conaghan J, Turek PJ. The relative viability of human spermatozoa from the vas deferens, epididymis and testis before and after cryopreservation. Hum Reprod. 1999;14(12):3048-51.
45. Wilcox AJ, Weinberg CR, Baird DD. Timing of sexual intercourse in relation to ovulation. Effects on the probability of conception, survival of the pregnancy, and sex of the baby. N Engl J Med. 1995;333(23):1517-21.
46. Jeyendran RS, Van der Ven HH, Perez-Pelaez M, et al. Development of an assay to assess the functional integrity of the human sperm membrane and its relationship to other semen characteristics. J Reprod Fertil. 1984;70(1):219-28.
47. Evenson DP, Jost LK, Marshall D, et al. Utility of the sperm chromatin structure assay as a diagnostic and prognostic tool in the human fertility clinic. Hum Reprod. 1999;14:1039-49.
48. Zini A, Bielecki R, Phang D, et al. Correlations between two markers of sperm DNA integrity, DNA denaturation and DNA fragmentation, in fertile and infertile men. Fertil Steril. 2001;75:674-7.
49. Ahmadi A, Ng SC. Fertilizing ability of DNA-damaged spermatozoa. J Exp Zool. 1999;284:696-704.
50. Cho C, Jung-Ha H, Willis WD, Goulding EH, Stein P, Xu Z, et al. Protamine 2 deficiency leads to sperm DNA damage and embryo death in mice. Biol Reprod. 2003;69:211-7.
51. Aitken RJ, Clarkson JS, Fishel S. Generation of reactive oxygen species, lipid peroxidation, and human sperm function. Biol Reprod. 1989;41(1):183-97.
52. Aitken RJ, Clarkson JS, Hargreave TB, et al. Analysis of the relationship between defective sperm function and the generation of reactive oxygen species in cases of oligozoospermia. J Androl. 1989;10(3):214-20.
53. Aitken RJ, Irvine DS, Wu FC. Prospective analysis of sperm-oocyte fusion and reactive oxygen species generation as criteria for the diagnosis of infertility. Am J Obstet Gynecol. 1991;164(2):542-51.
54. Agarwal A, Sharma RK, Nallella KP, et al. Reactive oxygen species as an independent marker of male factor infertility. Fertil Steril. 2006;86(4):878-85.
55. Marchetti C, Obert G, Deffosez A, et al. Study of mitochondrial membrane potential, reactive oxygen species, DNA fragmentation and cell viability by flow cytometry in human sperm. Hum Reprod. 2002;17(5):1257-65.
56. Agarwal A, Allamaneni SS, Nallella KP, et al. Correlation of reactive oxygen species levels with the fertilization rate after in vitro fertilization: a qualified meta-analysis. Fertil Steril. 2005;84(1):228-31.
57. Agarwal A, Makker K, Sharma R. Clinical relevance of oxidative stress in male factor infertility: an update. Am J Reprod Immunol. 2008;59(1):2-11.
58. Oehninger S, Blackmore P, Morshedi M, et al. Defective calcium influx and acrosome reaction (spontaneous and progesterone-induced) in spermatozoa of infertile men with severe teratozoospermia. Fertil Steril. 1994;61(2):349-54.

59. Liu DY, Baker HW. Disordered zona pellucida-induced acrosome reaction and failure of in vitro fertilization in patients with unexplained infertility. Fertil Steril. 2003;79(1):74-80.

60. Consensus workshop on advanced diagnostic andrology techniques. ESHRE (European Society of Human Reproduction and Embryology) Andrology Special Interest Group. Hum Reprod. 1996;11(7):1463-79.

61. Quintero I, Ghersevich S, Caille A, et al. Effects of human oviductal in vitro secretion on spermatozoa and search of sperm-oviductal proteins interactions. Int J Androl. 2005;28(3):137-43.

62. Fénichel P, Donzeau M, Farahifar D, et al. Dynamics of human sperm acrosome reaction: relation with in vitro fertilization. Fertil Steril. 1991;55(5):994-9.

63. Cross NL, Morales P, Overstreet JW, et al. Two simple methods for detecting acrosome-reacted human sperm. Gamete Res. 1986;15(3):213-26.

64. Henkel R, Müller C, Miska W, et al. Determination of the acrosome reaction in human spermatozoa is predictive of fertilization in vitro. Hum Reprod. 1993;8(12):2128-32.

65. Katsuki T, Hara T, Ueda K, et al. Prediction of outcomes of assisted reproduction treatment using the calcium ionophore-induced acrosome reaction. Hum Reprod. 2005;20(2):469-75.

66. Yanagimachi R. Penetration of guinea-pig spermatozoa into hamster eggs in vitro. J Reprod Fertil. 1972;28:477-80.

67. Yanagimachi R, Yanagimachi H, Rogers B. The use of zona-free animal ova as a test-system for the assessment of the fertilizing capacity of human sperma tozoa. Biol Reprod. 1976;15:471-6.

68. Rogers B, Brentwood J. Capacitation, acrosome reaction and fertilization. In: Zaneveld L, Chattterton T, (Eds). Biochemistry of mammalian reproduction. 1982. p. 203.

69. Cummins JM, Pember SM, Jequier AM, et al. A test of the human sperm acrosome reaction following ionophore challenge. Relationship to fertility and other seminal parameters. J Androl. 1991;12:98-103.

70. Gopalkrishnan K, Hinduja IN, Anand Kumar TC. Assessment of mitochondrial activity of human spermatozoa: motility/viability in fertile/infertile men. Mol Androl. 1991;3:243-50.

Chapter 2

Cryopreservation of Semen Samples

Pallavi Menon, Carol Rubina D'Souza

INTRODUCTION

The techniques used to stabilize cells at cryogenic temperatures are referred to as cryopreservation. Advances in this field have enabled the maintenance of cell types including male and female gametes and embryos as well. The conventional obstacles to reproduction such as death, age, nonsynchronous maturation and many as such have become insignificant with the progress in the field of cryobiology. At extremely low temperatures like -196°C, there is no evident biochemical activity[1] due the lack of adequate thermal energy for the chemical reactions and the deficit of liquid water essential for metabolic processes.[2] A successful cryopreservation technique involves maintenance of the postthaw structural and functional integrity of the frozen cells. Considerable survival of frozen cells postthaw was attained only after the finding and use of cryoprotective agents.[3] Among the mammalian cells, spermatozoa were the first to be successfully cryopreserved.[3] With a large surface area or volume ratio, human spermatozoa are relatively simple cells with a high permeability to water. This ensures rapid osmotic equilibrium when exposed to cryoprotectants (CPAs), facilitating a superior cryoresistance. The appreciable number of simple protocols have resulted in cryopreservation of spermatozoa forming an integral part of assisted reproductive technology (ART) providing the opportunity for future fertility under various circumstances. In 1953, Bunge and his group reported the first human birth which was the result of artificial insemination (AI) of cryopreserved semen.[4]

The techniques of sperm cryopreservation have gained popularity due to its varied applications including in the field of fertility preservation for cancer patients. Before the initiation of gonadotoxic chemotherapy or radiation,[5] pelvic or testicular surgeries which may lead to testicular failure or ejaculatory dysfunction, patients are advised to cryostore semen sample for future use. Patients with nonmalignant diseases such as diabetes, autoimmune disorders, multiple sclerosis, spinal cord disease or injury which lead to testicular damage can benefit from sperm cryopreservation too.[6] Also, to avoid repeated aspirations and biopsies in azoospermic patients, who have undergone percutaneous epididymal sperm aspiration (PESA) or testicular sperm aspiration (TESA), storage of sperm by cryopreservation, is favorable.[7]

Semen cryopreservation also facilitates donor samples to be quarantined to ensure prevention of transmitting infectious agents to recipients such as human immunodeficiency virus (HIV), hepatitis B virus (HBSAg), etc.[8] Furthermore, patients undergoing ART procedures, routinely have to cryostore the semen samples to avoid inconveniences caused due to failed ejaculation as a consequence of stress or inability to be physically present to provide semen sample on the day of oocyte retrieval.[9]

The generic steps involved in semen cryopreservation include, dilution, cryoprotection, cooling and freezing, storage and thawing.[10] The most commonly used methods for cryopreservation are vitrification and slow freezing. Literature confirms that the success of cryopreservation, despite the technique used, is strongly determined by the initial quality of the sample to be frozen.[11] During the process of cryopreservation, cells undergo transformation in their physical and chemical structures, as there is a drastic temperature drop from +37°C to –196°C. Almost 95% of cellular water content is lost, resulting in increased concentration of solutes, which could trigger an osmotic shock. The potential intracellular ice crystallization and mechanical deformation caused by extracellular ice, may contribute to the cell death. Osmotic shock could hamper the cell survival during the thawing procedure due to uncontrollable swelling and ice recrystallization.[12] Therefore, poor quality spermatozoa are more susceptible to cryoinjury.[13,14]

CRYOPROTECTANTS

Cryoprotectants are low-molecular weight chemical components, which provide defense to the cells from freezing damage or ice crystal formation by decreasing the freezing point of materials. CPAs are broadly classified into two groups, (1) penetrating and (2) nonpenetrating depending on their mode of action.

1. *Penetrating CPAs* function by readily permeating the spermatozoa through the plasma membrane and thereby act intracellularly and extra-cellularly. This class of CPAs follows the osmolarity gradient while moving across the plasma membrane. These molecules prevent ice crystal forma-tion by forming hydrogen bonds with water. Examples include dimethyl sulfoxide (DMSO), dimethylacetaldehyde, propylene glycol, ethylene, methanol and glycerol. These CPAs stabilize the plasma membrane proteins and reduce the concentration of electrolytes.[15] In the scenario of semen freezing, glycerol is commonly used.

2. *Nonpenetrating CPAs* are large molecules that remain and act only extra-cellularly. They create an osmolarity gradient by extracting the water content from within the cell and thereby dehydrating the intracellular space. Prolonged exposure and at high temperatures these molecules could be toxic to the cells, which is prevented by using them in combination with

Table 2.1: Summary of permeating and nonpermeating cryoprotectants and their characteristics.

	Mechanism of action	Names
Permeating	• Permeating cryoprotectants are compounds that readily permeated the plasma membranes of cells • Their movements across the membranes follow the osmolarity gradient • These molecules form hydrogen bonds with water molecules and prevent ice crystallization	• Dimethyl sulfoxide (DMSO), propylene glycol and glycerol • Glycerol is commonly used for semen freezing
Nonpermeating	• Nonpermeating cryoprotectants are larger molecules that remain extracellular • These create osmolarity gradient by drawing water from within the cell, thus dehydrating the intracellular space • Can be toxic to the cells at higher temperatures and after prolonged exposure • Used in combination with the penetrating cryoprotectants to prevent cytotoxicity	• Sucrose, raffinose and glycine

(DNA: Deoxyribonucleic acid; SCSA: Sperm chromatin structure assay; TUNEL: Terminal deoxynucleotidyl transferase-mediated deoxyuridine triphosphate (dUTP) nick end labeling).

the penetrating CPAs. Examples include sucrose, raffinose, glycine, albumins, dextrans, egg yolk citrate, hydroxyethyl, polyethylene glycols (PEG) and polyvinylpyrrolidone (PVP). These CPAs minimize intracellular crystallization by increasing the viscosity of the sample (Table 2.1).

TECHNIQUES FOR CRYOPRESERVATION

The common practice for routine cryopreservation of spermatozoa involves exposure of straws or vials to liquid nitrogen vapor followed by direct plunging into liquid nitrogen. This results in differences in cooling rates among different straws or vials causing a significant fall in survival and motility after thawing.[16] This procedure even after being replaced by automated cryobiology freezers, the motility of the spermatozoa after a freeze-thaw cycle is only 50–60%.[17-19] The reduction in the motility could be due to the atypical response of the spermatozoa to different cooling rates. This kind of insensitivity could be an attribution of its unique structure involving, large surface area to volume ratio, small cytoplasmic volume with high protein concentration and low water content, high cellular permeability to water and CPAs and presence of a heterogeneous mixture of sperm that vary in shape, maturation status and functional potential. The two most commonly used techniques for routine semen cryopreservation are (1) slow freezing and (2) vitrification.

Slow Freezing

This technique allows the cells in a medium to be cooled below the freezing point, was first proposed by Behrman and Sawada.[20] There is a brief preequilibration of cells in CPA solution followed by slow, and gradual controlled cooling at optimized rates. The entire procedure is carried out with the use of special programmable cell freezing equipments and requires about 3–6 hours for completion (Figs. 2.1A to C).

The temperature of the cells is reduced to a supercooled state ice crystal formation that is initiated by a process called seeding. As the size of the ice crystal increases, the water in the solution solidifies. This leads to an increase in the solute concentration in the extracellular medium which leads to the expulsion of intracellular water. The result is the dehydration of the cell, resulting in an increase in the intracellular solute concentration, which further lowers the freezing point of the cell to approximately −35°C. As the cell is devoid of any water content at this stage, freezing of the cells at this temperature has negligible ice crystal formation. The rate of cooling determines the rate at which the water exits the cell. Rapid cooling rates do not enable the complete expulsion of cellular water leading to intracellular ice crystal formation detrimental to the cells. Very slow cooling if cells lead to severe volume shrinkage resulting in high intracellular solute concentration. This has an adverse impact on the lipid-protein complexes of the cell membranes. Also these cells are prone to be affected by chilling injury. Hence optimization of the cooling rate and CPAs concentration is essential to avoid intracellular ice crystallization and high solute concentration which are the main events of cellular cryoinjury. The success of the slow cooling procedure is determined by the attainment of the optimal balance between the rate at which the water can exit the cell and the rate at which it is cooled before its conversion into ice.[21]

Vitrification

The term vitrification was first proposed by Luyet and it translates to glass formation, and transition from liquid to solid in the absence of crystallization.[22] This technique was developed in order to overcome the inadequacy

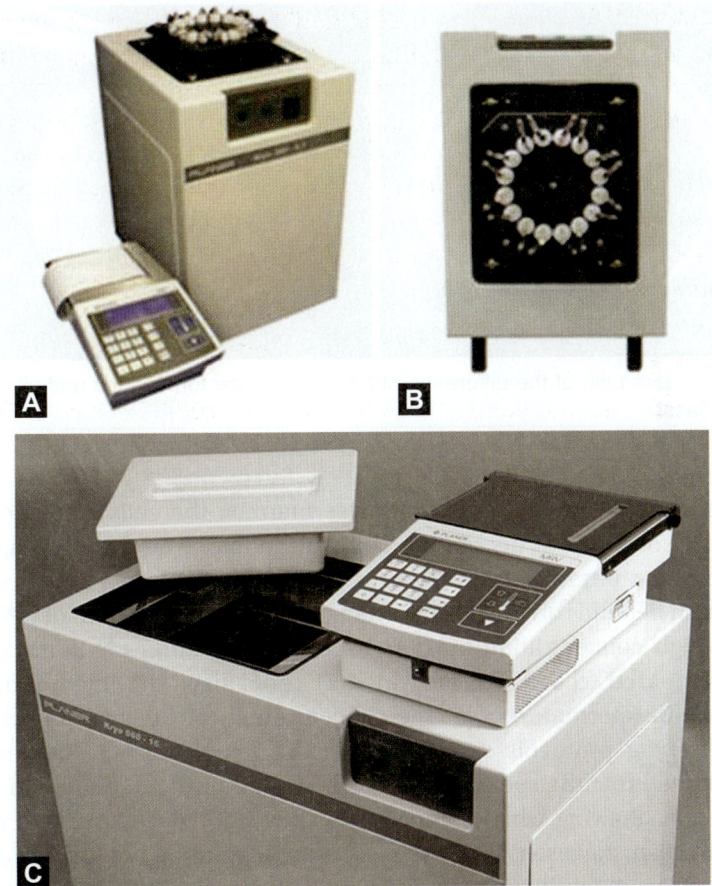

Figs. 2.1A to C: An example of programmable freezers from Planner (models Kryo 360-1.7, Kryo 360-3.3 and Kryo 560-16).

of slow freezing. The solidification of a solution occurs at low temperature, not by ice crystallization but by elevation in its viscosity using high cooling rates of 15,000–30,000 C/min. During vitrification, the viscosity of the cytosol becomes much greater until the molecules are immobilized and it attains the properties of a solid (Fig. 2.2).[23]

Vitrification involves exposure of the cells to high concentration of CPAs for a brief period at room temperature, followed by rapid cooling by exposure to liquid nitrogen. The initial preequilibration of the cells is in a CPA solution of lower concentration, leads to dehydration of the cells and permeation of CPAs. This is then followed by very short incubation in higher concentration of CPA solution followed by swift plunging into liquid nitrogen. The high osmolarity of CPAs leads to complete dehydration of the cell. By the time the cells are immersed in liquid nitrogen, they are nearly devoid of any water and hence there is no ice crystal formation. While warming, the process

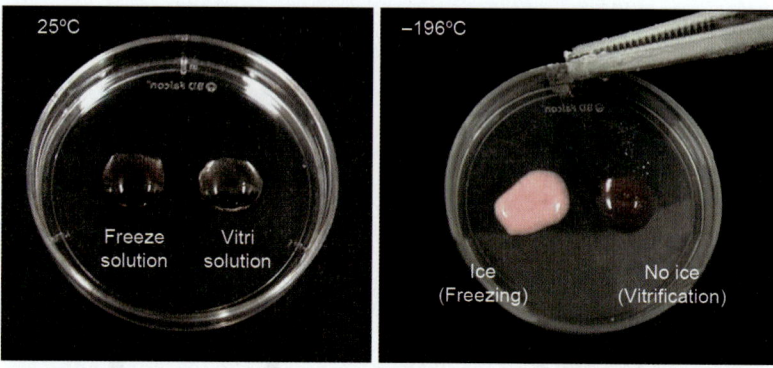

Fig. 2.2: An example of the difference of freezing, hence forming ice and vitrification, forming glass.

of vitrification is reversed. In a stepwise manner, the cells are exposed to hypotonic solutions of decreasing concentrations of nonpenetrating CPAs to remove the intracellular CPAs and gradually rehydrate. The success of vitrification depends on the rate of cooling and the concentration of CPA used.

The high concentration of CPAs used in vitrification medium (30–50% when compared to slow freezing media) could have detrimental osmotic effects on the spermatozoa.[24-26] The concentrations of CPAs used in conventional freezing protocols resulted in severe toxic effects.[27] Studies have demonstrated that the spermatozoa vitrified without CPAs resulted in higher motility after thawing when compared to conventional freezing with CPAs.[28] The study also suggested that use of very rapid cooling and warming rates along with very small specimen size with different carrier systems [open pulled straw (OPS), grids and cryoloops] support the vitrification of the spermatozoa. Evenson and his group demonstrated the integrity of sperm deoxyribonucleic acid (DNA) even at rapid cooling rate.[29]

Survival of the spermatozoa in the absence of permeable CPA could be due to the presence of large quantity of osmotically inactive water bound to the macromolecular structures like DNA, histones, and hyaluronidase.[30] The presence of high-molecular weight components in the spermatozoa could affect the viscosity and glass transition temperature of the intracellular cytosol.[31]

Freeze-drying or Lyophilization of Spermatozoa

The uninterrupted supplies of liquid nitrogen to ensure the frozen samples are maintained add to the cost factor of semen cryopreservation. Considering this, attempts were made to develop techniques to store semen samples for long-term without liquid nitrogen. Lyophilization or freeze-drying is a preservation technique which allows the sperm to be stored at

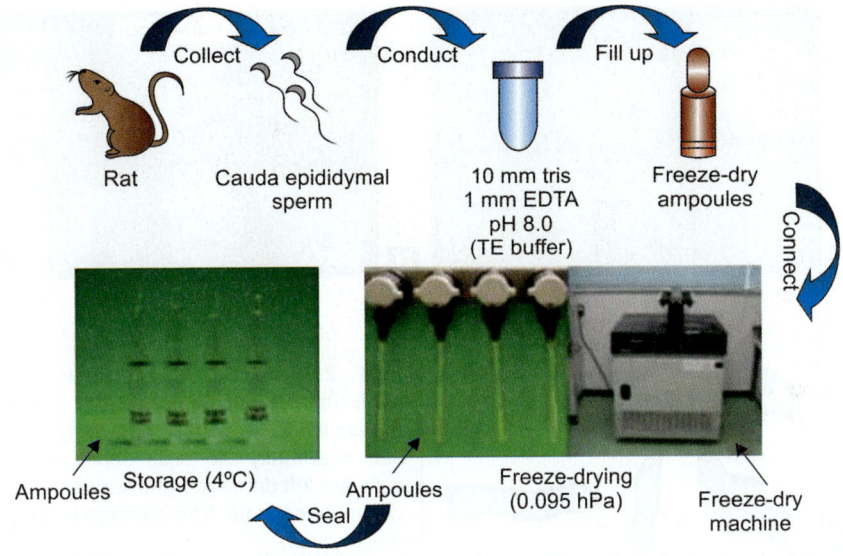

Fig. 2.3: Diagram of the sperm freeze-drying method in animal models. (EDTA: Ethylenediaminetetraacetic acid).

suprazero temperatures by sublimation of ice (Fig. 2.3). The quality of the products thus acquired is not altered during the drying process and can be easily rehydrated.[32] Though the DNA of the lyophilized sperm has been shown to remain intact, the other sperm structures are irreversibly damaged.[33] Though live births in several animal species have been reported[34] by this technique, lyophilization of human sperm is still an experimental technique which is not offered to patients due to lack of supportive literature.

DETRIMENTAL EFFECT OF SEMEN CRYOPRESERVATION

When compared to other cells, spermatozoa appear to be less susceptible to cryoinjury which is attributed to the low water content and high membrane fluidity. Nevertheless, cryopreservation could still have deleterious impact on the structural and functional aspects of the sperm (Figs. 2.4A to C).[35]

Effect of Cryopreservation on Deoxyribonucleic Acid Integrity

There is literature to support the fact that amendment in the DNA integrity of human sperm is noted following cryopreservation.[13,36-38] However, there are also studies that challenge this concept and claim no effect is seen.[39-42] This disagreement between studies could be sample size, the freezing-

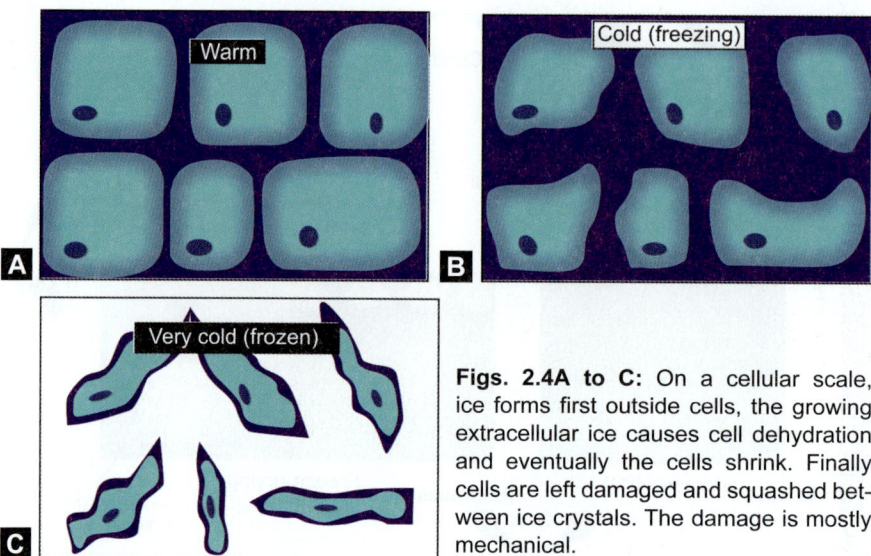

Figs. 2.4A to C: On a cellular scale, ice forms first outside cells, the growing extracellular ice causes cell dehydration and eventually the cells shrink. Finally cells are left damaged and squashed between ice crystals. The damage is mostly mechanical.

thawing protocol in use, sperm preparation techniques before or during cryopreservation and the use of diverse tests to assess the sperm DNA integrity (Table 2.2).

Effect of Cryopreservation on Motility and Viability

The plasma membrane of the spermatozoa is the prime site where cryoinjury occurs.[10,43,44] The mitochondria which is essential for sperm motility, is placed along the midpiece between the plasma membrane and the nine fibrous columns, this is assumed to have similar vulnerability to cryoinjury as the plasma membrane (Fig. 2.5).[45]

The maximum energy is derived from the adenosine triphosphate (ATP) molecules which are synthesised either by glycolysis in the cytoplasm[46] or through oxidative phosphorylation in the mitochondria.[47] Therefore any damage to the plasma membrane or mitochondria may lead to decline in the motility.[45] The same study also showed a significant reduction in the number of viable sperm after cryopreservation.

Effect of Cryopreservation on Fertilizing Ability

Cryopreservation also has been shown to have adverse impact on the fertilizing ability of the spermatozoa. In a study, it was suggested that the alterations in the plasma membrane of the spermatozoa due to the process of cryopreservation made the spermatozoa more susceptible to their milieu and thereby making them partially capacitated postthaw.[44] This cryocapacitation reduces the life span of spermatozoa *in vivo* and powerfully decreasing the efficiency of the entire population.

Table 2.2: Different cryopreservation methods and the DNA damage.

Authors	Test to evaluate DNA integrity	Cryopreservation method	"Does the freezing-thawing procedure induce sperm DNA damage?"
Hamamah et al.	Acridine orange staining and Feulgen-DNA quantitative microspectrophotometry	Unspecified	Yes
Span'o et al.	SCSA + Acridine orange staining	Equilibration at 37°C, freezing in liquid nitrogen vapor at −80°C and then storage in liquid nitrogen at −196°C	Yes
Hammadeh et al.	Acridine orange staining	Computerized slow-stage freezer + static liquid nitrogen vapor	Yes
Donnelly et al.	Comet assay	Equilibration at 37°C, freezing in liquid nitrogen vapor at −80°C and then storage in liquid nitrogen at −196°C	Yes
Gandini et al.	Acridine orange staining	Equilibration at 37°C, freezing in liquid nitrogen vapor at −80°C and then storage in liquid nitrogen at −196°C	Yes
de Paula et al.	TUNEL assay	Use of freezer at −20°C, freezing in liquid nitrogen vapor, then storage in liquid nitrogen at −196°C	Yes
Petyim and Choavaratana	Acridine orange staining	Freezing with liquid nitrogen vapor + computerized program freezer	Yes
Nagamwuttiwong and Kunathikom	Acridine orange staining	Freezing with liquid nitrogen vapor	Yes
Dejarkom and Kunathikom	Acridine orange staining	Computerized controlled rate freezing	Yes
Thomson et al.	TUNEL assay	Use of programmable freezer	Yes

Contd...

Contd...

Authors	Test to evaluate DNA integrity	Cryopreservation method	Does the freezing-thawing procedure induce sperm DNA damage?
Thomson et al.	TUNEL assay	Sample frozen with and without cryoprotectant by slow controlled-rate method using a programmable freezer	Yes
Zribi et al.	TUNEL assay	Equilibration at 37°C, freezing in liquid nitrogen vapor at −80°C, then storage in liquid nitrogen at −196°C	Yes
Donnelly et al.	Comet assay	Equilibration at 37°C, freezing in liquid nitrogen vapor at −80°C, then storage in liquid nitrogen at −196°C	Yes, but semen from fertile men appears to be more resistant to freezing damage
Kalthur et al.	Comet assay + acridine orange staining	Equilibration at 37°C, freezing in liquid nitrogen vapor at −80°C, then storage in liquid nitrogen at −196°C	Yes, but morphologically abnormal sperms seems to be less resistant to freezing damage
Ahmad et al.	Comet assay	Freezing with static phase vapor cooling procedure	Yes, but the sperm DNA integrity of frozen samples of fertile men is higher
Høst et al.	Immunoperoxidase detection of digoxigenin-labeled genomic DNA	Conventional cryopreservation	No
Steele et al.	Comet assay	Freezing in liquid nitrogen vapor	No
Duru et al.	TUNEL assay + annexin V	Equilibration at 37°C, freezing in liquid nitrogen vapor at −80°C, then storage in liquid nitrogen at −196°C	No
Isachenko et al.	Comet assay	Programmable slow freezing + vitrification	No
Paasch et al.	TUNEL assay + flow cytometric kit for apoptosis	Equilibration at 37°C, freezing in liquid nitrogen vapor at −80°C, then storage in liquid nitrogen at −196°C	No

(DNA: Deoxyribonucleic acid; SCSA: Sperm chromatin structure assay; TUNEL: Terminal deoxynucleotidyl transferase-mediated deoxyuridine triphosphate (dUTP) nick end-labeling).

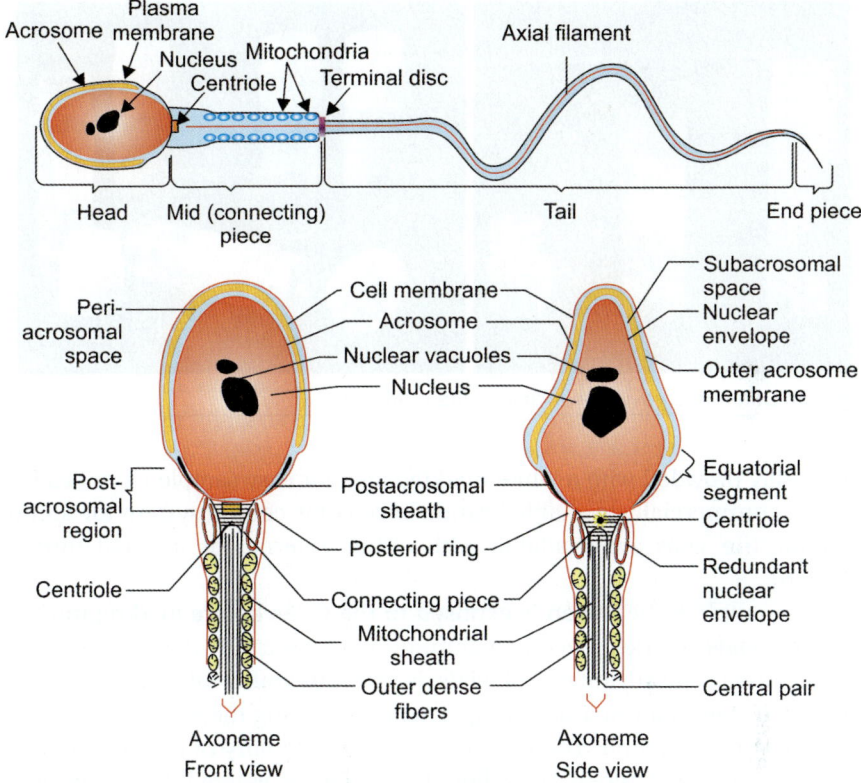

Fig. 2.5: Schematic representation of human spermatozoa.

DEVICES USED IN SEMEN CRYOPRESERVATION

The devices used for the storage of the frozen semen sample depend on various factors including the freezing protocol in use and the type of sperm sample to be frozen. They are broadly classified into two categories: (1) biological carriers and (2) nonbiological carriers.

1. *Biological carriers*: It include empty zonae of various species and Volvox globator algae.
2. *Nonbiological carriers*: It include cryovials, straws, 5 mm copper loops, cryoloops, calcium alginate beads, intracytoplasmic sperm injection (ICSI) pipettes, microdroplets on dry ice or plastic dish and agarose gel microspheres.

Vials

The most commonly used device for semen cryopreservation is the cryovials. These are usually made of specially formulated polypropylene and commercially available in various volumes ranging from 0.5 mL up to 5 mL. These

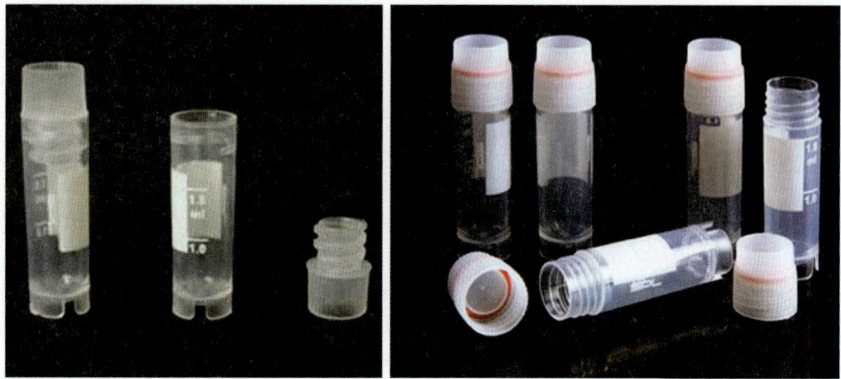

Fig. 2.6: Different cryovials available in the market.

are usually provided with a white marking area for easy sample identification. Several commercially available brands have color-coding system for identification. The vials are available with either external or internal threads (Fig. 2.6).

The sample to be frozen is exposed to the CPAs before loading into the vials. The vials are then placed on aluminium canes inside the storage tanks.

The major disadvantage of vials is the possibility of liquid nitrogen entering inside as a result of improper sealing, making the sample vulnerable to cross-contamination. There is also a high probability of the vial bursting during the thawing process, if the liquid nitrogen has entered the empty space inside the vial during freezing.

Straws

Freezing of semen samples in aliquots or storages of surgically retrieved spermatozoa are preferably done using straws. The usage of straws as carriers is very simple and easily applicable. The mixture of spermatozoa and CPAs is loaded into straws, which are then sealed before freezing. This provides a sterile system for storage.

The major disadvantage in this practice is the loss of sample due to adherence to the straws making it incompatible for storing severely impaired samples (Figs. 2.7A to D).

Empty Zona Pellucida

With the introduction of the concept of single sperm cryopreservation by Cohen et al., usage of empty zona as a pocket book to store individually selected sperm became the most widely used technique for freezing.[48]

Individually selected sperm are deposited into an empty zona with an ICSI pipette,[48,49] and then the zona are equilibrated with CPAs prior to loading into straws. The usage of empty zonae is beneficial in cases of severe

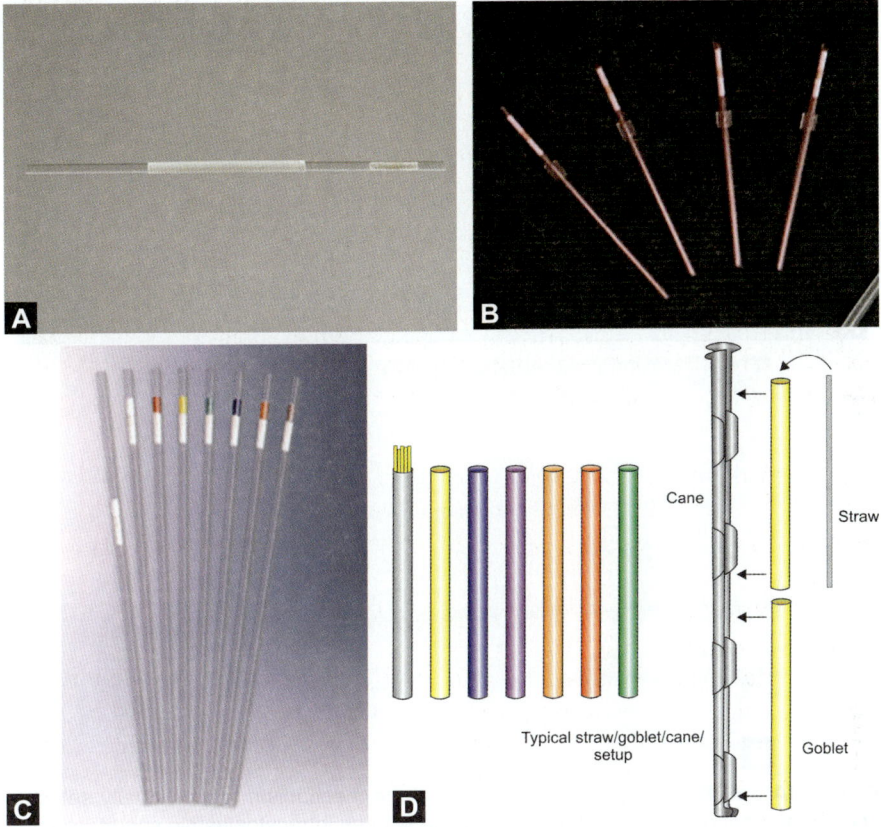

Figs. 2.7A to D: Different straws available in the market.

oligozoospermia or azoospermia. Also the addition and removal of CPAs without the loss of dilution of the spermatozoa enclosed within the zona can be easily achieved. The major disadvantage of this technique is the risk of biological contamination (Figs. 2.8A and B).

Microdroplets

To overcome the loss of sperm through adherence carriers the direct cryopreservation of sperm in microdroplets was introduced in 2000.[50,51] Aliquots of 50 or 100 μL of the spermatozoa and CPA mixture are placed on the surface of dry ice or cold stainless steel plate and then plunged into liquid nitrogen. These aliquots or pills can be removed as per requirement and thawed for use.

The major disadvantage of this practice is the risk of cross-contamination. In addition, the shape and size of the steel plate in use could cause hindrance during handling and storage in liquid nitrogen tanks or conventional freezers (Fig. 2.9).

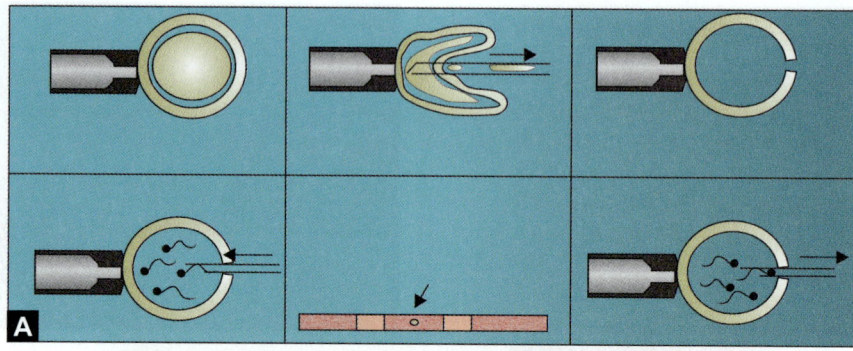

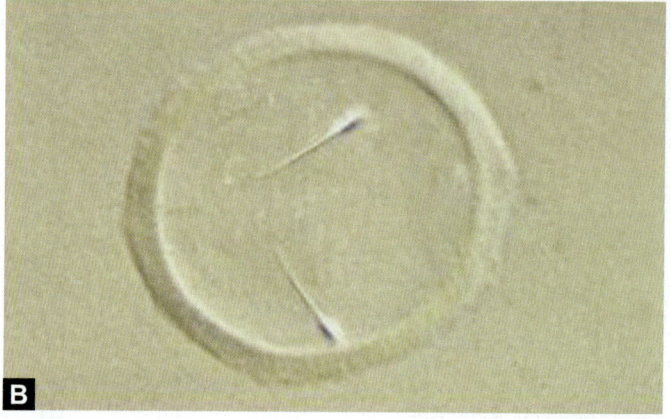

Figs. 2.8A and B: Empty zona pellucida and the mechanism to individually selected sperms and deposit them into an empty zona with an intracytoplasmic sperm injection (ICSI) pipette.

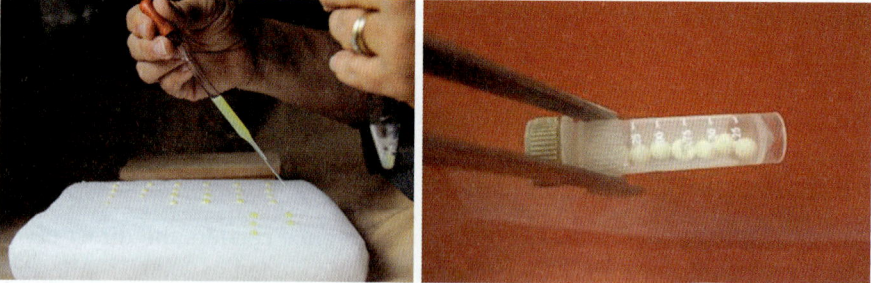

Fig. 2.9: With the microdroplets technique, aliquots of 50 or 100 µL of the spermatozoa and cryoprotectant (CPA) mixture are placed on the surface of dry ice or cold stainless steel plate and then plunged into liquid nitrogen.

Intracytoplasmic Sperm Injection Pipettes

Freezing of spermatozoa can be done using ICSI pipette as a sterile carrier.[52,53] Between 5 and 50 spermatozoa, either surgically retrieved or ejaculated can

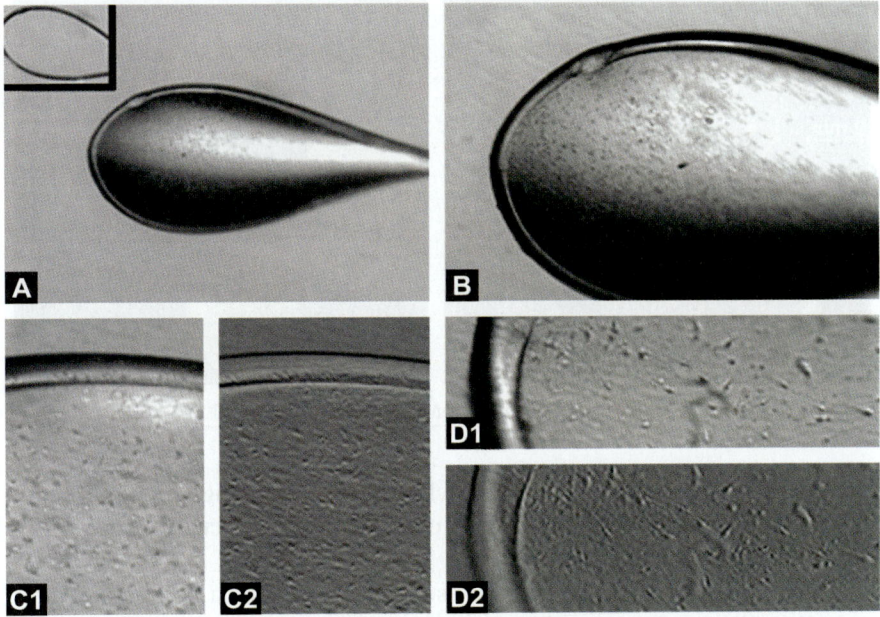

Figs. 2.10A to D: In this figure it can be seen the empty cryoloop prior to sperm inoculation. [Inoculated cryoloops at 3100 (A), 3200 (B), 3400 (C1) and 3640 (D1)]. To enhance visualization of individual spermatozoa, embossed photographs of 3400 and 3640 are shown in C2 and D2 respectively.
Source: Schuster TG, Keller LM, Dunn RL, et al. Ultra-rapid freezing of very low numbers of sperm using cryoloops. Hum Reprod. 2003;18(4):788-95.

be stored in each pipette. This technique is relatively simple and convenient system.

The disadvantage is that it is not a feasible practice for long-term storage. Due to the fragility of the ICSI pipettes, it can be easily broken resulting in loss of sample and risk of cross-contamination.

Cryoloop

Cryoloop was first introduced as a device for embryo freezing.[54] Later on this was used as a potential device to cryopreserve small volumes[27,40,55,56] and small numbers of spermatozoa (Figs. 2.10A to D).[57] Cryoloop serves as an excellent device for vitrification due to the diminutive volume of fluids (1/10–1/100th of a microliter) enabling rapid freezing rates. Apart from this, the inert, and nonbiological nature of the cryoloop which is made of nylon material helps to avoid problems associated with the usage of vessels of biological origin. As these are commercially available, no additional preparation is required. Cryoloops are easier to handle and store as compared to various other devices.

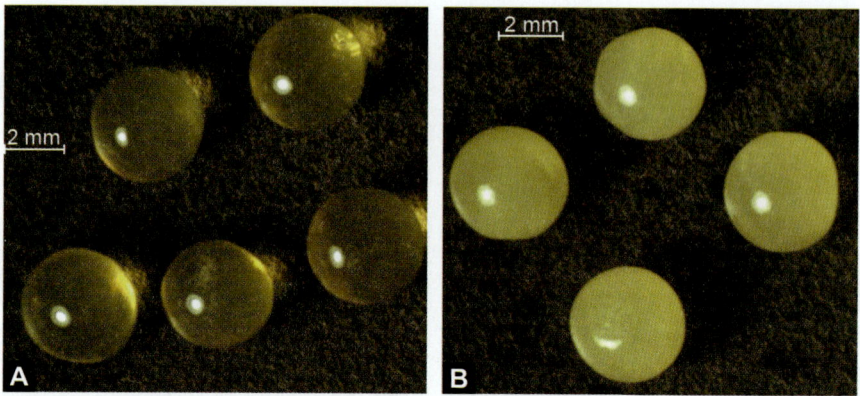

Figs. 2.11A and B: Alginate beads used for sperm cryopreservation.

The major disadvantage of this technique is that being an open system, there is a high-risk of cross-contamination due to direct exposure of the sample to liquid nitrogen.

There are lesser known devices used for spermatozoa cryopreservation including, Volvox globator spheres, alginate beads and agarose microspheres:

- Volvox globator algal colonies are held tightly in a sphere-like structure into which spermatozoa are injected. The exposure of the spermatozoa to the genetic material of the algae which may be introduced to the oocyte during ICSI and the constant availability of the algal material are the concerns
- Alginate beads are prepared from a nontoxic polysaccharide derived from different species of brown seaweed. The retention of alginic acid on the sperm surface resulted in reduced motility postthaw makes it unfavorable for use (Figs. 2.11A and B)
- The spermatozoa can also be stored in agarose microspheres, which is a nonbiological carrier. However, the clinical approach of this technique is not well evaluated and documented (Figs. 2.12A and B).

DONOR SEMEN SAMPLES

With the alarming increase in male infertility, various techniques such as testicular sperm extraction (TESE)-ICSI have evolved, which help patients with obstructive azoospermia. However, patients with nonobstructive azoospermia have no technique proven to be helpful. Studies suggest that patients with azoospermia have a genetic disposition to the condition which could be transmitted to subsequent generations. In such cases of severe male infertility, patients could be counseled for usage of donor sperm as an approach to infertility treatment.[58] Usage of fresh donor semen is almost always avoided for the fear transmitting common infectious diseases or any genetic disorders. However, in certain countries, it is legitimate for the semen donor to

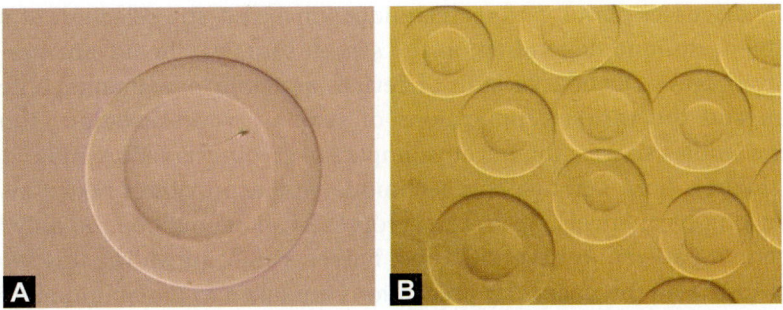

Figs. 2.12A and B: Solitary spermatozoa placed into agarose microsphere by similar to ICSI technique and with the same microtools can be frozen by conventional methods (DIC 40x).
(DIC: Differential interference contrast; ICSI: Intracytoplasmic sperm injection).

be known to the couple or the recipient women. The screening process for donors is painstaking as it includes the acquisition of the complete medical and sexual history, psychological and physical assessment, and examination of blood, urine and semen samples to screen for pathogens, such as hepatitis B and C, HIV, venereal disease research laboratory test for syphilis, cytomegalovirus and pathogens for other sexually transmitted diseases. Also genetic screening is performed for heritable diseases depending upon the ethnicity of the donor. This screening is necessary to protect the recipient and the future offspring. Regulatory bodies such as US Food and Drug Administration (FDA) require only the anonymous donors to undergo these through screening process. Many countries have age restrictions for sperm donors. The minimum age is usually 18 years and considering the age-related genetic risks, the recommended upper age limit for the semen donor is more than 40 years.

After the recruitment and screening of donors, it is advised to retest them after a required quarantine interval, which is a minimum of 180 days. During this period, the samples are cryopreserved and stored. The samples are released for the use of recipients only after the repeated test reports indicate negative results.

The samples from potential donors are collected by masturbation. The sample is then subjected to semen analysis for the macroscopic and microscopic assessment of the sample. This is then concentrated into aliquots and frozen. The postfreezing or thawing semen parameters are assessed. Donors whose postfreeze or thaw semen parameters meet a minimum standard are selected.

CONCLUSION

Today, with the advancement in the field of cryobiology, multiple options are available for cryopreservation of human spermatozoa. This chapter briefly discusses about various techniques involved, the selection of most suitable technique depending on the semen samples, the advantages and disadvantages of diverse variants of devices available for semen cryopreservation and the various applications of semen cryopreservation. Though several studies suggest the negative impact of cryopreservation, monitoring the children born through this technique would provide a better insight to the long-term effects. As semen cryopreservation could be the only help for certain patients to have their own babies, clinics providing this service must ensure all the necessary precautions are taken to maintain the frozen samples.

REFERENCES

1. Chian RC. Cryobiology: an overview. In: Chian RC, Quinn P (Eds). Fertility Cryopreservation. Cambridge: Cambridge University Press; 2010. pp. 1-9.
2. Mazur P. Freezing of living cells: mechanisms and implications. Am J Physiol. 1984;247(3 Pt 1):C125-42.
3. Polge C, Smith AU, Parkes AS. Revival of spermatozoa after vitrification and dehydration at low temperature. Nature. 1949;164(4172):666.
4. Bunge RG, Keettel WC, Sherman JK. Clinical use of frozen semen: report of four cases. Fertil Steril. 1954;5(6):520-9.
5. Sanger WG, Olson JH, Sherman JK. Semen cryobanking for men with cancer—criteria change. Fertil Steril. 1992;58(5):1024-7.
6. Anger JT, Gilbert BR, Goldstein M. Cryopreservation of sperm: indications, methods and results. J Urol. 2003;170(4 Pt 1):1079-84.
7. Donnelly ET, McClure N, Lewis SE. Cryopreservation of human semen and prepared sperm: effects on motility parameters and DNA integrity. Fertil Steril. 2001;76(5):892-900.
8. Morris GJ, Acton E, Avery S. A novel approach to sperm cryopreservation. Hum Reprod. 1999;14(4):1013-21.
9. Fabbri R, Ciotti P, Di Tommaso B, et al. Tecniche di crioconservazione riproduttiva. Rivista Italiana di Ostetricia e Ginecologia. 2004;3:33-41.
10. Hammerstedt RH, Graham JK, Nolan JP. Cryopreservation of mammalian sperm: what we ask them to survive. J Androl. 1990;11(1):73-88.
11. Hammadeh ME, Askari AS, Georg T et al. Effect of freeze-thawing procedure on chromatin stability, morphological alteration and membrane integrity of human spermatozoa in fertile and subfertile men. Int J Androl.1999;22:155-62.
12. Woods EJ, Benson JD, Agca Y, et al. Fundamental cryobiology of reproductive cells and tissues. Cryobiology. 2004;48(2):146-56.
13. Kalthur G, Adiga SK, Upadhya D, et al. Effect of cryopreservation on sperm DNA integrity in patients with teratospermia. Fertil Steril. 2008;89(6):1723-7.
14. Kopeika E, Kopeika J. Variability of sperm quality after cryopreservation in fish. In: Alavi SM, Cosson JJ, Coward K, Rafiee G (Eds). Fish Spermatology. Oxford: Alpha Science Ltd; 2008.
15. Arakawa T, Carpenter JF, Kita YA, et al. The basis for toxicity of certain cryoprotectants: a hypothesis. Cryobiology. 1990;27(4):401-15.
16. Raju GAR, Krishna KM, Prakash GJ, et al. Vitrification: an emerging technique for cryopreservation in assisted reproduction programmes. Embryo Talk. 2006; 1(4):210-27.

17. Henry MA, Noiles EE, Gao D, et al. Cryopreservation of human spermatozoa IV. The effect of cooling rate and warming rate on the maintenance of motility, plasma membrane integrity, and mitochondrial function. Fertil Steril. 1993; 60(5):911-8.

18. Mortimer D. Current and future concepts and practices in human sperm cryo-banking. Reprod Biomed Online. 2004;9(2):134-51.

19. Almlid T, Hofmo PO. A brief review of frozen semen applications under Norwegian AI swine conditions. Repord Domest Anim;31:169-73.

20. Behrman SJ, Sawada Y. Heterologous and homologous inseminations with human semen frozen and stored in a liquid-nitrogen refrigerator. Fertil Steril. 1966;17(4):457-66.

21. Joshi AJ. A Review and Application of Cryoprotectant: The Science of Cryonics. PharmaTutor. 2016;4(1):12-8.

22. Luyet BJ. The vitrification of organic colloids and of protoplasm. Biodynamica. 1937;1(29):1-14.

23. Fahy GM. Vitrification: a new approach to organ cryopreservation. In: Meryman HT (Ed). Transplantation: Approaches to Graft Rejection. New York: Alan R. Liss; 1986. pp. 305-35.

24. Holt WV. Alternative strategies for the long-term preservation of spermatozoa. Reprod Fertil Dev. 1997;9(3):309-19.

25. Katkov II, Katkova N, Critser JK, et al. Mouse spermatozoa in high concentra-tions of glycerol: chemical toxicity vs osmotic shock at normal and reduced oxygen concentration. Cryobiology. 1998;37(4):325-38.

26. Mazur P, Katkov II, Katkova N, et al. The enhancement of the ability of mouse sperm to survive freezing and thawing by the use of high concentrations of glycerol and the presence of an Escherichia coli membrane preparation (Oxy-rase) to lower the oxygen concentration. Cryobiology. 2000;40(3):187-209.

27. Nawroth F, Isachenko V, Dessole S, et al. Vitrification of human spermatozoa without cryoprotectants. Cryo Letters. 2002;23(2):93-102.

28. Isachenko E, Isachenko V, Katkov II, et al. Vitrification of human spermatozoa without cryoprotectants: review of problem and practical success. Reprod BioMed Online. 2003;6:191-200.

29. Evenson DP, Jost LK, Baer RK, et al. Individuality of DNA denaturation patterns in human sperm as measured by the sperm chromatin structure assay. Reprod Toxicol. 1991;5(2):115-25.

30. Gao D, Mazur P, Critser JK. Fundamental cryobiology of mammalian sperma-tozoa. In: Karow AM, Critser JK (Eds). Reproductive Tissue Banking Scientific Principles. New York: Academic Press; 1997. pp. 263-328.

31. Isachenko E, Isachenko V, Katkov II, et al. DNA integrity and motility of human spermatozoa after standard slow freezing versus cryoprotectant-free vitrifica-tion. Hum Reprod. 2004;19(4):932-9.

32. Krokida MK, Karathanos VT, Maroulis ZB. Effect of freeze-drying conditions on shrinkage and porosity of dehydrated agricultural products. J Food Eng. 1998; 35(4):369-80.

33. Gianaroli L, Magli MC, Stanghellini I, et al. DNA integrity is maintained after freeze-drying of human spermatozoa. Fertil Steril. 2012;97(5):1067-73.

34. Gil L, Olaciregui M, Luño V, et al. Current status of freeze-drying technology to preserve domestic animals sperm. Reprod Domest Anim. 2014;49 (Suppl 4): 72-81.

35. Watson PF. The causes of reduced fertility with cryopreserved semen. Anim Reprod Sci. 2000;60-61:481-92.

36. Thomson LK, Fleming SD, Aitken RJ, et al. Cryopreservation-induced human sperm DNA damage is predominantly mediated by oxidative stress rather than apoptosis. Hum Reprod. 2009;24(9):2061-70.
37. Zribi N, Feki Chakroun N, El Euch H, et al. Effects of cryopreservation on human sperm deoxyribonucleic acid integrity. Fertil Steril. 2010;93(1):159-66.
38. Meamar M, Zribi N, Cambi M, et al. Sperm DNA fragmentation induced by cryopreservation: new insights and effect of a natural extract from Opuntia ficus-indica. Fertil Steril. 2012;98(2):326-33.
39. Duru NK, Morshedi MS, Schuffner A, et al. Cryopreservation-Thawing of fractionated human spermatozoa is associated with membrane phosphatidylserine externalization and not DNA fragmentation. J Androl. 2001;22(4): 646-51.
40. Isachenko V, Isachenko E, Katkov II, et al. Cryoprotectant-free cryopreservation of human spermatozoa by vitrification and freezing in vapor: effect on motility, DNA integrity, and fertilization ability. Biol Reprod. 2004;71(4):1167-73.
41. Kadirvel G, Kumar S, Kumaresan A. Lipid peroxidation, mitochondrial membrane potential and DNA integrity of spermatozoa in relation to intracellular reactive oxygen species in liquid and frozen-thawed buffalo semen. Anim Reprod Sci. 2009;114(1-3):125-34.
42. Vutyavanich T, Piromlertamorn W, Nunta S. Rapid freezing versus slow programmable freezing of human spermatozoa. Fertil Steril. 2010;93(6):1921-8.
43. Parks JE, Graham JK. Effects of cryopreservation procedures on sperm membranes. Theriogenology. 1992;38(2):209-22.
44. Watson PF. Recent developments and concepts in the cryopreservation of spermatozoa and the assessment of their post-thawing function. Reprod Fertil Dev. 1995;7(4):871-91.
45. O'Connell M, McClure N, Lewis SE. The effects of cryopreservation on sperm morphology, motility and mitochondrial function. Hum Reprod. 2002;17(3): 704-9.
46. Ford WC, Rees JM. The bioenergetics of mammalian sperm motility. In: Gagnon C (Ed). Controls of Sperm Motility: Biological and Clinical aspects. Boca Raton: CRC Press; 1990. pp. 175-202.
47. Mahadevan M, Trounson AO. Effect of cooling, freezing and thawing rates and storage conditions on preservation of human spermatozoa. Andrologia. 1984; 16(1):52-60.
48. Cohen J, Garrisi GJ, Congedo-Ferrara TA, et al. Cryopreservation of single human spermatozoa. Hum Reprod. 1997;12(5):994-1001.
49. Borini A, Sereni E, Bonu MA, et al. Freezing a few testicular spermatozoa retrieved by TESA. Mol Cell Endocrinol. 2000;169(1-2):27-32.
50. Gil-Salom M, Romero J, Rubio C, et al. Intracytoplasmic sperm injection with cryopreserved testicular spermatozoa. Mol Cell Endocrinol. 2000;169(1-2):15-9.
51. Quintans CJ, Donaldson MJ, Asprea I, et al. Development of a novel approach for cryopreservation of very small numbers of spermatozoa. Hum Reprod. 2000;15:99.
52. Gvakharia M, Adamson GD. A method of successful cryopreservation of small numbers of human spermatozoa. Fertil Steril. 2001;76(3):S101.
53. Sohn JO, Jun SH, Park LS, et al. Comparison of recovery and viability of sperm in ICSI pipette after ultra rapid freezing or slow freezing. Fertil Steril. 2003;80 (Suppl 3):S128.
54. Lane M, Bavister BD, Lyons EA, et al. Containerless vitrification of mammalian oocytes and embryos. Nat Biotechnol. 1999;17(1):1234-6.

55. Schuster TG, Keller LM, Dunn RL, et al. Ultra-rapid freezing of very low numbers of sperm using cryoloops. Hum Reprod. 2003;18(4):788-95.
56. Isachenko V, Isachenko E, Montag M, et al. Clean technique for cryoprotectant-free vitrification of human spermatozoa. Reprod Biomed Online. 2005;10(3): 350-4.
57. Desai NN, Blackmon H, Goldfarb J. Single sperm cryopreservation on cryoloops: an alternative to hamster zona for freezing individual spermatozoa. Reprod Biomed Online. 2004;9(1):47-53.
58. Botchan A, Hauser R, Gamzu R, et al. Results of 6139 artificial insemination cycles with donor spermatozoa. Hum Reprod. 2001;16(11):2298-304.

Chapter 3

New Techniques for Sperm Selection in the Andrology Laboratory

Cristina González-Ravina, Alberto Pacheco, Irene Rubio Palacios, Javier Herrero Zapata

INTRODUCTION

Male infertility is a relatively common condition that affects approximately 30–40% of the male population. Although a majority of such patients produces sufficient numbers of spermatozoa to achieve conception, fertility is compromised because these cells are functionally deficient and could influence both the fertilizing potential of the spermatozoa and their ability to promote normal embryonic development as a consequence of high levels of deoxyribonucleic acid (DNA) damage in the paternal genome.

Semen samples consist of cellular mixtures suspended in seminal plasma composed of precursor germ cells, subpopulations of viable and nonviable spermatozoa, debris and multiple leukocyte subtypes. During the ejaculation process, the human male deposits millions of spermatozoa in the woman's vagina, near the cervical orifice, from where they begin a competitive race through the genital tract until they reach and fertilize the oocyte in the fallopian tube. Until a few years ago, it was thought that the enormous amount of sperm ejaculated in the female genital tract competed from the beginning to reach the oocyte and fertilize it. However, it is known that only a few spermatozoa are able to reach the fallopian tubes, and even fewer are able to fertilize the oocyte (Fig. 3.1).

When assisted reproduction techniques first appeared, sperm selection protocols were initially based on sperm separation from seminal plasma and retrieval of motile spermatozoa. However, since spermatozoa with nuclear DNA damage have the ability to fertilize the oocyte, and depending on the level of fragmentation, give rise to repeat miscarriage in the recipient woman, or to generate embryos with uncertain prognosis in future neonates, in the last years new techniques of sperm selection have been developed focusing on the isolation of functional spermatozoa. This is really important as it is recognized that the spermatozoa are more than a mere DNA delivery vehicle to the oocyte, and play a role far beyond the fertilization process by contributing paternal messenger ribonucleic acids (mRNAs), which it is believed to be crucial for normal early and late embryonic development.[1]

In order to develop new methodologies that would help to improve the currently low live birth rates achieved by assisted reproductive technologies

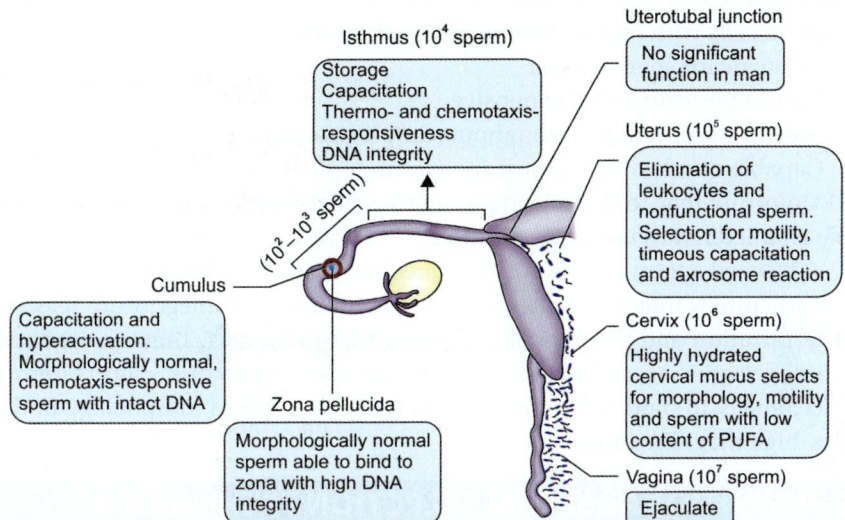

Fig. 3.1: Sites of sperm selection in the human female. Estimated numbers of spermatozoa in the respective sections of the female genital tract are given in brackets. Soon after deposition in the vagina, spermatozoa move out of the seminal plasma and enter the highly hydrated cervical mucus where sperm selection for morphology and motility takes place. Spermatozoa that are selected here are characterized by a low plasma membrane content of PUFA. Subsequently, spermatozoa are transported through the uterus where male germ cells are selected for motility and timely capacitation. Dysfunctional spermatozoa are eliminated. After passing the uterotubal junction, which has in contrast to numerous animal species, no significant function in man, spermatozoa enters the isthmus of the fallopian tube. In the isthmus, spermatozoa can be stored for up to 5 days. In the isthmus and the cumulus, spermatozoa are selected for capacitation, thermo- and chemotaxis-responsiveness and DNA integrity. Finally, after passing through the cumulus, spermatozoa bind to the zona pellucida where another morphological selection takes place. Moreover, male germ cells are further selected for zona-binding ability and DNA integrity.

(DNA: Deoxyribonucleic acid; PUFA: Polyunsaturated fatty acid).

Source: Henkel R. Sperm preparation: state-of-the-art—physiological aspects and application of advanced sperm preparation methods. Asian J Androl. 2012;14(2):260-9.

(ARTs), it has been of great relevance to analyze how the selection of functional spermatozoa with low level of DNA fragmentation by the female organism is carried out. While it is true that some of the processes are more or less controlled, the exact mechanism by which this process is regulated in women is still unknown (Fig. 3.1). In any case, what is clear is that the techniques developed should be focused on selecting spermatozoa with good functional capacity and integral nuclear DNA.

The new techniques of sperm selection are based on two fundamental principles: (1) greater precision in the morphological analysis of spermatozoa, and (2) an analysis focused on molecular characteristics associated with functionality and genomic integrity. To date an ideal protocol for selection of sperm cells with high fertilizing ability should be:

- Nontoxic for spermatozoa
- Easy to perform and inexpensive
- Able to support high-throughput sample processing
- Capable of selecting the best sperm subpopulation for ARTs.

Unfortunately, to date no single sperm selection protocol meets all desirable characteristics mentioned earlier.[2]

Advanced sperm selection techniques are thought to improve the chance that structurally intact and mature sperm with high DNA integrity are selected for fertilization and theoretically improve ART outcomes. These procedures include selection according to surface charge, sperm apoptosis, sperm birefringence, ability to bind to hyaluronic acid (HA), and sperm morphology under ultra-high magnification.

CONVENTIONAL SPERM SELECTION TECHNIQUES: ADVANTAGES AND DISADVANTAGES

Semen preparation techniques are intended to separate sperm from seminal plasma containing decapacitating substances, prostaglandins and lymphocytes as well as to remove dead spermatozoa, leukocytes, round cells and infectious agents. The purpose of capacitation is to make the population of spermatozoa morphologically normal and of better motility, separated from the rest of the components that often interfere with their capacity of fertilization. Adequate processing of the sample will influence the fertilizing capacity of spermatozoa, both *in vivo* and *in vitro*, and will be fundamental for the success of assisted reproduction treatments.

A variety of sperm preparation techniques have been proven to select spermatozoa that are characterized by superior motility and morphology and are capable of fertilizing the oocyte. Among them, the double density gradient centrifugation (DGC) and the swim-up procedure are currently used as standard preparation techniques.[3,4] The capacitation process is necessary so that the spermatozoon will be able to cross the layer of cumulus cells surrounding the oocyte and once there, suffer the acrosomal reaction that allows it to cross the oocyte cover and fuse with the membrane. Only small fractions of the spermatozoa (less than 10% in humans) at some point reach the capacitated state. Both the cells of the cluster and the zona pellucida are the last two barriers to selection of optimal and morphologically normal functional spermatozoa.

The sperm migration or swim-up method is easy and very cost-effective. It is the most physiological sperm selection procedure, and is based on spermatozoa self-propelled active movement from a cell pellet into an overlaying medium. The disadvantage of this method is that the immature spermatozoa and the rest of the cells remain in contact throughout the process with the mature spermatozoa and may produce adverse effects on them. In addition, many of the motile spermatozoa may be trapped at the bottom of the sediment and never reach the culture medium. Only a small fraction of total motile sperm is recovered, therefore its use is mostly restricted to ejaculates with high sperm counts and good motility.[5]

The sperm DGC method is less physiological than the swim-up procedure, and is mainly used for semen with low parameters and cryopreserved sperm samples. The density gradients currently used colloidal suspension of silica particles covalently attached to silane molecules, which are used discontinuously in isotonic solutions at different concentrations. It is recommended to use volumes of 0.5–1 mL of each concentration gradient to prepare the layers. After centrifuging, highly motile sperm cells are enriched in the soft pellet at the bottom of the tube. This method is based on the selection of spermatozoa that can overcome the difficulty of density gradients and reach the bottom of the tube, besides acting as a filter for seminal plasma, round cells, detritus and those spermatozoa with nonprogressive motility:

- Mature spermatozoa are compacted cells and reach the highest density gradient (at the bottom of the tube)
- Seminal plasma remains floating on the lower density gradient
- Immature and dead spermatozoa are located at the interface between the two gradients.

In conclusion, conventional sperm preparation techniques, namely, swim-up and DGC, are not efficient enough to produce sperm populations free of DNA damage, because these techniques are not physiological and not modeled on the stringent sperm selection processes taking place in the female genital tract. By employing conventional sperm preparation strategies for ART, natural sperm selection processes taking place at various levels of the female genital tract (Fig. 3.1) are bypassed to varying extents. To improve the sperm selection, methodologies is crucial since the intracytoplasmic sperm injection (ICSI) became the gold standard procedure in ART; a single spermatozoa is selected by the technician based solely on motility and morphology parameters, and therefore, optimal selection of these gametes is mandatory. Thus, we should emphasize the need for more accurate sperm markers of fertilizing and normal developmental potential. However, while some of the advanced sperm selection methods are of value in specific clinical ART settings, further evaluation of most of them are needed before universally implement them in ART.

MAGNETIC-ACTIVATED CELL SORTING TECHNIQUE

Principle of the Technique

Magnetic-activated cell sorting (MACS, Miltenyi Biotec™) is a cell separation technique based on the use of 50 nm superparamagnetic particles that are conjugated to highly specific antibodies against a particular antigen on the cell surface that is used to discriminate the cells in which is present or not. Due to their small size, the superparamagnetic particles do not activate cells and will not saturate cell surface epitopes; besides, they are nontoxic and biodegradable, so they can be used for clinical purpose. After labeling with the specific antibody, samples must be poured into a specific column that is placed onto a very strong magnet. The column contains a matrix composed of ferromagnetic spheres that amplify the magnetic field by 10,000-fold, thus inducing a high gradient within the column, allowing the isolation of cells that are only minimally labeled, and leaving enough epitopes free for concurrent antibody staining. The space between the spheres is several times larger than sperm cells, allowing them to freely flow through the column. Moreover, magnetically labeled cells are held in suspension within the column and do not actually 'bind' the column matrix. This suspension minimizes stress on the cells and allows for efficient sterile washing by avoiding cell aggregation. For that reason, MACS technology can be used to perform a positive (with cells retained into the column) or negative (with cells flowed through the column) cell selection.

Although this technique is valid for any membrane marker present in the cell (in fact, it is routinely used in hematology or immunology), in human reproduction the technique only has at present clinical application for the separation of nonapoptotic cells from a semen sample.

Magnetic-activated Cell Sorting and Apoptosis

Apoptosis is a highly regulated physiological process that is crucial to maintain testicular cell homeostasis, and to eliminate those sperm cells that have been generated with meiotic errors during spermatogenesis. This process can be deregulated by different intrinsic (alterations during spermatogenesis, meiotic errors) and/or extrinsic factors (drugs, pharmacological treatments) causing an increase of apoptotic sperm cells in the ejaculate that, if they are used in an ART treatment, can reduce the probabilities to obtain a pregnancy.

One of the early events in the apoptotic cascade is the externalization of phosphatidylserine residues of the plasma membrane, so its detection on the cell surface serves to the recognition of apoptotic cells and their separation from the other spermatozoa with higher fertilization potential. Annexin V is a calcium-dependent phospholipid binding protein (PBP) with high affinity for phosphatidylserine;[6] for that reason, this molecule has been the chosen candidate to detect apoptotic (i.e. annexin V-positive) cells in MACS technology.[7]

Published studies showed that the use of MACS together with DGC when preparing a human sperm sample reduces the percentage of apoptotic sperm after preparation and improves sperm motility and viability.[8,9] In addition, some works have described an increase of several sperm functional parameters by using MACS selection technique, showing that annexin V-negative sperm fraction has less nucleus DNA fragmentation and is of higher morphological quality compared to the annexin V-positive sperm fraction;[10,11] other authors have shown that MACS sperm selection improves the acrosome reaction in couples with unexplained infertility.[12] Finally, an improvement of sperm motility and other functional parameters has been described when a combination of conventional sperm separation procedures plus MACS technique is used in thawed sperm samples.[13]

Magnetic-activated Cell Sorting Technique and Assisted Reproductive Technology Results

Some works have been published using this technique of cell separation in intrauterine insemination (IUI) treatments, showing that MACS technique can significantly improve the pregnancy rate in IUI.[14,15]

However, most of the published studies that use of this sperm selection technique have been performed in *in vitro* fertilization (IVF) or ICSI cycles. In some of them, the results showed that the technique does not offer significant improvements in reproductive outcome when unselected males were used for the cycles,[16] but it may have clinical utility when there is a male factor associated, as shown in a published meta-analysis.[17]

Indeed, it seems especially useful in cases of samples with high levels of sperm DNA fragmentation. In this sense, several publications have correlated the use of MACS with a significant decrease in both apoptotic markers and sperm DNA fragmentation in which pregnancies were obtained.[18,19] In another study performed by Lukaszuk et al. a pregnancy is described in a couple undergoing an ICSI treatment with spermatozoa isolated by testicular sperm aspiration (TESA) and further MACS selection in order to reduce sperm DNA fragmentation, suggesting that the use of MACS can be considered as valid support in cases where a high percentage of fragmented DNA is observed in the sample.[20]

It is also important to mention that a recent published article has confirmed that the use of the MACS technique has no adverse obstetric effects[21] confirming the safety use of this technique in ART.

INTRACYTOPLASMIC MORPHOLOGICALLY SELECTED SPERM INJECTION

Principle of the Technique

In a daily clinical practice, the selection of the spermatozoa to perform an ICSI cycle is solely based on motility and morphology criteria carried out by

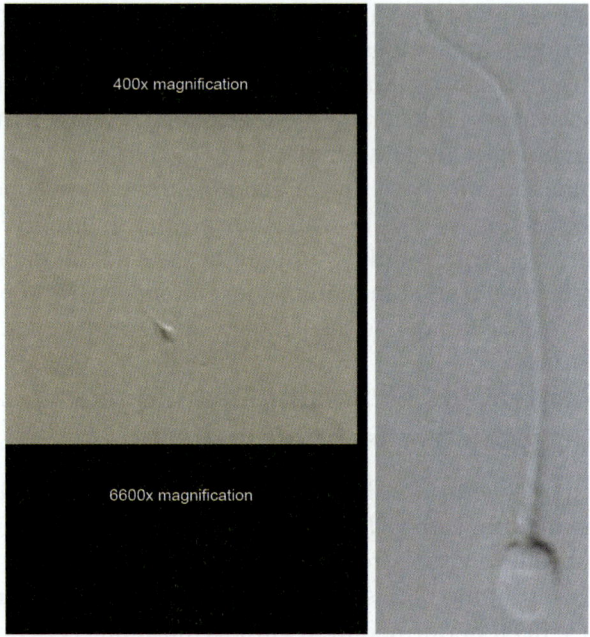

400x magnification

6600x magnification

Fig. 3.2: Morphological differences in the observation of spermatozoa in normal optic (400x level of magnification) and Nomarski optics used for motile sperm organelle morphology examination (MSOME) (6600x level of magnification).

an optic microscopy under 400× magnification. Although it is widely described that sperm morphology is related to embryo quality and the probability of pregnancy, due to the small size of sperm cells, at this level of magnification only gross morphological defects can be observed.[22] An increase in the magnification level would allow a more detailed analysis of sperm morphology, such as the presence of vacuoles or other anomalies of sperm head or midpiece, and therefore a better selection of the best spermatozoa to be used for the ICSI cycle. In this sense, Bartoov and colleagues described in 2001 a pregnancy by using a new optic system that increased to 6000X the level of magnifications. It allowed also the selection of spermatozoa based on motile sperm organelle morphology examination (MSOME),[23] and then by performing an ICSI cycle using this sperm selection technique. It was called intracytoplasmic morphologically selected sperm injection (IMSI). This new optic allows the visualization of much denser specimens because the projected image is three-dimensional, describing new sperm morphological characteristics, as the number and size of vacuoles on the sperm head (Fig. 3.2). Thanks to this optic, new morphological classification criteria have been established, although there is no agreement in the classification system, nor in the clinical consequences that can have the new observed morphological characteristics.

On the other hand, the main disadvantages of this technique are the high cost of the equipment required and the time consuming of its application. It is important to keep in mind that the time taken to perform sperm selection through MSOME may impair sperm viability and have subsequent deleterious effects on embryo quality.

Intracytoplasmic Morphologically Selected Sperm Injection and Assisted Reproductive Technology Results

Although there have been many publications since its development that have shown results in IMSI cycles, the utility of routine use of IMSI is still under controversial.

In any case, there are many data of cycles performed with IMSI that suggest that the presence of vacuoles in the sperm nucleus adversely affects the reproductive outcome. Different works indicate that MSOME can improve clinical outcomes in assisted reproduction cycles, with an increase of fecundation rate, and also an increase of the number of good quality embryos and of the obtained blastocysts.

Some works have described that IMSI increases the implantation rate in couples with male factor infertility and in cases of advanced maternal age, and therefore should be the method of choice for these cases.[24,25] In agreement of these data, other works suggest that IMSI should have a clear role as a routine procedure in every IVF laboratory.[26]

On the contrary, others groups suggest that there are not enough randomized studies to confirm the effectiveness of IMSI and therefore its use should be limited strictly in cases of severe male factor infertility and repeated implantation failures following ICSI,[27] or when there is at least one previous failed ICSI cycle.[28]

In conclusion, IMSI may have clinical utility in selected cases, such as recurrent implantation failure following ICSI and severe male factor infertility,[28] so it is crucial to select the cases to be included and that can in fact benefit from it.

PHYSIOLOGICAL INTRACYTOPLASMIC SPERM INJECTION

Principle of the Technique

The formation of hyalvronic acid (HA) binding sites on the sperm plasma membrane is one of the signs of sperm maturity that has been used as a basis for a sperm binding assay.[29,30] Early studies have revealed that the percentage of sperm bound to HA reflect their maturational status and function, and therefore can be used for fertility diagnosis as well as for the selection of functional spermatozoa for ICSI. This method of sperm selection is highly specific and has minimal safety concerns.[31]

To date, there are two methods for HA binding in use, namely, (1) the physiological ICSI (PICSI) dish (hyaluronan-coated chamber) and the hyaluronan-containing medium. Both methods are commercially ready to use systems that have received official recognition for conformity with health and safety requirements in the European Union (EU) and the United States (US).

The first of them is a PICSI dish, which consists of a petridish with spots of immobilized HA on it (Midatlantic Diagnostic, Mount Laurel, NJ, USA). With this selection assay, one drop of a spermatozoa suspension is placed on top of these spots of HA and incubated for 15 min at 37°C. Subsequently, the freely moving spermatozoa are removed by gently rinsing the HA droplet and removing the nonbound sperm. After this, the bound spermatozoa attached to the dish are picked up with an ICSI pipette (hence PICSI).

The other method consists of a viscous hyaluronan-containing medium (Sperm Slow, MediCult, Jyllinge, Denmark). In this assay, a 5 mL droplet of density gradient prepared spermatozoa is connected with a pipette tip to a 5 mL droplet of Sperm Slow medium by dragging the suspension into contact and incubated for 15 min at 37°C under oil. Afterwards, spermatozoa bound to HA at the interface of the two droplets are selected with an ICSI pipette.[32]

In both cases, as HA is a natural occurring compound present in cervical mucus, cumulus cells and follicular fluid, the binding method is considered to have minimal biosafety risks for both the embryo and the patient.

Main Described Applications of Physiological ICSI Technique

As previously mentioned, the human oocyte is surrounded by HA, which acts as a natural selector of spermatozoa. For this reason, human sperm that express HA receptors and bind to HA are expected to have normal shape, minimal DNA fragmentation, better progressive motility, nonreacted acrosomes as well as lower frequency of chromosomal aneuploidies.[31,33]

Intracytoplasmic sperm injection, introduced over 25 years ago, is widely used in assisted reproduction technique treatments;[34] however, the optimal technique for selecting the spermatozoa for insemination is yet to be determined.[35]

Current sperm selection techniques, such as DGC and swim-up, depend on sedimentation or migration of the sperm, and unfortunately important sperm characteristics, such as apoptosis, DNA integrity, membrane maturation and ultrastructure are not targeted by these techniques.[35] Current research seeks to improve ICSI outcome by isolating mature, structurally intact and nonapoptotic spermatozoa with high DNA integrity. This method (HA binding) is based on membrane maturity. It has been described that only mature spermatozoa that express receptors specific to HA can fertilize the oocyte. For this reason, this technique has been recommended in order to improve the selection of the optimal spermatozoa for ICSI and therefore obtain better clinical outcomes reducing the risks for genetic complications associated with the use of abnormal spermatozoa.[36] However, it is important to know that this added step of selection will require embryologists to invest more time into preparatory steps during ICSI.

Physiological ICSI and Assisted Reproductive Technology Results

Use of HA binding assays in PICSI cycles to improve clinical outcomes has been studied, although none of the studies had sufficient statistical power. The proportion of sperm capable of binding to HA had no correlation with fertilization, cleavage, good quality embryos, and miscarriage and pregnancy rates in couples undergoing IVF.[37] Consistently, patients with clinical pregnancies had a percentage of HA-bound sperm that was comparable to those without pregnancy.[37]

A recent systematic review and meta-analysis has been published in order to clarify if this binding selection method is beneficial in patients undergoing assisted reproduction treatments. In the selected articles, the main outcomes were fertilization rate and clinical pregnancy rate, and the secondary outcomes included cleavage rate, embryo quality, implantation rate, spontaneous abortion and live birth rate.[36] The use of HA binding sperm selection technique yielded no improvement in fertilization and pregnancy rates. Meta-analytic pooling of the data revealed no association between sperm selection technique and pregnancy rate, however, one prospective study demonstrated improved embryo quality in the HA binding group ($p = 0.005$).[38] The conclusion is that evidence does not support routine use of HA binding assays in all ICSI cycles, and the identification of patients that might benefit from this technique needs further study.

OTHER APPROACHES IN SPERM SELECTION

In addition to the techniques mentioned earlier, there are other emerging approaches for sperm selection that are currently in a development phase, such as Raman spectroscopy, electric charge-based selection method, and sperm chemotactic-based method.

Techniques Based on Deoxyribonucleic Acid Integrity (Raman Spectroscopy)

It is well-established that a high sperm DNA fragmentation index can be negatively associated with embryo quality.[39] Moreover, high DNA fragmentation can be positively associated with an increase of pregnancy loss, confirming the importance of chromatin packaging in maintaining a viable pregnancy.[40]

For that reason, several test have been performed [Terminal deoxynucleotidyl transferase-mediated deoxyuridine triphosphate (dUTP) nick end-labeling (TUNEL), sperm chromatin structure assay (SCSA), sperm chromatin dispersion (SCD), and Comet assay] to study the DNA integrity in a semen sample. All of them are diagnostic tools that can be only used to know the level of sperm DNA fragmentation in a specific sample, and therefore there is no possibility to use the same sample to isolate viable spermatozoa with high DNA integrity for a reproduction treatment.

In this sense, Raman microspectroscopy, the combination of Raman spectroscopy and confocal microscopy is a new technique that can solve this problem. This technique can give information of the composition and localization of different internal structures of the cell without its manipulation.[41] The study published by Sanchez V et al. showed that Raman microspectroscopy is able to identify individual spermatozoa with oxidative DNA damage to a degree comparable to the most dependable currently available technique. The utility of the technique for both clinical and andrology research is its ability to not only to identify sperm with physiologically damaged DNA but also to do this in a noninvasively and nondestructively manner,[42] permitting the use of this spermatozoa with high DNA integrity to be used or the ICSI treatment. Although Raman microspectroscopy still requires further validation, this technique may potentially provide a means of assessing the DNA status of a living sperm.[43]

Techniques Based on Electric Charge (Electrophoresis Separation)

The negative electrical charge of the spermatozoon depends largely on the expression of various glycocalyx proteins, especially gp20 or CD52, which is a sialoglycoprotein present in the sperm surface. This sialoglycoprotein is added during the passage of the spermatozoa through the epididymis and its expression levels appear to be positively correlated with the morphology, DNA integrity and functional status of the cell. Based on these characteristics of the sperm cells, several selection systems have been developed focused on the isolation and separation of those cells with higher negative charge. The most known system is the microelectrophoresis using specific devices that was firstly developed by Ainsworth et al. in 2005.[44] This device is composed of four chambers: two outer, filled with buffer, and two inner chambers (for inoculation of sample and collection, separated by a polycarbonate membrane). After application a current of 75 mA and variable voltage, the selected sperm population with high negative electric charge is collected from the inner compartment. Several works have been published by using this technique, showing that the selected populations are correlated with better morphology and with low-levels of DNA damage,[44] and the first pregnancy reported by using this system was published in 2007.[45]

Techniques Based on Microgradients

One of the physiological processes of sperm selection is the attraction of the spermatozoa to the proximity of the egg mediated by chemical gradients, especially progesterone secreted by oocyte cumulus cells. As only a small proportion of capacitated spermatozoa are capable of responding to these gradients, it has been hypothesized that those spermatozoa with a greater capacity to migrate to chemoattractants will be those with better functional characteristics. Based on this principle, different devices that produce microgradients of chemoattractants have been developed.[46-48] However, the impact of using these devices to isolate chemotaxis selected sperm on ART outcomes is currently unknown.

CONCLUSION

Reproductive specialists are constantly looking for methods to improve treatment success rates. Considering the central role of the male gamete, finding a way to select the adequate spermatozoon is clearly warranted.

In natural reproduction, sperm selection is a necessary step to achieve a pregnancy. Conventional techniques of sperm selection (swim-up and density gradients) are based primarily on sperm motility, although other sperm parameters may be indirectly improved. On the contrary, the new techniques of sperm selection are based on the analysis of functional characteristics, trying to mimic what happens physiologically. Between them, there are techniques that improve the global sperm population, such as MACS or microgradients, while other techniques are focused on the individual selection of spermatozoa to be used in ART, such as IMSI, PICSI or Raman spectroscopy.

The data obtained so far, although sometimes conflicting, seem to indicate that these techniques may be useful in selected infertile cases, especially when there is an associated male factor, such as MACS and IMSI, or in cases of repetitive abortion, such as PICSI. Even so, although the results obtained so far are promising are still necessary more prospective and randomized studies to draw more consistent conclusions.

REFERENCES

1. Barroso G, Valdespin C, Vega E, et al. Developmental sperm contributions: fertilization and beyond. Fertil Steril. 2009;92(3):835-48.
2. Ortega NM, Bosch P. Methods for sperm selection for in vitro fertilization. In: Friedler S (Ed). In Vitro Fertilization-Innovative Clinical and Laboratory Aspects. Croatia: InTech; 2012.
3. Henkel RR, Schill WB. Sperm preparation for ART. Reprod Biol Endocrinol. 2003;1:108.
4. Henkel R. Sperm preparation: state-of-the-art—physiological aspects and application of advanced sperm preparation methods. Asian J Androl. 2012;14(2): 260-9.

5. Mahadevan M, Baker G. Assessment and preparation of semen for in vitro fertilization. In: Wood C, Trounson A (Ed). Clinical In Vitro Fertilization. Berlin: Springer-Verlag; 1984. pp. 83-97.

6. Arends MJ, Wyllie AH. Apoptosis: mechanisms and roles in pathology. Int Rev Exp Pathol. 1991;32:223-54.

7. Grunewald S, Paasch U, Glander HJ. Enrichment of non-apoptotic human spermatozoa after cryopreservation by immunomagnetic cell sorting. Cell Tissue Bank. 2001;2(3):127-33.

8. Said TM, Agarwal A, Grunewald S, et al. Evaluation of sperm recovery following annexin V magnetic-activated cell sorting separation. Reprod Biomed Online. 2006;13(3):336-9.

9. Said TM, Agarwal A, Zborowski M, et al. Utility of magnetic cell separation as a molecular sperm preparation technique. J Androl. 2008;29(2):134-42.

10. Hoogendijk CF, Kruger TF, Bouic PJ, et al. A novel approach for the selection of human sperm using annexin V-binding and flow cytometry. Fertil Steril. 2009; 91(4):1285-92.

11. Bucar S, Gonçalves A, Rocha E, et al. DNA fragmentation in human sperm after magnetic-activated cell sorting. J Assist Reprod Genet. 2015;32(1):147-54.

12. Lee TH, Liu CH, Shih YT, et al. Magnetic-activated cell sorting for sperm preparation reduces spermatozoa with apoptotic markers and improves the acrosome reaction in couples with unexplained infertility. Hum Reprod. 2010;25(4): 839-46.

13. Said TM, Grunewald S, Paasch U, et al. Effects of magnetic-activated cell sorting on sperm motility and cryosurvival rates. Fertil Steril. 2005;83(5):1442-6.

14. Khalid SN, Qureshi IZ. Effect of magnetic selected sperm on fertilization and embryo development: an animal model study. Fertil Steril. 2011;96(3):S169.

15. Romany L, Meseguer M, Garcia-Herrero S, et al. Magnetic activated sorting selection (MACS) of non-apoptotic sperm (NAS) improves pregnancy rates in homologous intrauterine insemination (IUI). preliminary data. Fertil Steril. 2010; 94(4):S14.

16. Romany L, Garrido N, Motato Y, et al. Removal of annexin V-positive sperm cells for intracytoplasmic sperm injection in ovum donation cycles does not improve reproductive outcome: a controlled and randomized trial in unselected males. Fertil Steril. 2014;102(6):1567-75.

17. Gil M, Sar-Shalom M, Melendez Sivira Y, et al. Sperm selection using magnetic activated cell sorting (MACS) in assisted reproduction: a systematic review and meta-analysis. J Assist Reprod Genet. 2013;30(4):479-85.

18. Dirican EK, Ozgün OD, Akarsu S, et al. Clinical outcome of magnetic activated cell sorting of non-apoptotic spermatozoa before density gradient centrifugation for assisted reproduction. J Assist Reprod Genet. 2008;25(8):375-81.

19. Herrero MB, Delbes G, Chung JT, et al. Case report: the use of annexin V coupled with magnetic activated cell sorting in cryopreserved spermatozoa from a male cancer survivor: healthy twin newborns after two previous ICSI failures. J Assist Reprod Genet. 2013;30(11):1415-9.

20. Lukaszuk K, Wcislo M, Liss J, et al. First Pregnancy, Somatic and Psychological Status of a 4-Year-Old Child Born following Annexin V TESA Sperm Separation. AJP Rep. 2015;5(2):e105-8.

21. Romany L, Garrido N, Cobo A, et al. Obstetric and perinatal outcome of babies born from sperm selected by MACS from a randomized controlled trial. J Assist Reprod Genet. 2017;34(2):201-7.

22. De Vos A, Van de Velde H, Bocken G, et al. Does intracytoplasmic morphologically selected sperm injection improve embryo development? A randomized sibling-oocyte study. Hum Reprod. 2013;28(3):617-26.

23. Bartoov B, Berkovitz A, Eltes F. Selection of spermatozoa with normal nuclei to improve the pregnancy rate with intracytoplasmic sperm injection. N Engl J Med. 2001;345(14):1067-8.

24. Setti AS, Figueira RC, Braga DP, et al. Intracytoplasmic morphologically selected sperm injection is beneficial in cases of advanced maternal age: a prospective randomized study. Eur J Obstet Gynecol Reprod Biol. 2013;171(2):286-90.

25. Setti AS, Paes de Almeida Ferreira Braga D, Iaconelli A, et al. Twelve years of MSOME and IMSI: a review. Reprod Biomed Online. 2013;27(4):338-52.

26. Berkovitz A, Eltes F, Lederman H, et al. How to improve IVF-ICSI outcome by sperm selection. Reprod Biomed Online. 2006;12(5):634-8.

27. Boitrelle F, Guthauser B, Alter L, et al. High-magnification selection of spermatozoa prior to oocyte injection: confirmed and potential indications. Reprod Biomed Online. 2014;28(1):6-13.

28. Ebner T, Shebl O, Oppelt P, et al. Some reflections on intracytoplasmic morphologically selected sperm injection. Int J Fertil Steril. 2014;8(2):105-12.

29. Jakab A, Sakkas D, Delpiano E, et al. Intracytoplasmic sperm injection: a novel selection method for sperm with normal frequency of chromosomal aneuploidies. Fertil Steril. 2005;84(6):1665-73.

30. Huszar G, Sbracia M, Vigue L, et al. Sperm plasma membrane remodeling during spermiogenetic maturation in men: relationship among plasma membrane beta 1,4-galactosyltransferase, cytoplasmic creatine phosphokinase, and creatine phosphokinase isoform ratios. Biol Reprod. 1997;56(4):1020-4.

31. Huszar G, Ozenci CC, Cayli S, et al. Hyaluronic acid binding by human sperm indicates cellular maturity, viability, and unreacted acrosomal status. Fertil Steril. 2003;79 Suppl 3:1616-24.

32. Parmegiani L, Cognigni GE, Bernardi S, et al. Comparison of two ready-to-use systems designed for sperm-hyaluronic acid binding selection before intracytoplasmic sperm injection: PICSI vs. Sperm Slow: a prospective, randomized trial. Fertil Steril. 2012;98(3):632-7.

33. Ye H, Huang GN, Gao Y, et al. Relationship between human sperm-hyaluronan binding assay and fertilization rate in conventional in vitro fertilization. Hum Reprod. 2006;21(6):1545-50.

34. Mansour R, Ishihara O, Adamson GD, et al. International Committee for Monitoring Assisted Reproductive Technologies world report: Assisted Reproductive Technology 2006. Hum Reprod. 2014;29(7):1536-51.

35. Said TM, Land JA. Effects of advanced selection methods on sperm quality and ART outcome: a systematic review. Hum Reprod Update. 2011;17(6):719-33.

36. Beck-Fruchter R, Shalev E, Weiss A. Clinical benefit using sperm hyaluronic acid binding technique in ICSI cycles: a systematic review and meta-analysis. Reprod Biomed Online. 2016;32(3):286-98.

37. Tarozzi N, Nadalini M, Bizzaro D, et al. Sperm-hyaluronan-binding assay: clinical value in conventional IVF under Italian law. Reprod Biomed Online. 2009;19 Suppl 3:35-43.

38. Parmegiani L, Cognigni GE, Ciampaglia W, et al. Efficiency of hyaluronic acid (HA) sperm selection. J Assist Reprod Genet. 2010;27(1):13-6.

39. Avendaño C, Oehninger S. DNA fragmentation in morphologically normal spermatozoa: how much should we be concerned in the ICSI era? J Androl. 2011;32(4):356-63.

40. Ioannou D, Miller D, Griffin DK, et al. Impact of sperm DNA chromatin in the clinic. J Assist Reprod Genet. 2016;33(2):157-66.

41. Mallidis C, Wistuba J, Bleisteiner B, et al. In situ visualization of damaged DNA in human sperm by Raman microspectroscopy. Hum Reprod. 2011;26(7):1641-9.

42. Sánchez V, Redmann K, Wistuba J, et al. Oxidative DNA damage in human sperm can be detected by Raman microspectroscopy. Fertil Steril. 2012;98(5):1124-9.

43. Mallidis C, Sanchez V, Wistuba J, et al. Raman microspectroscopy: shining a new light on reproductive medicine. Hum Reprod Update. 2014;20(3):403-14.

44. Ainswoth C, Nixon B, Aitken RJ. Development of a novel electrophoretic system for the isolation of human spermatozoa. Hum Reprod. 2005;20(8):2261-70.

45. Ainswoth C, Nixon B, Jansen RP, et al. First recorded pregnancy and normal birth after ICSI using electrophoretically isolated spermatozoa. Hum Reprod. 2007; 22(1):197-200.

46. Chung Y, Zhu X, Gu W, et al. Microscale integrated sperm sorter. Methods Mol Biol. 2006;321:227-44.

47. Xie L, Ma R, Han C, et al. Integration of sperm motility and chemotaxis screening with a microchannel-based device. Clin Chem. 2010;56(8):1270-8.

48. Gatica LV, Guidobaldi HA, Montesinos MM, et al. Picomolar gradients of progesterone select functional human sperm even in subfertile samples. Mol Hum Reprod. 2013;19(9):559-69.

Chapter 4

From the Gamete to the Zygote

Alberto Tejera, Belén Aparicio, Mª José de los Santos

INTRODUCTION

The impact of oocyte morphology on further embryo development as well as on implantation is not clear, being the subject of debate. Even so, it is generally recognized that certain type of oocyte morphology alterations can have a negative effect on further fertilization and development, and consequently, on the outcome. Another controversial issue is the effect of pronuclear score on the embryo development and its relation with the embryo quality and implantation.

This chapter assesses the influence of oocyte phenotypes and some fertilization events (pronuclear score and symmetry) using time-lapse technology in implanted and nonimplanted embryos. Just in cases of several abnormalities of the oocytes (high number of vacuoles or heavy cluster) the fertilization rate is affected, but the rest of the phenotypes did not affect the fertilization ability, as well as the embryo quality.

The zygote score did not differ between implanted and none implanted embryos, and according to PN symmetry, those zygotes with unequal size of pronuclei gave rise to embryos with low implantation (13%) while those zygotes with equal or similar pronuclear size generated embryos with higher implantation (22%).

CUMULUS-OOCYTE COMPLEX

The mature cumulus-oocyte complex (COC) is composed of the secondary oocyte [which is arrested at metaphase II (MII)] surrounded by a multilayer of specialized granulosa cells called cumulus cells (CCs). They possess highly specialized transzonal cytoplasmic projections that penetrate through the zona pellucida (ZP) and form gap junctions at their tips with the oocyte.[1] The gap junctions will allow paracrine factors and low-molecular weight factors to freely travel in both directions.[2,3]

Since fully grown oocytes from late antral follicle to preovulatory follicle are meiotically competent, after stimulation and ovulation triggering, the majority of the aspirated follicles will contain nuclear mature "MII" oocytes. However, before arrival of mature oocytes to laboratories, oocytes have had to initiate a rather long journey from the arrested phase of the diplotene stage of prophase I, to MII oocytes.[4,5] Endocrinological inactive primordial follicles are capable to generate mature oocytes at ovulation process. During the last phase of follicular growth, hormones will act on the oocyte, releasing the G2 arrest and causing the oocyte to progress through a receptive configuration for fertilization.

After puberty, follicular enclosed oocytes will need to pass through a series of follicular growing phases, the first phase is not hormone-dependent and the second is dependent on them.[6] This journey lasts around 180 days and is not easy for oocytes to progressively gain oocyte competence.[4] During this long travel, different processes are triggered giving rise to the expression of a new set of genes, cytoplasmic organization, reorganization and formation of new organelles, and creation of the glycoprotein layer of the ZP. For example, it has been shown that the presence of endocytic vacuoles, reorganization of organelles [like the mitochondria-smooth endoplasmic reticulum (M-SER) aggregates] or the appearance of necrotic areas emerge in the final part of maturation.[7] Other processes such as the transformation of the Golgi apparatus into Golgi-derived vesicles called cortical granules (CG) occurs during the early stages of oocyte growth.[8] Also, ooplasma may also accumulate lipid droplets, multivesicular and crystalline bodies, which may remain until ovulation and may play a role during fertilization and further embryo development.

Luteinizing hormone (LH) surge a cascade of events is leads to further CC proliferation and expansion by mediating the synthesis of hyaluronic acid and organization of and stable cellular matrix. The degree of expansion of the CCs has been proposed as an indicator of the nuclear maturation stage of the oocytes, however, objective criteria of assessment oocyte quality are lacking and not always exists a direct correlation between degree of expansion and nuclear maturity.

Generally speaking the oocyte CCs complexes can be divided into three main categories with regards of the degree of expansion and nuclear maturity of the enclosed oocytes:

1. Grade 1 (containing MII oocytes): CCs with even distribution and a much expanded appearance.
2. Grade 2 [containing metaphase I (MI) oocytes]: CCs with a dense matrix and an intermediate degree of expansion.
3. Grade 3 oocytes [containing germinal vesicle (GV) oocytes]: CCs very compacted and dark.

Once the oocytes have been stripped from the surrounded layer of CCs, it becomes easy to observe the morphology of the denuded oocyte.

OOCYTE

From a broad general agreement, although a morphological normal MII[9] oocyte should be in spherical form, and have no a large perivitelline space, a homogenous cytoplasm with no inclusions and ZP of around 15–20 µm thick, physiological variation throughout oocyte growth may cause differences in oocyte phenotypes, and consequently, in their morphologies. Some aspects occurred during follicular stimulation process and oocyte growth could affect to the different oocyte dimorphisms. For example, the hormonal follicular environment seems to be related to the incidence of specific oocyte morphological features, such as polar body fragmentation, a large perivitelline space and presence of cytoplasmic inclusions. Interestingly one curious point is that for some authors, the so-called "normal oocyte phenotype" is actually the least recently used. As a result between 60–70% of the oocytes from stimulated cycles present one or more phenotypic alterations.[10,11]

Assessment of Oocyte Phenotypic Characteristics

Oocyte phenotypes can be classified by morphological categories based on the cytoplasmic and extracytoplasmic attributes observed; van Blerkom and Alikani previously described most of them.[12] In their study, oocytes were grouped into 12 classes as follows:

1. *Normal (N) oocytes*: With homogenous or very slightly granulated cytoplasm, a nonfragmented, normal size polar body and without an overlarge perivitelline space, a normal ZP
2. Oocytes with altered necrotic bodies (NBs) in the cytoplasm
3. Oocytes with refractile bodies (RBs)
4. Oocytes with homogenous very granular cytoplasm (HGC)
5. Oocytes with severe centrally located granular cytoplasm (CLGC)
6. Oocytes with SER
7. Oocytes with vacuoles (VACs)
8. Oocytes with multiple (M) abnormalities
9. Oocytes with a large perivitelline space (LPS)
10. Oocytes with abnormal polar bodies (PBs)
11. Elongated (E) oocytes
12. Oocytes with debris (Db) in the perivitelline space.

    Moreover, oocytes were grouped also according to the appearance of the ZP:

- Oocytes with normal ZP (nZP)
- Oocytes with an elongated ZP (eZP)
- Oocytes with a pigmented ZP (pZP) or dark ZP (dZP)
- Oocytes with a thick ZP (thZP)
- Oocytes with a thin ZP (tZP)
- Oocytes with an evident bilayered ZP (bZP)
- Oocytes with a irregular thickness ZP (irZP)
- Oocytes with a rough inner ZP (izrZP).

    A brief description of each of these phenotypic characteristics assessed in the oocytes have been given here.

Refractile and Necrotic Bodies

Both these kinds of phenotypes include a variety of cytoplasmic features that are considered small necrotic areas of around 10 μm in size, and composed of lipid droplets that can be located isolated or in groups.[13,14]

Homogenous Granular and Centrally Located Granular Cytoplasm

In some cases, one can appreciate the granulation in the cytoplasm, which is located homogeneously or centrally. When this is the case (CLGC) it is diagnosed as being a larger, dark, and granular area. This phenotype may correspond to the central location of organelles in the cytoplasm. Severity of granulation is based on the diameter of the granular area and depth.

Smooth Endoplasmic Reticulum

This dimorphism is the result of a massive accumulation of tubular type SER clusters.[15] Even though we do not really have a clear explanation for the mechanisms that allow to the appearance of SER aggregates, different groups have observed a positive effect between presence of SER and serum estradiol concentrations on the day of ovulation induction, as well as concentrations of antimullerian hormone.[16-18]

Vacuoles

One of the most common oocyte dimorphism is cytoplasmic vacuolization. VACs are, according to Van Blerkom, membrane-bound cytoplasmic inclusions filled with fluid that is similar to perivitelline fluid. The incidence involves 5–12% of oocytes, and the size and number may vary. Appearance of VACs can be spontaneous or through the fusion of preexisting vesicles which derive from the Golgi apparatus or the SER.[19]

Large Perivitelline Space

This dimorphism can be clearly visualized under an inverted microscope due to an increase in the perivitelline space, and there is no contact, so the oocyte seems to float within the interior of the ZP. Some authors have reported that an increase in the perivitelline space can be related to extreme oocyte maturation.[20,21]

First Polar Body

It seems that the morphology of the first PB (fPB) changes within first hours of in vitro culture and, consequently, may vary depending on the observation time.[22] Different dimorphisms are related to the fPB, such as number or fragmentation. However, apart from the very large fPB, the impact and effect of this dimorphism on the development potential of this oocyte is not clear.

Cellular Debris in the Perivitelline Space

The presence of cellular Db in the perivitelline space is considered an extra-cytoplasmic abnormality. Even though there is currently no scientific evidence for the influence of this dysmorphism on the oocyte, and it cannot be quantified or measured, some authors have related this kind of dysmorphism to internal ZP deterioration, while others have observed that the presence of detritus may correspond to a sign of an "overdose" of gonadotropins used in stimulation protocols.[23]

Experts from the Istanbul consensus have expressed that given the limited knowledge and controversial topic of biological significance of the most of oocytes dimorphisms, their primary concern is focused in those oocyte phenotypes relevant to the result. In other words, those dimorphisms with greater impact on embryo development, e.g. oocytes with severe central granularity, called cluster oocytes, oocytes with a SER, oocytes with VACs more than 14 µm, and oocytes with big PBs.[24] Many articles regard to oocyte dysmorphisms and their relation to adverse *in vitro* fertilization (IVF) outcomes have been published. Even though extensive reviews have been performed[25,26] a consensus about the predictive value to consider an oocyte with poor or good quality based merely on its morphology is lacking.

Embryo Kinetics of Dysmorphic Oocytes

This section will show the association of oocyte morphology with the fertilization and embryos cleavage event, as well as the influence of zygote score pronuclear to embryo implantation.

In the chapter published by Aparicio and de los Santos[27] they included a study in which the morphology of 5252 oocytes was analyzed. The results showed that the highest proportion corresponded to "normal category", as expected (38.3%), followed by OR (25%), AC (12.1%), fPB (10%), LPS (6.6%), M (5.9%) and PB (1.6%). The ZP phenotypes of the oocytes resulting from this study population were distributed as follows: 1.3% dZP, 0.6% hZP, 3% eZP, 4.5% tZP, 3.2% thZP, 2.1% irZP, 0.2% mZP, 72.7% nZP, 0.6% pZP, and 0.9% bZP. Only three types of oocyte morphologies showed statistically lower fertilization ability compared to normal oocytes. These oocytes were those with multiples abnormalities (66.0%), those with VACs (64.3%), and the heavily granulated ones (68.15%), whereas the normal oocytes had a 78.6% fertilization rate (Table 4.1). Fertilization was also similar regardless of type of ZP (normal and abnormal). When analyzing the correlation between embryo quality and oocyte morphology, the average percentage of good quality embryos founded was 50%. The embryo quality was not affected by oocyte morphological categories, obtaining similar percentages in different phenotypes (Table 4.1), and the same embryo quality was achieved considering

Table 4.1: Distribution of oocyte dysmorphisms, fertilization ability and embryo quality. Only fertilization rates were significant different among some types of oocyte dysmorphisms.

Oocyte phenotype	Phenotype distribution	Fertilization n (5%)	OR CI 95%	GQ embryos n (%)	OR CI 95%
Normal	3456 (66.9%)	2715 (78.6%)		1368 (50.4%)	
NB	91 (1.8%)	66 (72.5%)	0.72 (0.41–1.27)	39 (59.1%)	0.43–1.26
RB	249 (4.8%)	198 (79.5%)	1.06 (0.77–1.46)	100 (50.5%)	1.47–1.52
HGC	285 (5.5%)	194 (68.1%)*	0.58* (0.45–0.76)	95 (48.7%)	0.37–1.17
CLGC	266 (5.2%)	202 (75.9%)	0.86 (0.63–1.15)	108 (53.5%)	0.51–2.15
SER	76 (1.5%)	57 (75.0%)	0.82 (0.48–1.39)	33 (57.9%)	0.33–1.80
VAC	42 (0.8%)	27 (64.3%)*	0.49* (0.26–0.93)	12 (44.4%)	0.38–1.39
M	53 (1.0%)	35 (66.0%)*	0.53* (0.30–0.94)	13 (36.4%)	0.41–1.35
LPS	434 (6.6%)	297 (74.6%)	0.82 (0.63–1.06)	141 (47.5%)	0.23–1.47
PB	136 (2.6%)	104 (76.5%)	0.89 (0.59–1.33)	52 (50%)	0.38–1.26
E	48 (0.9%)	35 (72.9%)	0.74 (0.39–1.40)	18 (51.4%)	0.17–1.1
A	54 (1.0%)	41 (77.4%)	0.93 (0.49–1.78)	12 (29.3%)	0.13–0.71
Db	62 (1.2%)	45 (72.6%)	0.72 (0.45–1.15)	20 (44.4%)	0.26–1.28

*$P < 0.05$

(CI: Confidence interval; CLGC: Centrally located granular cytoplasm; Db: Debris; E: Elongated; HGC: Homogenous very granular cytoplasm; LPS: Large perivitelline space; M: Multiple; NB: Necrotic body; OR: Odds ratio; PB: Polar body; RB: Refractile body; SER: Smooth endoplasmic reticulum; VAC: Vacuole).

the shape of ZP (Table 4.2). Similarly, when the kinetics parameters were evaluated, no discrepancies were seen among all the phenotypes analyzed (Table 4.3), or between the embryos originated from oocytes with normal or abnormal ZPs (Table 4.4).

Table 4.2: Distribution of zona pellucida morphology, fertilization ability and embryo quality. Regarding fertilization and embryo quality, no significant differences were observed among the groups.

Zona pellucida phenotypes	Zona pellucida distribution	Fertilization n (%)	OR CI 95%	GQ embryos N (%)	OR CI 95%
nZP	4312 (81.6%)	3329 (77.4%)		1678 (50.4%)	
eZP	152 (3.0%)	116 (76.3%)		52 (44.8%)	0.48–6.65
tZP	172 (3.3%)	135 (78.5%)	0.74–5.65	74 (54.5%)	0.46–8.69
thZP	276 (5.3%)	221 (80.1%)	0.40–4.57	101 (45.7%)	0.42–5.41
IrZP	42 (0.8%)	29 (69.0%)	0.84–6.91	16 (57.1%)	0.34–4.59
Dark ZP	16 (0.3%)	10 (62.5%)	0.61–5.36	4 (4.0%)	0.54–7.63
BZP	52 (1.0%)	36 (69.2%)	0.74–6.42	19 (52.8%)	0.48–6.65
izrZP	141 (2.7%)	106 (75.2%)	0.65–5.68	62 (57.5%)	0.46–7.70

(bZP: Bilayered ZP; CI: Confidence interval; eZP: Elongated ZP; IrZP: Irregular ZP; IzrZP: Rough inner ZP; nZP: Normal ZP; OR: Odds ratio; tZp: Thin ZP; thZP: Thick ZP; ZP: Zona pellucida).

Fertilization Initial Stages

After the oocytes have been inseminated by intracytoplasmic sperm injection (ICSI) of conventional IVF, some of them will become fertilized.

Sperm Preparation

Although the male gamete is morphologically complete, is not functional; in other words, is not able to fertilize the egg by itself. In order to do it, the gamete needs to be prepared; this implies a number of changes or modifications aimed at increasing their motility and their ability to fertilize. *In vivo*, such changes take place during migration of sperm through the female genital tract and *in vitro*, by processing the sperm sample in the laboratory and later culture in a medium with an appropriate concentration of Ca^{2+}, and HCO_3^- and other factors contributing to sperm capacitation.[28,29]

Some of the changes that occur during sperm preparation include an increase in fluidity of the plasma membrane (mainly due to loss of cholesterol and reorientation of the molecules that compose the lipid bilayer), changes in the state of tyrosine phosphorylation of certain sperm proteins, hyperpolarization of membrane potential and increased intracellular pH and Ca^{2+} levels. Aimed all to the acquisition of hyperactivity, finally the sperm acquire a fast movement *in situ* and a large lateral displacement of the head

Table 4.3: Kinetic timings including some early fertilization events and the most relevant cleavage morphokinetic parameters in each type of oocyte dysmorphism.

Oocyte phenotype	tPB2	tPNa	tPNf	t2	cc2	s2	t5
Normal	3.5 (3.4–3.6)	7.9 (7.7–8.0)	23.3 (22.8–23.6)	26.0 (25.6–26.4)	12 (11.6–12.5)	3.9 (3.6–4.2)	47.7 (46.8–48.5)
NB	3.4 (2.8–3.9)	8.2 (7.3–9.2)	24.4 (22.2–26.7)	24.4 (22.2–26.7)	11.7 (8.7–14.8)	4.2 (1.6–6.7)	43.6 (38.6–48.7)
RB	3.5 (3.2–3.7)	7.9 (7.2–8.6)	23.0 (21.5–24.5)	25.2 (23.8–26.5)	12.0 (10.3–13.7)	3.5 (2.2–4.8)	46.5 (42.9–50.0)
HGC	3.9 (3.3–4.6)	8.5 (7.8–9.2)	24.9 (22.8–27.2)	25.8 (24.3–27.3)	11.8 (9.8–13.6)	4.8 (3.4–6.2)	46.8 (44.1–49.6)
CLGC	3.8 (3.5–4.0)	8.3 (7.7–8.9)	22.9 (21.4–24.3)	27.1 (25.2–28.9)	12.6 (11.1–14.1)	3.7 (2.5–4.9)	50.1 (46.7–53.3)
SER	3.9 (3.2–4.7)	7.2 (6.4–7.9)	22.5 (19.9–25.1)	25.3 (21.8–29.9)	12.3 (9.7–14.9)	6.8 (2.2–11.4)	42.1 (37.0–47.0)
VAC	3.4 (2.4–4.3)	9.3 (6.9–11.8)	24.5 (19.2–29.7)	27.1 (24.1–30.1)	10.8 (5.4–16.2)	4.6 (0.5–8.6)	48.0 (41.6–64.3)
M	3.1 (2.6–3.6)	8.1 (6.1–10.1)	25.1 (21.3–28.8)	28.3 (26.7–30.1)	9.4 (4.2–14.6)	8.7 (0.5–16.9)	39.1 (24.1–64.1)
LPS	3.3 (3.1–3.5)	7.8 (7.4–8.4)	22.2 (21.1–23.9)	25.9 (24.9–26.9)	11.9 (10.9–12.9)	3.7 (2.6–4.7)	47.5 (45.1–50.0)
PB	3.3 (3.0–3.7)	8.5 (7.4–9.7)	25.9 (24.2–27.7)	26.3 (24.6–28.0)	11.9 (9.6–14.2)	3.8 (2.2–5.3)	45.5 (41.4–49.6)
E	3.8 (3.1–4.4)	7.5 (6.3–8.7)	25.0 (23.7–26.3)	25.7 (22.6–28.7)	13.4 (9.9–17.0)	1.2 (0.5–3.4)	52.5 (45.4–69.4)
A	3.6 (3.0–4.3)	7.3 (5.6–9.0)	25.2 (21.4–29.1)	25.6 (22.5–28.9)	11.6 (7.9–15.2)	2.8 (1.3–4.3)	44.9 (38.8–50.9)
Db	4.4 (3.6–5.2)	6.9 (5.4–8.5)	19.7 (19.9–25.1)	25.8 (23.3–28.2)	12.4 (8.5–16.2)	3.8 (1.4–6.0)	48.4 (42.9–63.8)

(CLGC: Centrally located granular cytoplasm; Db: Debris; E: Elongated; HGC: Homogenous very granular cytoplasm; LPS: Large perivitelline space; M: Multiple; NB: Necrotic body; PB: Polar body; RB: Refractile body; SER: Smooth endoplasmic reticulum; VAC: Vacuole).

Table 4.4: Kinetic timings in embryos with normal and abnormal zona pellucidas. Values between brackets are 95% confidence interval.

Zona pellucida phenotype	tPB2	tPNa	tPNf	t2	cc2	s2	t5
Normal Zp	3.5 (3.4–3.6)	7.9 (7.7–8.0)	23.3 (22.8–23.6)	26.2 (25.6–26.4)	11.9 (11.6–12.5)	4.0 (3.6–4.2)	47.5 (46.8–48.5)
Abnormal Zp	3.5 (2.8–4.3)	7.9 (7.9–8.5)	22.9 (20.9–24.9)	25.4 (23.9–26.8)	12.7 (8.7–14.8)	3.1 (2.3–4.1)	47.3 (44.1–50.3)

(ZP: Zona pellucida).

to facilitate their passage through the granulosa cells and penetration of the ZP.[30,31]

Interaction of Spermatozoon with the Zona Pellucida and Acrosome Reaction

Once the spermatozoon is prepared, it interacts with the oocyte ZP. This interaction is species-specific and a series of ZP glycoproteins are involved: ZP1, ZP2, ZP3 and ZP4. The initial adhesion sperm-ZP is mediated by ZP3, the receptor-ligand interaction results in an entry of Ca^{2+} through T-type channels and this increases the concentration of Ca^{2+}, which triggers the sperm acrosome reaction. This releases the contents of the acrosome vesicle, including enzymes such as acrosin, galactosyltransferase and hyaluronidase, to help the sperm to digest the ZP on its way to the plasma membrane of the oocyte to finally merge with it. ZP penetration by spermatozoon occurs therefore mechanically, facilitated by the pointed shape of the head and tail shaking and enzymatic action conducted by acrosome enzymes.[30]

Fusion between Membranes Oocyte-sperm

A transmembrane protein located in the plasma membrane of sperm catalyzes the fusion. When the sperm fuses with the plasma membrane of the oocyte, it activates cell signaling pathway of inositol phospholipids in the oocyte. This activation, in turn, generates a local increase in cytosolic Ca^{2+} concentration, which as a wave spreads throughout the cell. It seems that the increase of cytosolic calcium activates to oocyte and initiates the cortical reaction, in which the cortical granules release their contents by exocytosis. The enzymes released by the cortical reaction change the structure of ZP, which become hardened, so finally that spermatozoon cannot longer join it, forming a barrier to polyspermy. Among the changes taking place in the ZP, it is noteworthy ZP2 proteolytic degradation and hydrolysis of sugar groups on ZP3.[32,33]

Oocyte Activation

Oocyte activation occurs because of the fusion of two membranes, resulting in the resumption of meiosis with subsequent extrusion of the second PB and formation of female pronuclei (PN), while at the same time the head of the spermatozoon is decondensed to form the male PN which attracts the female PN adopting both a central position.

From now on, the development of the zygote begins after the haploid PN of spermatozoon and oocyte have contacted by mixing their chromosomes to form a diploid nucleus. Human embryos inherit the male centriole, whose function is the assembly of microtubules around the paternal nucleus and alignment of male PN to female PN, so that centriole defects could cause problems in the syngamy and subsequent embryonic development. The human embryo in addition to receiving the genetic heritage of the deoxyribonucleic acid (DNA) nucleus, receives the genetic heritage contained in the mitochondria. This mitochondrial genome is inherited only from the mother.

Fertilization Assessment

Despite is a process requiring many steps to be successfully completed; the fertilization assessment is a simple process. Oocytes will be considered that have been successfully fertilized, if they show the presence of two PN and two PBs. The presence of PN is not an absolute evidence of normal fertilization, because it cannot be determined that one has maternal origin and the other paternal. Likewise, the evaluation of the second PB can also be misleading, since the fPB is often fragmented and cause misinterpretations. Despite those facts, it continues to be one of the most useful systems for the fertilization assessment when you clearly observe two PBs and two PN centrally located, with even or similar sized, clearly defined by distinct membranes.

ZYGOTE

Since the zygote morphological attributes are associated with the time postfertilization, an agreement has been reached whereby zygote scoring should be carried through according to prefixed times postinsemination. Regarding the appearance time by the PN and CP, it has been studied that after conventional IVF, the PN formation occurs between 8 hours and 14 hours postinsemination (Capmany G. et al., 1996) and after ICSI between 3 hours and 13 hours postinjection.[34]

Recent data obtained by our group using the embryoscope confirm these time ranges, being 9.3 ± 2.3 h the average of appearance of the PN and 24.2 ± 3.3 h the average of disappearance of PN.[35]

Pronuclear Scoring

Regarding the predictive value of pronuclear scoring, it continues to puzzle, frequently debated during the last years with articles demonstrating a positive effect[36-40] and others that found no positive predictive value.[41,42] Pronuclear scoring refers to the annotation of different features of the zygote, such as the symmetry and alignment of the PN, taking into account the number and relative position of the nucleolar precursor bodies (NPBs) located in the PN. The Istanbul consensus established the classification of the zygotes according to the NPBs into four main categories assessed 17 ± 1 h after ICSI:

1. Z1 = Zygotes having 3–7 polarized NPB
2. Z2 = Zygotes with homogeneously dispersed NPB
3. Z3 = All the zygotes with a NPB distribution not included in groups 1, 2 or 4 (i.e. >7 polarized NPB, one PN polarized and the other dispersed or both dispersed but not homogeneously)
4. Z4 = Zygotes with only one or two NPB, as described by Gamiz et al. in 2003.

Concerning to the PN symmetry three classes were established: symmetry 1, 2 and 3, defined as equal size, similar size or very different size, respectively.[43]

As prescribed by the consensus[22] there are some features of PN to note, being considered as strongly atypical: broadly separated PN, PN of grossly different sizes, micronuclei and the presence of SER disks. Embryos from zygotes with different pronuclear sizes (> 4 µm difference) have been related to a high rate of embryonic developmental arrest, a high rate of multi-nucleation on day 2 of development and a greater percentage of chromosomal abnormalities.[44,45] So, according to consensus, there should be three categories on pronuclear scoring: (1) symmetrical (equivalent to Z1 and Z2), (2) nonsymmetrical (other aspects, including peripheral PN) and (3) abnormal (those pronuclei with 0 or 1 NPB, which have been associated with abnormal outcomes in animal models).[22]

Historically, it has always believed that equality in number and distribution of NPBs was sign of good prognosis or normality, while any inequality in number or distribution of the NPBs was considered to be abnormal. Since the burgeoning growth of time-lapse systems, it suggests us to call into question this general belief. Time-lapse technology provides extra information as the identification of the precise cell division timings. Focusing only on timing of early fertilization events, we can determine: the extrusion of the second polar body (tPB2), PN appearance (tPNa) and PN fading (tPNf), and some of the first divisions and intervals [division to 2 cells (t2), the duration of second cell cycle (cc2), the synchrony of divisions from the 2-cell to 4-cell stages (s2) and the division to 5 cells (t5)].[46]

Embryo Implantation Rate According to Pronuclear Score

In most cases both PN appeared simultaneously (96.4%), just in few instances (3.6%) one pronucleus appeared before the other. The analysis of the categorical fertilization events showed the following results: the distribution of the four Z-scores (Z1, Z2, Z3, and Z4) did not differ between implanted and nonimplanted embryos (Z1 = 23.7%, Z2 = 28.2%, Z3 = 21.1% and Z4 = 30.8%). Regarding score distribution Z1 and Z3 were the most majorities (41% and 40% respectively) and Z2 and Z4 were the lower proportion (18% and <1%). The percentage of implanting known implantation data (KID) embryos according to PN symmetry (1, 2, and 3) did not showed significant differences; those zygotes with equal or similar size (symmetry 1 and 2) reached to 22.1% and 22.5% implantation rate (IR) respectively, while those zygotes with different size (symmetry 3) just achieved a 13.3% of IR. The symmetry distribution was 58%, 39% and 3% respectively.[35]

KEY POINTS TO CONSIDER

The present chapter checked that just specific phenotypes, such as presence of multiple abnormalities, VACs and heavily granulated cytoplasms, could compromise the zygotes viability were being associated with a significant 10% decrease in fertilization ability, as described in previous chapter by our colleagues.[35] No differences were observed in the accurate timings related to fertilization events, such as tPB2, tPNa, and tPNf, which actually occurred within the optimal ranges previously established by our team[46] and were comparable and similar to the timing undertaken by the normal oocytes.

It should be noted that once fertilization has been passed, is very difficult to predict embryo quality using just the simple oocyte morphological assessment; this was proven by the fact that no significant differences were observed in the kinetic evaluation data of the embryos generated from different types of oocytes.[46] The influence of other types of phenotypes studied, such as necrotic and RBs, was not evident, showing the same cleavage pattern as the embryos originated from normal oocytes.

Regarding PN score the most usual Z-score was 1, followed by 3 and 2, with 7.4 being the lower pronuclear pattern achieved (1.2%). However, the implantation was not affected by Z-score. As is well known to everybody the pronuclear morphology is a dynamic process from first PN appearance until the fading out of the PN, so, we recommend the use of last image taken by a time-lapse system before pronuclear fade out as the best moment to assess the Z-score, when the diameter of each PN is biggest and pronuclear scoring could be evaluated with better preciseness.

All in all, the new approach to measure embryo cleavage timings of the embryos resulting from a variety of oocyte phenotypes shows that the great majority exhibit a similar pattern. Some categories of dimorphisms, such as presence of VACs and multiple abnormalities, have been significantly related to a lower fertilization rate, but once fertilization took place, both embryo development measurements were similar among groups, confirming that variations in oocytes morphology are not predictive of oocyte competence after ICSI.[46]

CONCLUSION

Briefly summarizing, a variety of specific anomalies (such as presence of multiple abnormalities, vacuoles and strongly grainy cytoplasm) affect seriously to fertilization process. The rest of dimorphisms might not affect to the oocyte health and consequently to the zygote. Regarding Kinetic evaluation the embryos resulting from different phenotypes studied showed no differences, getting the same cleavage pattern than normal oocytes.

In the end, the vast majority of phenotypes show a similar cleavage pattern. Only in severe cases were related to a poor fertilization, but once that part is overcome, cellular division timings were similar either way, reaffirming what we had already suspected: oocytes morphology lacks predictive value.

REFERENCES

1. Albertini DF, Combelles CM, Benecchi E, et al. Cellular basis for paracrine regulation of ovarian follicle development. Reproduction. 2001;121(5):647-53.
2. Canipari R. Oocyte-granulosa cell interactions. Hum Reprod Update. 2000;6 (3):279-89.
3. Feuerstein P, Cadoret V, Dalbies-Tran R, et al. Oocyte-cumulus dialog. Gynecol Obstet Fertil. 2006;34(9):793-800.
4. Brewer L, Corzett M, Balhorn R. Condensation of DNA by spermatid basic nuclear proteins. J Biol Chem. 2002;277(41):38895-900.
5. Boissonneault G. Chromatin remodeling during spermiogenesis: a possible role for the transition proteins in DNA strand break repair. FEBS Lett. 2002;514(2-3): 111-4.
6. Diaz I, Navarro J, Blasco L, et al. Impact of stage III-IV endometriosis on recipients of sibling oocytes: matched case-control study. Fertil Steril. 2000;74(1):31-4.
7. Jamnongjit M, Hammes SR. Oocyte maturation: the coming of age of a germ cell. Semin Reprod Med. 2005;23(3):234-41.
8. Liu DY, Baker HW. Defective sperm-zona pellucida interaction: a major cause of failure of fertilization in clinical in-vitro fertilization. Hum Reprod. 2000; 15(3):702-8.
9. Parks JE, Graham JK. Effects of cryopreservation procedures on sperm membranes. Theriogenology. 1992;38(2):209-22.
10. Laboratory manual of the WHO for the examination of human semen and sperm-cervical mucus interaction. Ann Ist Super Sanita. 2001;37(1):I-XII.
11. Anger JT, Gilbert BR, Goldstein M. Cryopreservation of sperm: indications, methods and results. J Urol. 2003;170(4 Pt 1):1079-84.

12. Van Blerkom J, Henry G. Oocyte dysmorphism and aneuploidy in meiotically mature human oocytes after ovarian stimulation. Hum Reprod. 1992;7(3): 379-90.

13. Ombelet W, Campo R. Affordable IVF for developing countries. Reprod Biomed Online. 2007;15(3):257-65.

14. Glasier A, Gebbie A. Contraception for the older woman. Baillieres Clin Obstet Gynaecol. 1996;10(1):121-38.

15. Kably Ambe A, Carballo Mondragon E, Karchmer Krivitsky S. Gamete laboratory. Determining factors of success in in-vitro fertilization. Ginecol Obstet Mex. 2001;69:172-9.

16. Tournaye H, Camus M, Goossens A, et al. Recent concepts in the management of infertility because of non-obstructive azoospermia. Hum Reprod. 1995;10 Suppl 1:115-9.

17. Matsumiya K, Namiki M, Kondoh N, et al. New indication of testis biopsy for azoospermia: a clinical study in Japanese patients. Int J Urol. 1994;1(2):177-80.

18. Raman JD, Schlegel PN. Testicular sperm extraction with intracytoplasmic sperm injection is successful for the treatment of nonobstructive azoospermia associated with cryptorchidism. J Urol. 2003;170(4 Pt 1):1287-90.

19. McLachlan RI, Rajpert-De Meyts E, Hoei-Hansen CE, et al. Histological evaluation of the human testis—approaches to optimizing the clinical value of the assessment: mini review. Hum Reprod. 2007;22(1):2-16.

20. Larson-Cook KL, Brannian JD, Hansen KA, et al. Relationship between the outcomes of assisted reproductive techniques and sperm DNA fragmentation as measured by the sperm chromatin structure assay. Fertil Steril. 2003;80(4): 895-902.

21. Benchaib M, Braun V, Lornage J, et al. Sperm DNA fragmentation decreases the pregnancy rate in an assisted reproductive technique. Hum Reprod. 2003;18 (5):1023-8.

22. Chehval MJ, Purcell MH. Deterioration of semen parameters over time in men with untreated varicocele: evidence of progressive testicular damage. Fertil Steril. 1992;57(1):174-7.

23. Bloch EH, Kafig E, Meryman HT, et al. A comparison of the surfaces of human erythrocytes from health and disease by in vivo light microscopy and in vitro electron microscopy. Angiology. 1956;7(6):479-94.

24. Hall LF, Neubert AG. Obesity and pregnancy. Obstet Gynecol Surv. 2005;60 (4):253-60.

25. Kruger TF, Acosta AA, Simmons KF, et al. New method of evaluating sperm morphology with predictive value for human in vitro fertilization. Urology. 1987;30(3):248-51.

26. Muldrew K, McGann LE. Mechanisms of intracellular ice formation. Biophys J. 1990;57(3):525-32.

27. Aparicio-Ruiz B, de los Santos MJ. Morphological cytoplasmic oocyte alterations: embryo kinetics of dysmorphic oocytes. In: Meseguer M (Ed). Time-Lapse Microscopy in In-Vitro Fertilization. Cambridge: Cambridge University Press; 2016.

28. Marin-Briggiler CI, Vazquez-Levin MH, Gonzalez-Echeverria F, et al. Effect of antisperm antibodies present in human follicular fluid upon the acrosome reaction and sperm-zona pellucida interaction. Am J Reprod Immunol. 2003;50 (3):209-19.

29. Gadella BM, Van Gestel RA. Bicarbonate and its role in mammalian sperm function. Anim Reprod Sci. 2004;82-83:307-19.

30. Visconti PE, Galantino-Homer H, Moore GD, et al. The molecular basis of sperm capacitation. J Androl. 1998;19(2):242-8.
31. Visconti PE, Kopf GS. Regulation of protein phosphorylation during sperm capacitation. Biol Reprod. 1998;59(1):1-6.
32. Evans JP. The molecular basis of sperm-oocyte membrane interactions during mammalian fertilization. Hum Reprod Update. 2002;8(4):297-311.
33. Evans JP, Florman HM. The state of the union: the cell biology of fertilization. Nat Cell Biol. 2002;4 Suppl:s57-63.
34. Payne D, Flaherty SP, Barry MF, et al. Preliminary observations on polar body extrusion and pronuclear formation in human oocytes using time-lapse video cinematography. Hum Reprod. 1997;12(3):532-41.
35. Aguilar J, Motato Y, Escribá MJ, et al. The human first cell cycle: impact on implantation. Reprod Biomed Online. 2014;28(4):475-84.
36. Tesarik J, Greco E. The probability of abnormal preimplantation development can be predicted by a single static observation on pronuclear stage morphology. Hum Reprod. 1999;14(5):1318-23.
37. Scott L, Alvero R, Leondires M, et al. The morphology of human pronuclear embryos is positively related to blastocyst development and implantation. Hum Reprod. 2000;15(11):2394-403.
38. Tesarik J, Junca AM, Hazout A, et al. Embryos with high implantation potential after intracytoplasmic sperm injection can be recognized by a simple, non-invasive examination of pronuclear morphology. Hum Reprod. 2000;15(6):1396-9.
39. Balaban B, Urman B, Isiklar A, et al. The effect of pronuclear morphology on embryo quality parameters and blastocyst transfer outcome. Hum Reprod. 2001;16(11):2357-61.
40. Scott L. Pronuclear scoring as a predictor of embryo development. Reprod Biomed Online. 2003;6(2):201-14.
41. Salumets A, Hydén-Granskog C, Suikkari AM, et al. The predictive value of pronuclear morphology of zygotes in the assessment of human embryo quality. Hum Reprod. 2001;16(10):2177-81.
42. James AN, Hennessy S, Reggio B, et al. The limited importance of pronuclear scoring of human zygotes. Hum Reprod. 2006;21(6):1599-604.
43. Sadowy S, Tomkin G, Munné S, et al. Impaired development of zygotes with uneven pronuclear size. Zygote. 1998;6(2):137-41.
44. Gámiz P, Rubio C, de los Santos MJ, et al. The effect of pronuclear morphology on early development and chromosomal abnormalities in cleavage-stage embryos. Hum Reprod. 2003;18(11):2413-9.
45. Munné S, Cohen J. Chromosome abnormalities in human embryos. Hum Reprod Update. 1998;4(6):842-55.
46. Meseguer M, Herrero J, Tejera A, et al. The use of morphokinetics as a predictor of embryo implantation. Hum Reprod. 2011;26(10):2658-71.

Chapter 5

Embryo Culture

Deven Patel, Preeti Shah, Aditi Kotdawala

INTRODUCTION

The ultimate goal of embryo culture in an assisted reproductive technology (ART) programme is to improve the quality of embryos developing in the laboratory and the chances of successful delivery of a healthy baby.

Culture conditions for human embryos have evolved over the past 3 decades.[1,2] In the natural environment, cleaving embryos develop in the fallopian tube, whereas the morulae and blastocysts in the uterine cavity. The success of clinical *in vitro* fertilization (IVF) was initially compromised by suboptimal culture conditions, resulting in impaired embryo development[3-5] and a subsequent loss of viability. There has been extensive research on the metabolism of *in vitro* fertilized embryos that have revealed that there are specific needs, depending on the developmental stage of the preimplantation embryo which has helped in improving the culture media system according to the oviduct and uterine milieu.[6-8] Over the last 10–15 years there have been major advancements in this area, with culture media developing from simple salt solutions into highly complex defined media, specifically designed to reduce stress to the embryo and maintain high pregnancy rates.

EVOLUTION OF EMBRYO CULTURE MEDIA

The idea introduced by Bernard in the late 1800s, that the immediate environment surrounding living tissues is an active one led, in turn, to the notion that organs and tissues could be studied outside their setting in a suitable fluid formulated to facilitate these studies.[9] It is an interesting aspect that the culture media evolved and used in the clinical setting were construed to support the development of somatic cell culture applications. The first success of fertilization of the human oocyte *in vitro* by Robert Edwards was accomplished in a simple, chemically defined media. These commercially available media were a modified Earle's balanced salt solution, and a modified Ham's F-10 or T6. They were supplemented with maternal serum thus converting them into biological media.[10,11] These varying compositions of culture media for clinical IVF appeared to be hardly different in their ability to support development of the human embryo *in vitro* for up to 48 hours or in subsequent pregnancy rates after transfer.[12] This led to a great deal of confusion concerning the formulation of embryo culture media and the role of individual components in embryo development. A culture medium is a foreign environment for the human embryo. Hence, the design of media is complicated, because the components must be selected, and their concentrations determined in order to minimize stress for the cultured embryo.[2,13,14]

An understanding of the role of culture media and their components is to some extent hampered by the routine inclusion of serum in human embryo culture media. Serum has the ability to both mask potential embryo toxins and suppress the beneficial effects of other medium components. In light of this, there has been considerable research into the development of serum-free embryo culture media. Such studies have been invaluable in the understanding of the embryo's requirements during the preimplantation period. Menezo et al.[15] broke with the tradition of using balanced salt solution and produced a medium containing amino acids (AAs) without the need of a serum supplement. Another medium specifically designed for human IVF was human tubal fluid (HTF).[16] HTF, supplemented with either whole serum or with serum albumin, gained great popularity for the use of day 2 or day 3 human embryo culture, and has remained in use ever since. It also became clear that early embryos show an evolving need for energy substrates, moving from a pyruvate-lactate preference, while the embryos are under maternal genetic control—to glucose-based metabolism after activation of the embryonic genome.[17,18] Media used to culture the mammalian preimplantation embryo generally fall into one of four types.

Simple Salt Solutions with Added Energy Substrates

These media were originally formulated to support the development of zygotes from certain inbred strains of mice and their F1 hybrids.[19] Examples of this type of media used in clinical IVF are M16,[20] T6,[20] Earle's,[11] CZB,[21] and potassium simplex optimization medium (KSOM).[22] Derived from such types of media were HTF medium,[15,23] and P1.[24] Such 'simple' media are usually supplemented with either whole serum or serum albumin, and are used for the cleavage stage embryo only, i.e. pronucleate oocyte to the 8-cell stage.

Complex Tissue Culture Media

These media are commercially available and are designed to support the growth of somatic cells in culture, e.g. Ham's F-10.[25,26] Such media are far more complex, containing AAs, vitamins, nucleic acid precursors, and transitional metals, and are usually supplemented with 5–20% serum. Importantly, such media were not formulated with the specific needs of the human embryo in mind, and they contain components which are now known to be detrimental to the developing embryo.

Simplex Optimized Media

This approach to formulate culture media depended on a computer program to generate successive media formulations based on the response of mouse embryos in culture.[27,28] Once a specific medium was formulated, tested, and blastocyst development analyzed, the computer program would then generate several more media formulations for use in the next series of cultures. This procedure was performed several times to generate media that supported high rates of blastocyst development of embryos derived from the oocytes of outbred mice (CF1) crossed with the sperm of an F1 hybrid male, and were termed SOM and KSOM. Such media were subsequently modified by another laboratory to include KSOM(AA)s.[29] This last phase of medium development was based on previous studies on the mouse embryo[26] and did not involve the simplex procedure. This single medium formulation, KSOM(AA), has been used to produce human blastocysts in culture.[30] In such types of media, the embryo therefore has to adapt to its surroundings as it develops and differentiates.

Sequential Media

This approach is learnt from the environment to which embryos are exposed *in vivo*.[18,31] It helps to understand the physiology and metabolism of the embryo in culture, in order to determine what causes intracellular stress to the embryo.[8,32-35] Examples of sequential media include G1/G2,[36-38] universal IVF medium and M3,[39] and P1 together with blastocyst medium.[40] Interestingly, medium M3 is a modification of Ham's F-10 and F-12, while blastocyst medium is a modification of Ham's F-10.

PHILOSOPHIES BEHIND HUMAN EMBRYO CULTURE MEDIA

The culture media preparation of preimplantation embryos is been influenced by two fundamentally different philosophies.[2,41] The growth of *in vitro* embryos is inferior to that of *in vivo* embryos, indicating that ART procedures create cellular and metabolic stress situations. Thus, the ART embryos are forced to spend energy, so that they can adapt to this foreign environment. Moreover, the culture media is an important factor for successful *in vitro* interactions between gametes and subsequent embryo development.[42] All the manufacturers of human embryo culture media tend to follow either the 'back-to-nature' (sequential media) or the 'let-the-embryo-choose' (single step media) philosophy.[43]

Sequential Culture "Back-to-Nature" Principle

The "back-to-nature" hypothesis mimics the changing needs of the developing zygote and embryo in a culture media that approximates the concentration to which the embryo is physiologically exposed.[42,43] The embryo is capable of actively controlling the ionic gradients, etc. and can regulate its internal environment. Thus as per embryo physiology, the preimplantation period can be subdivided in at least two phases: (1) pre and (2) postcompaction.[42] This breakdown of the preimplantation period is crucial for considering changes to medium formulations and the time when the embryonic genome activation takes place.[42]

Monoculture "Let-the-Embryo-Choose" Principle

This culture system design involves the simultaneous use of all the concentrations in a mixture because the effects of each component in the medium may depend on the concentrations of the other components.[43] As long as concentrations are within "tolerable ranges", the embryo itself will adapt and utilize whatever it requires.[2,43,44] This includes the group of media in which all the necessary substances for early embryological development are provided, and there is no need for a media change. Single-step formulation is applied throughout the *in vitro* development from fertilization to the blastocyst stage of the embryo.

Four protocols can be used for the culture from fertilization to the blastocyst stage in an ART laboratory:

1. Sequential media protocol, with an interrupted culture where two media of different compositions are used sequentially, change of medium occurs on day 3 of embryo culture.
2. Sequential media protocol with fresh medium change everyday.
3. Monoculture, uninterrupted culture using one medium throughout the 5 days of embryo culture.
4. Interrupted culture where a monoculture medium is used throughout but is renewed on day 3 of embryo culture.

KEY COMPONENTS OF ASSISTED REPRODUCTIVE TECHNOLOGY CULTURE MEDIA

Studies using the development of mammalian preimplantation embryos *in vitro* have played a major role in the understanding of preembryo physiology.[42,44-50] The most widely used models for understanding the human embryo have been the mouse and the cow. The composition of embryo culture systems can be broken down into water, ion, carbohydrates, AAs, vitamins, chelators, antioxidants, antibiotics, protein or macromolecules, hormones and growth factors, and buffer system. Each component has a crucial role to play in embryo development in culture, with focus on the pre and post-compaction stages.

Water

Water is the major component of any culture medium, making up around 99% of the content. The source and purity of water used for media preparation is a major factor in assuring the quality of media. The ability of embryos to develop in culture is positively correlated to water quality. Whittingham[20] has reported that *in vitro* development of 2-cell mouse embryos to the blastocyst was enhanced when the media was prepared using triple distilled water as opposed to double or single distilled water. It is recommended to use commercially available high quality water which is endotoxin tested (less than 0.1 IU/mL).

Cell Volume Regulation: Ions and Osmolytes

Clinical IVF media vary markedly as far as ionic basis are considered. Maintenance of a constant volume in the face of extracellular and intracellular osmotic perturbations is a critical problem faced by all cells. Most cells respond to swelling or shrinkage by activating specific metabolic or membrane transport processes that return cell volume to its normal resting state. These processes are essential for the normal function and survival of cells.[51] Surprisingly, the role of ions during the preimplantation development is not well understood. The osmotic pressure of oviduct fluid is more than 360 mOsmol.[52] However, the osmolarity of most commercially available ART culture media is lower at about 250–300 mOsmol. Unfortunately, it is difficult to interpret the effects of individual ions on embryo development and viability, as there are many subtle interactions which exist between ions, carbohydrates, and AAs. When the $NaCl^-$ concentration is forced up to 290 mOsmol, the development of the embryo is severely impaired.[53] Addition of extracellular AA, such as glycine, betaine, proline, alanine and hypotaurine (which act as organic osmolytes), protects the preimplantation embryo against hypertonicity and increases embryo development.[30,53,54]

Carbohydrates

Carbohydrates are present within the luminal fluids of the female reproductive tract. Their levels vary both between the oviduct and uterus and within the cycle.[18,55] Therefore, the developing embryo is exposed to gradients of carbohydrates as it develops. The early embryo shows a rather simplistic physiology and maintains only low levels of oxidative metabolism, whereas it exhibits a somatic cell-like physiology postcompaction using wider spectrum of nutrients. The biosynthetic rates increase, along with an increase in respiratory capacity and an ability to utilize glucose.[8,48] This involves a shift in the energy requirements at the time at which the embryonic genome is activated or at the postcompaction stage. Zygotes and subsequent cleavage stages prefer pyruvate as the primary source of energy, while the 8-cell stage embryo uses glucose.[56-58] Glucose is a key anabolic precursor and is required for the synthesis of triacylglycerol and phospholipids, and as a precursor for complex sugars and glycoproteins. Glucose also metabolized by the pentose phosphate pathway (PPP) generates ribose moieties required for nucleic acid synthesis.[59]

Amino Acids

It is well accepted that all 20 naturally occurring AAs are important for regulation of mammalian preimplantation development.[8,60] On one side, oviduct and uterine fluids contain significant levels of free AAs;[31,61,62] on the other side, oocytes and embryos possess specific transport systems for AAs[63] and maintain an endogenous pool of them.[64] From various reports, the physiological role of AAs in pre- and peri-implantation stages of embryonic development is now well-understood.[65] The carboxyl group acts as the energy source prior to embryonic genome activation of the embryo.[49] They have many other supportive roles in formation of biosynthetic precursor molecules,[66] osmolytes,[54] buffers of internal pH,[35] antioxidants[67] and chelators, especially for heavy metals.[68] One of the major component of culture media is AA group containing the sulphur, which helps in minimizing apoptosis, causative factor of monozygotic twinning.[69]

Chelators: Ethylenediaminetetraacetic Acid

Chelators of heavy metal ions in culture media enhance the development of preimplantation embryos. They have the ability to 'sequester' metal ions. The metal ions after binding with ethylenediaminetetraacetic acid (EDTA) remain in solution but their reactivity is diminished. EDTA helps in alleviating the 2-cell block in mice embryos.[69] It also helps in inhibiting premature utilization of glycolysis by cleavage stage embryos preventing any crabtree-like effect that can cause arrest in culture.[70] However, in postcompaction stage embryos, EDTA at a concentration of 0.1 mmol/L reduces blastocyst development and cell number.[71,72]

Impact of pH and Buffers

The pH only refers to hydrogen ion, and the pH of an aqueous solution is very dynamic. Association and dissociation of compounds and ions like sodium, potassium, magnesium, chloride, lactate and glycine regulate the balance of pH.[73,74] The culture media pH is maintained by the balance of carbon dioxide (CO_2) concentration and the concentration of bicarbonate in the media.

The intracellular pH (pHi) in human cleavage embryo cells is 7.2,[75] so an acceptable pH range for embryo culture media is usually set between pH 7.2 and 7.4. In postcompaction stage after formation of tight junctions between the cells, embryos appear to have more control over their pHi.[76,77] Hence, there is a trend to culture cleavage stage embryos in a slightly lower pH and morulae and blastocysts in a slightly higher pH (low-high paradigm).

The most commonly used buffer in commercially available culture media are [4-(2-hydroxyethyl)-1-piperazineethanesulfonic acid (HEPES) at 21 mmol/L] and 3-(N-morpholino)propanesulfonic acid (MOPS). Both buffers have a pKa value of 7.2, it is the closest of the zwitter ionic buffers to the pHi of embryos of 7.2. There is not much understanding about the impact of either of the buffers on embryo osmotic regulation.[78]

Macromolecules

Human serum albumin or synthetic serum serves as the common source of proteins in human embryo culture medium. It is usually added at 5–20% concentrations. All new generation media include synthetic serum as has known composition. Albumin helps in maintaining cell membrane stability and chelation of toxic components of culture components and water as well as the culture dishes. It also aids in capillary membrane permeability and osmoregulation. The presence of proteins in the culture media facilitates the manipulation of gametes and embryos.[8] However, the uses of any blood products involve the risk of potential contamination and infection of pre-implantation embryos.

Vitamins

All the commercially available media formulations contain vitamins. Although their effects on embryo development remain largely unknown both human[79] and mouse zygotes[19] form blastocysts in culture in the absence of vitamins. It may be the role of vitamin in the culture media is when they act in synergy with AAs to prevent distress in metabolism and loss of vitality induced by suboptimal culture conditions.[8,80] The addition of vitamins as antioxidants to the culture media containing glucose and phosphate help to prevent a loss in respiration and metabolic control.[81] The B-group vitamins are integral part of carbohydrate and AA metabolism; thereby certain vitamins may have an important role to play in embryo development especially in the presence of AAs.

Growth Factors

Mammalian embryos are naturally exposed to a complex mixture of growth factors that play a key role in growth and differentiation from the time of morula to blastocyst transition. However, defining their role and potential for improving *in vitro* preimplantation development is complicated by factors such as gene expression of both the factors and their receptors. The blastocyst expresses ligands and receptors for several growth factors, many of which can cross-react thus making it difficult to interpret the effect of single factors added to a culture media.[82,83]

Antibiotics

Embryo culture media are routinely supplemented with antibiotics to prevent bacterial contamination.[84] Nowadays, commonly used antibiotics are penicillin (β-lactam, 100 U/mL), streptomycin (aminoglycoside, 100 µg/mL) and gentamicin (aminoglycoside, 50 µg/mL). The antibacterial effect of penicillin is attributed to its disturbance of cell wall integrity through the inhibition of the synthesis of peptidoglycan. Penicillin has no direct toxic effects on the preimplantation embryo. Streptomycin and gentamicin disturb bacterial protein synthesis. However, the aminoglycosides show more toxic effects.[84]

CULTURE SYSTEMS

For the optimum embryo development *in vitro*, not just the composition of the culture media used, but also the physical parameter, such as the incubation environment and gas phase play an important role (Flowchart 5.1).

Flowchart 5.1 serves to illustrate the complex and interdependent nature of human IVF treatment. For example, the stimulation regimen used not only impacts oocyte quality (hence embryo physiology and viability), but can also affect subsequent endometrial receptivity. Furthermore, the health and dietary status of the patient can have a profound effect on the subsequent developmental capacity of the oocyte and embryo. The dietary status of patients attending IVF is typically not considered as a compounding variable, but growing data would indicate otherwise. In this schematic, the laboratory has been broken down into its core components, only one of which is the culture system. The culture system has in turn been broken down into its components, only one of which is the culture media. Therefore, it would appear rather simplistic to assume that by changing only one part of the culture system (i.e. culture media), that one is going to mimic the results of a given laboratory or clinic. A major determinant of the success of a laboratory and culture system is the level of quality control (QC) and quality assurance (QA) in place. For example, one should never assume that anything

Flowchart 5.1: A holistic analysis of human IVF.

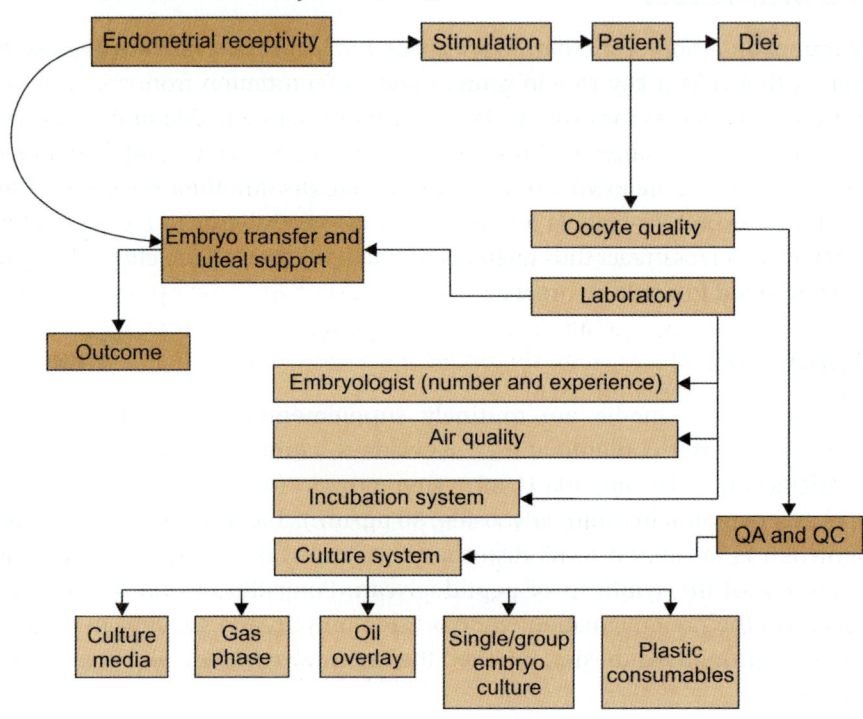

(IVF: *In vitro* fertilization; QC: Quality control; QA: Quality assurance).

coming into the laboratory that has not been pretested with a relevant bio-assay (for example, mouse embryo assay) is safe merely because a previous lot has performed satisfactorily. Only a small percentage of the contact supplies and tissue culture ware used in IVF come suitably tested. Therefore, it is essential to assume that everything entering the IVF laboratory without a suitable pretest is embryo toxic until proven otherwise.[85]

Oxygen Concentration

Studies on several types of mammalian embryo have demonstrated that culture at a reduced oxygen concentration results in enhanced development *in vitro*.[86] It has been observed that human blastocysts cultured in a low oxygen environment (5%) have significantly more cells than those cultured in a high oxygen environment (20%) (Gardner DK, unpublished data, 2006).[85] However, human and mouse embryos can grow at elevated oxygen concentrations and this has led to some confusion regarding the optimal concentration for embryo culture. The physiology of the reproductive tract and the beneficial effects of using a reduced oxygen concentrations determined in controlled studies indicate that to employ low oxygen concentrations appears prudent.

Carbon Dioxide

Carbon dioxide is not only required to maintain the pH of bicarbonate buffered medium, but is readily incorporated into protein and nucleic acids by the mouse embryo at all stages prior to implantation.[87] Culture systems for the preimplantation mammalian embryo routinely employ a CO_2 concentration of 5% coupled with a bicarbonate concentration of around 25 mm. It has been proposed that the beneficial effects of a high CO_2 concentration is due to a decrease in the pH of the medium as the beneficial effects of increased CO_2 could be replaced with a weak acid.[88] The optimal concentration of CO_2 for human embryo development has yet to be determined; however the CO_2 concentration is related to pH of the medium which also needs to be considered.

Temperature

Temperature fluctuations at the early cleavage stages have been demonstrated to decrease the subsequent development potential of embryos *in vitro*. Exposure of human oocytes to room temperature has been reported to induce damage to the meiotic spindle.[89] It would therefore seem advisable to maintain a constant temperature of 37°C when handling human oocytes and embryos.

Incubator or Incubation Chamber

As discussed earlier, for optimal development of human embryos *in vitro* it is important to maintain both the pH of the medium and temperature. The choice and use of incubators is therefore paramount for the success of an IVF program. Several studies have determined that embryo development *in vitro* is increased by restricting the opening of an incubator.[90] The use of incubators that have multiple chambers within the single incubator chamber can also reduce fluctuations in temperature and CO_2 levels induced by frequent door openings.

Light

Several studies have investigated the effect of exposure to visible light on the development of mammalian preimplantation embryos *in vitro*. In the human, implementation of an oocyte collection system employing low light at low oxygen concentration resulted in significantly increased rates of blastocyst formation of spare embryos and increased pregnancy and live birth rates when embryos were transferred on days 2–4 of culture.[91] Therefore, it would seem prudent to perform all oocyte and embryo collections and manipulations under low illumination.

Incubation Volume, Embryo Grouping and Oil Overlay

Within the lumen of the female reproductive tract, the developing embryo is exposed to microliter volumes of fluid.[92] In contrast, the embryo grown in vitro is subject to relatively large volumes of medium up to 1 mL. Consequently, any autocrine factor(s) produced by the developing embryo will be diluted and may therefore become ineffectual. Of greatest significance is the observation that decreasing the incubation volume significantly increases embryo viability[93] due to an increase in inner cell mass (ICM) development.[94,95] In order to culture in such reduced volumes (20–50 mL), an oil overlay is required. Although the use of an oil overlay is time-consuming, it prevents the evaporation of media, thereby reducing the harmful effects of increase in osmolality, and reduces changes in pH caused by a loss of CO_2 from the medium when culture dishes are taken out of the incubator for embryo examination. Furthermore, it has been proposed that an overlay of mineral oil can actually act as a trap for potential embryo toxins.[96]

As it is shown in Figure 5.1, as per the *in vivo* exposure of gradients of nutrients and environment to embryo in the female reproductive tract, culture media is tailored accordingly. During the precompaction stage, embryo has low biosynthetic activity, thus preferring pyruvate as the primary source of nutrition compared to high biosynthetic activity exhibiting post-compacting embryo preferring glucose. The AA availability also changes from

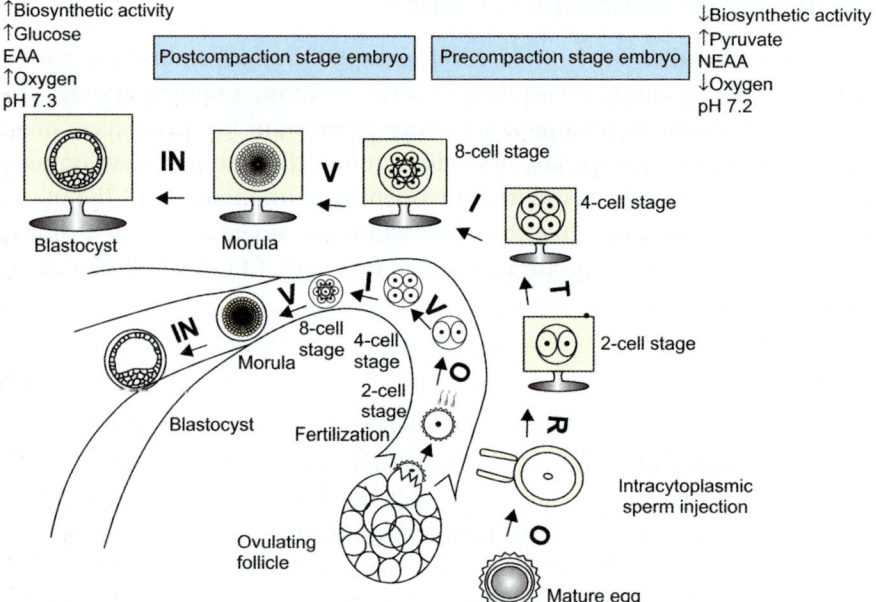

Fig. 5.1: Stage-specific requirements of developing preimplantation embryo. (EAA: Essential amino acid; NEAA: Nonessential amino acid).

primarily nonessential AA (NEAA) to essential AA (EAA), as it passes from fallopian tube during the precompaction stage to the uterus in the post-compaction stage. Female reproductive tract shows hypoxic condition in the fallopian tube compared to uterus, which may suggest that precompaction stage embryo may require lower oxygen concentration compared to post-compaction stage when embryo starts utilizing glucose as primary energy substrate.

QUALITY CONTROL

Mouse Bioassay

The QC of commercial media includes pH, osmolality, sterility, endotoxin tests and the mouse embryo assay (MEA). The preimplantation mouse embryo is the most widely used bioassay for medium components, culture media, and equipment used in clinical IVF. The medium can usually pass the MEA, if it supports development of more than or equal to 80% of mouse embryos to blastocyst stage. Using mice for testing media for human embryos has been the focus of discussion due to conflicting reports in the literature of its suitability as a bioassay.[97,98] The apparent contradiction of these studies can be resolved by taking into account the different stages of development used at the start of culture, the types of media used, and the supplementation of medium with protein. Furthermore, all studies used blastocyst development as the sole criterion for assessing embryo develop-ment, which is a poor indicator of embryo quality and does not reflect developmental potential.[99,100] A far more sensitive and quantitative parameter is blastocyst cell number.[77] A practical mouse embryo bioassay is to culture the zygote for 96 hours in protein-free medium. The rationale for using protein-free medium is that serum or serum albumin can chelate toxins, such as heavy metal ions, present in the medium. The presence of proteins would there-fore hide any potential detrimental effects of the medium. One can readily obtain 80% blastocyst development on day 5, but it is important also to note how many embryos formed blastocysts in the afternoon of day 4 (i.e. on time development), and what is the cell number of resultant blastocysts.[85,101]

Using such an approach to testing, one can pick up subtle problems that can exist with any media, or more typically with any contact supplies. However, the mouse model should be used with caution as it presents obvious differences in reproductive physiology compared with humans[102] and there is no standardization of the day the culture should start, the mouse strain, number of embryos, etc. Efforts to increase its sensitivity include one cell as the starting point,[101,103] zona-free embryos,[104] the inclusion of posi-tive controls,[105] accurate sample size calculations[106] and assessment of multiple endpoints and of blastocyst cell number.[85,105]

The ultimate QC on all media for IVF is their ability to support human embryo growth. It is obviously unethical to use human embryos for this purpose. A possible solution would be the use of triploid embryos as an assay of media quality, as these cannot be replaced in the prospective mother. Therefore vigilant monitoring of embryo development within the IVF laboratory is not only essential, but should be considered as part of the laboratory's overall QC system.

Sperm Bioassay

An alternative method to the mouse embryo bioassay is to use sperm motility as a method to detect potential embryo toxins. This assay utilizes both the number of motile sperm and degree of motility to determine the suitability of media to support embryo development. An advantage of this test is that it can be performed in 4–6 hours as opposed to the several days for the embryo bioassay. However, its sensitivity is very low, as human sperms are able to maintain their motility in very adverse culture conditions. Unfortunately, there is little clinical data on the applicability of such tests.

CONCLUSION

Unlike the dynamic changes in the environment of female reproductive tract, most conventional culture media systems are static in nature, where single system is used for the entire preimplantation period. Therefore, embryos have different requirements over the growing period those are reflected in the physiology and energy metabolism.[8,47,107] We also need to consider the other problems of a static culture media generation of potential toxins over the time. Thus, the change of media over the time through the development of zygote to blastocyst is required rather than using single media is necessary to support the development and differentiation. Again the recent reports support using single media throughout the growth with competitive results like sequential media.

We also need to remember that unlike the *in vivo* conditions, ART culture media contain only a subset of parts resulting in the continuous stressed condition for growing embryo. Any suboptimal condition forces the embryo to undergo adaptations, which may lead to lower pregnancy and higher abortion rates. It is evident that all necessary steps in ART as part of the treatment of infertility can influence the epigenetic programming during early development.[108] Thus, it is essential that the best level of QC exists in the laboratory and optimal environmental conditions are maintained for the development of the preimplantation embryo.

REFERENCES

1. Biggers JD. Pioneering mammalian embryo culture. In: Bavister BD (Ed). The Mammalian Preimplantation Embryo: Regulation of Growth and Differentiation *in Vitro*. New York: Plenum Press; 1987. pp. 1-22.
2. Bigger JD. Thoughts on embryo culture conditions. Reprod Biomed Online. 2002; 4 Suppl 1:30-8.
3. Bowman P, McLaren A. Cleavage rate of mouse embryos *in vivo* and *in vitro*. J Embryol Exp Morphol. 1970;24(1):203-7.
4. Harlow GM, Quinn P. Development of preimplantation mouse embryos *in vivo* and *in vitro*. Aust J Biol Sci. 1982;35(2):187-93.
5. Edwards RG. Causes of early embryonic loss in human pregnancy. Hum Reprod. 1986;1(3):185-98.
6. Biggers JD. Fundamentals of the design of culture media that support human preimplantation development. In: Van Blerkom J (Ed). Essential IVF. Norell: Kluwer Academic Press; 2003. pp. 291-332.
7. Leese HJ. The formation and function of oviduct fluid. J Reprod Fertil. 1988; 82(2):843-56.
8. Gardner DK. Changes in requirements and utilization of nutrients during mammalian preimplantation embryo development and their significance in embryo culture. Theriogenology. 1998;49(1):83-102.
9. Freshney RI. Culture of Animal Cells: A Manual of Basic Technique, 4th edition. New York: Wiley-Liss; 2000. p. 600.
10. Edwards RG. Test-tube babies, 1981. Nature. 1981;293(5830):253-6.
11. Edwards RG, Purdy JM, Steptoe PC, et al. The growth of human preimplantation embryos *in vitro*. Am J Obstet Gynecol. 1981;141(4):408-16.
12. Staessen C, Van den Abbeel E, Janssenswillen C, et al. Controlled comparison of Earle's balanced salt solution with Ménézo B2 medium for human in-vitro fertilization performance. Hum Reprod. 1994;9(10):1915-9.
13. Barnett DK, Bavister BD. What is the relationship between the metabolism of preimplantation embryos and their developmental competence? Mol Reprod Dev. 1996;43(1):105-33.
14. Gardner DK, Lane M. Embryo culture systems. In: Trounson AO, Gardner DK (Eds). Handbook of *In Vitro* Fertilization, 2nd edition. Boca Raton: CRC Press; 1999. pp. 205-64.
15. Menezo Y, Testart J, Perrone D. Serum is not necessary in human *in vitro* fertilization, early embryo culture, and transfer. Fertil Steril. 1984;42(5):750-5.
16. Quinn P, Kerin JF, Warnes GM. Improved pregnancy rate in human *in vitro* fertilization with the use of a medium based on the composition of human tubal fluid. Fertil Steril. 1985;44(4):493-8.
17. Gardner DK, Lane M, Calderon I, et al. Environment of the preimplantation human embryo *in vivo*: metabolite analysis of oviduct and uterine fluids and metabolism of cumulus cells. Fertil Steril. 1996;65(2):349-53.
18. Leese HJ, Barton AM. Production of pyruvate by isolated mouse cumulus cells. J Exp Zool. 1985;234(2):231-6.
19. Whitten WK, Biggers JD. Complete development *in vitro* of the pre-implantation stages of the mouse in a simple chemically defined medium. J Reprod Fertil. 1968;17(2):399-401.
20. Whittingham DG. Culture of mouse ova. J Reprod Fertil Suppl. 1971;14:7-21.
21. Chatot CL, Ziomek CA, Bavister BD, et al. An improved culture medium supports development of random-bred 1-cell mouse embryos *in vitro*. J Reprod Fertil. 1989;86(2):679-88.

22. Lawitts JA, Biggers JD. Joint effects of sodium chloride, glutamine, and glucose in mouse preimplantation embryo culture media. Mol Reprod Dev. 1992;31 (3):189-94.

23. Quinn P. Enhanced results in mouse and human embryo culture using a modified human tubal fluid medium lacking glucose and phosphate. J Assist Reprod Genet. 1995;12(2):97-105.

24. Carrillo AJ, Lane B, Pridman DD, et al. Improved clinical outcomes for *in vitro* fertilization with delay of embryo transfer from 48 to 72 hours after oocyte retrieval: use of glucose- and phosphate-free media. Fertil Steril. 1998;69(2): 329-34.

25. Ham RG. An improved nutrient solution for diploid Chinese hamster and human cell lines. Exp Cell Res. 1963;29:515-26.

26. Gardner DK, Lane M. Amino acids and ammonium regulate mouse embryo development in culture. Biol Reprod. 1993;48(2):377-85.

27. Lawitts JA, Biggers JD. Optimization of mouse embryo culture media using simplex methods. J Reprod Fertil. 1991;91(2):543-56.

28. Lawitts JA, Biggers JD. Culture of preimplantation embryos. Methods Enzymol. 1993;225:153-64.

29. Ho Y, Wigglesworth K, Eppig JJ, et al. Preimplantation development of mouse embryos in KSOM: augmentation by amino acids and analysis of gene expression. Mol Reprod Dev. 1995;41(2):232-8.

30. Biggers JD, Racowsky C. The development of fertilized human ova to the blastocyst stage in KSOM(AA) medium: is a two-step protocol necessary? Reprod Biomed Online. 2002;5(2):133-40.

31. Gardner DK, Leese HJ. Concentrations of nutrients in mouse oviduct fluid and their effects on embryo development and metabolism *in vitro*. J Reprod Fertil. 1990;88(1):361-8.

32. Gardner DK, Pool TB, Lane M. Embryo nutrition and energy metabolism and its relationship to embryo growth, differentiation, and viability. Semin Reprod Med. 2000;18(2):205-18.

33. Edwards LJ, Williams DA, Gardner DK. Intracellular pH of the mouse preimplantation embryo: amino acids act as buffers of intracellular pH. Hum Reprod. 1998;13(12):3441-8.

34. Lane M, Gardner DK. Understanding cellular disruptions during early embryo development that perturb viability and fetal development. Reprod Fertil Dev. 2005;17(3):371-8.

35. Lane M. Mechanisms for managing cellular and homeostatic stress *in vitro*. Theriogenology. 2001;55(1):225-36.

36. Gardner DK. Mammalian embryo culture in the absence of serum or somatic cell support. Cell Biol Int. 1994;18(12):1163-79.

37. Gardner DK, Lane M. Development of viable mammalian embryos *in vitro*: evolution of sequential media. In: Cibelli R, Lanza K, Campbell AK, West MD (Eds). Principles of Cloning. San Diego: Academic Press; 2002. p. 187.

38. Barnes FL, Crombie A, Gardner DK, et al. Blastocyst development and birth after in-vitro maturation of human primary oocytes, intracytoplasmic sperm injection and assisted hatching. Hum Reprod. 1995;10(12):3243-7.

39. Bertheussen K, Forsdahl F, Maltau JM. *In vitro* fertilization. New media for embryo culture to the blastocyst stage. In: Gomel V, Leung PC (Eds). *In Vitro* Fertilization and Assisted Reproduction. Bologna: Monduzzi Editore; 1997. pp. 199-204.

40. Behr B, Milki AA, Giudice LC, et al. High yield blastocyst culture and transfer: a new approach using P1 and blastocyst medium in reduced O$_2$ environment. Fertil Steril. 1998;70(3 Suppl 1):S98.

41. Biggers JD. Reflections on the culture of the preimplantation embryo. Int J Dev Biol. 1998;42(7):879-84.

42. Gardner DK, Lane M. Culture and selection of viable blastocysts: a feasible proposition for human IVF? Hum Reprod Update. 1997;3(4):367-82.

43. Summers MC, Biggers JD. Chemically defined media and the culture of mammalian preimplantation embryos: historical perspective and current issues. Hum Reprod Update. 2003;9(6):557-82.

44. Biggers JD, Summers MC. Choosing a culture medium: making informed choices. Fertil Steril. 2008;90(3):473-83.

45. Whitten WK. Culture of tubal mouse ova. Nature. 1956;177(4498):96.

46. Brinster RL. Studies on the development of mouse embryos *in vitro*. IV. Interaction of energy sources. J Reprod Fertil. 1965;10(2):227-40.

47. Leese HJ. Metabolism of the preimplantation mammalian embryo. Oxf Rev Reprod Biol. 1991;13:35-72.

48. Rieger D. Relationships between energy metabolism and development of early mammalian embryos. Theriogenology. 1992;37(1):75-93.

49. Bavister BD. Culture of preimplantation embryos: facts and artefacts. Hum Reprod Update. 1995;1(2):91-148.

50. Bavister BD. Glucose and culture of human embryos. Fertil Steril. 1999;72(2): 233-4.

51. McManus ML, Churchwell KB, Strange K. Regulation of cell volume in health and disease. N Engl J Med. 1995;333(19):1260-6.

52. Borland RM, Biggers JD, Lechene CP, et al. Elemental composition of fluid in the human Fallopian tube. J Reprod Fertil. 1980;58(2):479-82.

53. Biggers JD, Lawitts JA, Lechene CP. The protective action of betaine on the deleterious effects of NaCl on preimplantation mouse embryos *in vitro*. Mol Reprod Dev. 1993;34(4):380-90.

54. Van Winkle LJ, Haghighat N, Campione AL. Glycine protects preimplantation mouse conceptuses from a detrimental effect on development of the inorganic ions in oviductal fluid. J Exp Zool. 1990;253(2):215-9.

55. Nichol R, Hunter RH, Gardner DK, et al. Concentrations of energy substrates in oviductal fluid and blood plasma of pigs during the peri-ovulatory period. J Reprod Fertil. 1992;96(2):699-707.

56. Leese HJ, Barton AM. Pyruvate and glucose uptake by mouse ova and preimplantation embryos. J Reprod Fertil. 1984;72(1):9-13.

57. Leese HJ, Biggers JD, Mroz EA, et al. Nucleotides in a single mammalian ovum or preimplantation embryo. Anal Biochem. 1984;140(2):443-8.

58. Leese HJ, Conaghan J, Martin KL, et al. Early human embryo metabolism. Bioessays 1993;15(4):259-64.

59. Reitzer LJ, Wice BM, Kennell D. The pentose cycle. Control and essential function in HeLa cell nucleic acid synthesis. J Biol Chem. 1980;255(12):5616-26.

60. Biggers JD, McGinnis LK, Lawitts JA. One-step versus two-step culture of mouse preimplantation embryos: is there a difference? Hum Reprod. 2005;20 (12): 3376-84.

61. Casslén BG. Free amino acids in human uterine fluid. Possible role of high taurine concentration. J Reprod Med. 1987;32(3):181-4.

62. Miller JG, Schultz GA. Amino acid content of preimplantation rabbit embryos and fluids of the reproductive tract. Biol Reprod. 1987;36(1):125-9.

63. Van Winkle LJ. Amino acid transport in developing animal oocytes and early conceptuses. Biochim Biophys Acta. 1988;947(1):173-208.

64. Schultz GA, Kaye PL, McKay DJ, et al. Endogenous amino acid pool sizes in mouse eggs and preimplantation embryos. J Reprod Fertil. 1981;61(2):387-93.

65. Chatot CL, Tasca RJ, Ziomek CA. Glutamine uptake and utilization by preimplantation mouse embryos in CZB medium. J Reprod Fertil. 1990;89(1):335-46.

66. Crosby IM, Gandolfi F, Moor RM. Control of protein synthesis during early cleavage of sheep embryos. J Reprod Fertil. 1988;82(2):769-75.

67. Liu Z, Foote RH. Development of bovine embryos in KSOM with added superoxide dismutase and taurine and with five and twenty percent O_2. Biol Reprod. 1995;53(4):786-90.

68. Lindenbaum A. A survey of natural occurring chelating ligands. Adv Exp Med Biol. 1973;40:67-77.

69. Cassuto G, Chavrier M, Menezo Y. Culture conditions and not prolonged culture time are responsible for monozygotic twinning in human *in vitro* fertilization. Fertil Steril. 2003;80(2):462-3.

70. Gardner DK, Lane M. The 2-cell block in CF1 mouse embryos is associated with an increase in glycolysis and a decrease in tricarboxylic acid (TCA) cycle activity: alleviation of the 2-cell block is associated with the restoration of *in vivo* metabolic pathway activities. Biol Reprod. 1993;49(Suppl 1):152.

71. Abramczuk J, Solter D, Koprowski H. The beneficial effect EDTA on development of mouse one-cell embryos in chemically defined medium. Dev Biol. 1977;61(2):378-83.

72. Gardner DK, Lane MW, Lane M. Bovine blastocyst cell number is increased by culture with EDTA for the first 72 h of development from the zygote. Theriogenology. 1997;47:278.

73. Bavister BD, McKiernan SH. Regulation of hamster embryo development *in vitro* by amino acids. In: Bavister BD (Ed). Preimplantation Embryo Development. New York: Springer-Verlag; 1992. pp. 57-72.

74. Ducibella T, Anderson E. Cell shape and membrane changes in the eight-cell mouse embryo: prerequisites for morphogenesis of the blastocyst. Dev Biol. 1975;47(1):45-58.

75. Lane M, Boatman DE, Albrecht RM, et al. Intracellular divalent cation homeostasis and developmental competence in the hamster preimplantation embryo. Mol Reprod Dev. 1998;50(4):443-50.

76. Lane M, Bavister BD. Calcium homeostasis in early hamster preimplantation embryos. Biol Reprod. 1998;59(4):1000-7.

77. Gardner DK, Lane M. Culture and selection of viable blastocysts: a feasible proposition for human IVF? Hum Reprod Update. 1997;3(4):367-82.

78. Swain JE. Optimizing the culture environment in the IVF laboratory: impact of pH and buffer capacity on gamete and embryo quality. Reprod Biomed Online. 2010;21(1):6-16.

79. Bavister BD. Preimplantation Embryo Development. New York: Springer-Verlag; 1993. p. 184.

80. Lane M, Gardner DK. Amino acids and vitamins prevent culture-induced metabolic perturbations and associated loss of viability of mouse blastocysts. Hum Reprod. 1998;13(4):991-7.

81. Lane M, Gardner DK. Embryo culture medium: which is the best? Best Pract Res Clin Obstet Gynaecol. 2007;21(1):83-100.

82. Bulgurcuoglu S, Özsait B, Attar E. Büyüme Faktörlerinin Oosit ve Embriyo Gelisimi Üzerindeki Etkisi. Artemis. 2003;4:18-26.

83. Richter KS. The importance of growth factors for preimplantation embryo development and in-vitro culture. Curr Opin Obstet Gynecol. 2008;20(3): 292-304.

84. Lemeire K, Van Merris V, Cortvrindt R. The antibiotic streptomycin assessed in a battery of *in vitro* tests for reproductive toxicology. Toxicol *In Vitro*. 2007;21 (7):1348-53.

85. Gardner DK. *In Vitro* Fertilization: A Practical Approach. New York: CRC Press; 2006. p. 528.

86. Thompson JG, Simpson AC, Pugh PA, et al. Effect of oxygen concentration on in-vitro development of preimplantation sheep and cattle embryos. J Reprod Fertil. 1990;89(2):573-8.

87. Graves CN, Biggers JD. Carbon dioxide fixation by mouse embryos prior to implantation. Science. 1970;167(3924):1506-8.

88. Carney EW, Bavister BD. Regulation of hamster embryo development *in vitro* by carbon dioxide. Biol Reprod. 1987;36(5):1155-63.

89. Gardner DK, Lane M. Alleviation of the '2-cell block' and development to the blastocyst of CF1 mouse embryos: role of amino acids, EDTA and physical parameters. Hum Reprod. 1996;11(12):2703-12.

90. Pickering SJ, Braude PR, Johnson MH, et al. Transient cooling to room temperature can cause irreversible disruption of the meiotic spindle in the human oocyte. Fertil Steril. 1990;54(1):102-8.

91. Noda Y, Goto Y, Umaoka Y, et al. Culture of human embryos in alpha modification of Eagle's medium under low oxygen tension and low illumination. Fertil Steril. 1994;62(5):1022-7.

92. Leese HJ. The formation and function of oviduct fluid. J Reprod Fertil. 1988;82 (2):843-56.

93. Lane M, Gardner DK. Effect of incubation volume and embryo density on the development and viability of mouse embryos *in vitro*. Hum Reprod. 1992;7 (4):558-62.

94. Gardner DK, Lane MW, Lane M. Development of the inner cell mass in mouse blastocyst is stimulated by reducing the embryo: incubation volume ratio. Hum Reprod. 1997;12(1):132.

95. Ahern TJ, Gardner DK. Culturing bovine embryos in groups stimulates blastocyst development and cell allocation to the inner cell mass. Theriogenology. 1998;49(1):194.

96. Miller KF, Goldberg JM, Collins RL. Covering embryo cultures with mineral oil alters embryo growth by acting as a sink for an embryotoxic substance. J Assist Reprod Genet. 1994;11(7):342-5.

97. Weiss TJ, Warnes GM, Gardner DK. Mouse embryos and quality control in human IVF. Reprod Fertil Dev. 1992;4(1):105-7.

98. Gerrity M. Mouse embryo culture bioassay. In: Wolf DP (Ed). *In Vitro* Fertilization and Embryo Transfer. New York: Plenum Publishers; 1988. p. 57.

99. Gardner DK, Sakkas D. Mouse embryo cleavage, metabolism and viability: role of medium composition. Hum Reprod. 1993;8(2):288-95.

100. Lane M, Gardner DK. Selection of viable mouse blastocysts prior to transfer using a metabolic criterion. Hum Reprod. 1996;11(9):1975-8.

101. Scott LF, Sundaram SG, Smith S. The relevance and use of mouse embryo bioassays for quality control in an assisted reproductive technology program. Fertil Steril. 1993;60(3):559-68.

102. Ménézo YJ, Hérubel F. Mouse and bovine models for human IVF. Reprod Biomed Online. 2002;4(2):170-5.

103. Davidson A, Vermesh M, Lobo RA, et al. Mouse embryo culture as quality control for human *in vitro* fertilization: the one-cell versus the two-cell model. Fertil Steril. 1988;49(3):516-21.
104. Montoro L, Subias E, Young P, et al. Detection of endotoxin in human *in vitro* fertilization by the zona-free mouse embryo assay. Fertil Steril. 1990;54(1):109-12.
105. Dubin NH, Bornstein DR, Gong Y. Use of endotoxin as a positive (toxic) control in the mouse embryo assay. J Assist Reprod Genet. 1995;12(2):147-52.
106. Hendriks JC, Teerenstra S, Punt-Van der Zalm JP, et al. Sample size calculations for a split-cluster, beta-binomial design in the assessment of toxicity. Stat Med. 2005;24(24):3757-72.
107. Lane M, Gardner DK. Lactate regulates pyruvate uptake and metabolism in the preimplantation mouse embryo. Biol Reprod. 2000;62(1):16-22.
108. Rivera RM, Stein P, Weaver JR, et al. Manipulation of mouse embryos prior to implantation result in aberrant expression of imprinted genes on day 9.5 of development. Hum Mol Genet. 2008;17(1):1-14.

Chapter 6

Embryo Selection and Transfer

Anisha Uberoi, Himani Agnihotri

INTRODUCTION

Ever since the inception of *in vitro* fertilization (IVF), accurate selection of embryos with high implantation potential has been an integral part of the practice. The quality of embryos and their rate of development may vary across different clinics. This may be attributed to the inherent potential of the embryo itself, the IVF method or the culture medium used.

Embryo assessment before transfer in IVF or intracytoplasmic sperm injection (ICSI) helps to select the most viable embryo during culture by evaluating the embryo at specific time points from day 1 zygote to day 3 embryos or day 5 blastocyst, thereby increasing the pregnancy rates (PRs).

Morphological parameters have been the basis of selecting the most viable embryo or blastocyst for transfer globally. The parameters influencing the selection of good quality embryos are as follows:

- Pronuclear (PN) morphology
- Polar body (PB) structure and placement
- Appearance of cytoplasm [vacuoles, necrotic bodies, smooth endoplasmic reticulum (SER), granularity, etc.] and zona pellucida (ZP)
- Number, symmetry, fragmentation and multinucleation of blastomeres on day 2 and day 3 of embryo culture
- Compaction of blastomeres and expansion of blastocoel on day 5.

MORPHOLOGICAL ASSESSMENT

Accurate selection of embryos for transfer is of paramount importance. Thus, it is highly crucial to evaluate the quality of embryo at appropriate time in the laboratory (Table 6.1).

Fertilization Assessment (Day 1)

Fertilization can be assessed by the presence of two PBs and two centrally located juxtaposed pronuclei (PNs) [which contains nucleolar precursor bodies (NPBs) equatorially aligned] that are even sized with distinct membranes. Ideal features shared by the zygote are illustrated in Figure 6.1:

Table 6.1: Standardized timing relative to insemination time-based on the Istanbul consensus workshop.[27]

Assessment	Timing (hours postinsemination)	
Fertilization (Day 1)	16–19 hpi	ICSI at 13.00: 5–8 am
Day 2	44–47 hpi	9–12 am
Day 3	67–71 hpi	8–12 am
Day 5	116–120 hpi	8–12 am
Day 6	140–144 hpi	8–12 am

(ICSI: Intracytoplasmic sperm injection).

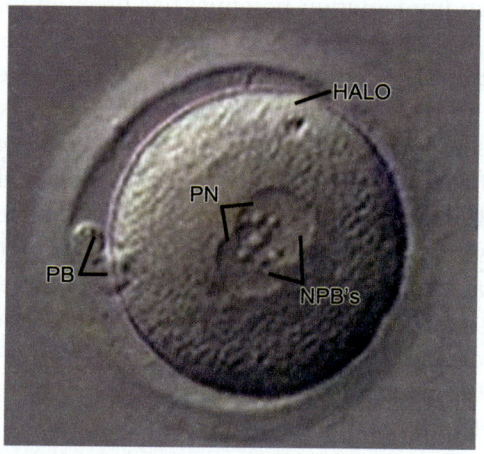

Fig. 6.1: Zygote showing 2 PN, 2 PB and Halo.
(NPBs: Nucleolar precursor bodies; PB: Polar body; PN: Pronuclear).

- The cytoplasm should be heterogeneous with a cortical halo effect on the peripheral side. Studies have reported higher quality embryos (60.9%) in zygotes with halo in comparison to zygotes without a halo (52.2%).[1,2]
- Number of NPBs in both the nuclei should not differ by three.[3]
  This PN scoring should be performed 16–19 hour postinsemination.

There are numerous systems in literature which classify zygotes based on the size, number and distribution of nucleoli within the nuclei.

Garello and his colleagues established a correlation between the orientation of PNs relative to the PBs and the embryo quality, thus angle β plays a crucial role while evaluating the zygote.[4]

- Angle β: The angle between a line drawn through the axis of the PNs and the position of the furthest PB
- Generally, the angle β should be less than 50°.

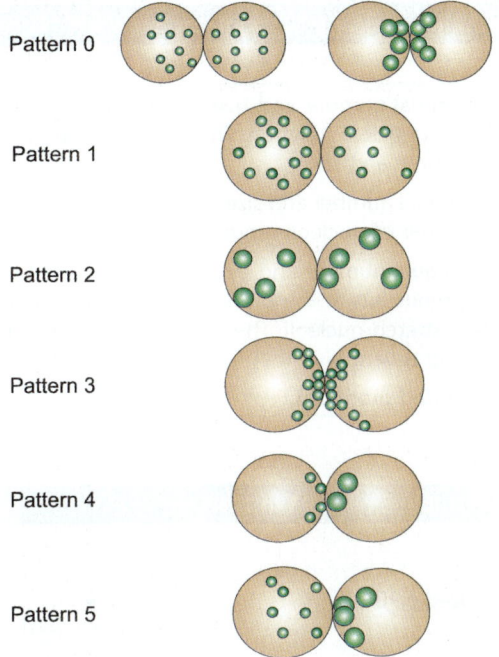

Pattern 0

Pattern 1

Pattern 2

Pattern 3

Pattern 4

Pattern 5

Fig. 6.2: Zygote classification according to Tesarik and Greco, 1999.

The grading system recommended by Tesarik and Greco classifies the zygotes (day 1) based on six patterns of PN, wherein pattern 0 corresponds to normal zygotes and patterns 1–5 represent the varying irregularities in the zygote (Fig. 6.2).[3]

According to the model proposed by Scott and his colleagues, zygotes are classified according to PN morphology labeled with grades corresponding to their quality.[5] The Z-score describes the number, size, and position of the nucleoli and the equality between the nuclei for these characteristics (Box 6.1).

According to Association for the Study of the Biology of Reproductive (ASEBIR) grading, zygotes are classified based on the PN symmetry and the distribution of NPB within the PN. Ideally, in a zygote the PN should be of the same size, have 3–7 polarized NPBs and a cytoplasmic halo (Tables 6.2 and 6.3).[6]

Presence of more than or equal to 3 PN or 1 PN after IVF or ICSI is the most common anomaly seen on day 1 (Fig. 6.3), caused by dispermy in IVF and by parthenogenetic activation of oocytes due to mechanical or chemical factors during ICSI.[7,8]

Cleavage Stage Embryos (Day 2 and Day 3)

Cleavage stage embryos range from 2-cell stage to the compacted morula composed of 8–16 cells. Ideally, on day 2 and on day 3, the number of

Box 6.1: Z-scoring for pronuclear (PN) zygote by Scott and his colleagues.

Definition

Z1 Equal pronuclei. Equal number and size of nucleoli, aligned in both pronuclei at the pronuclear junction. The absolute number of nucleoli ranges between three and seven.

Z2 Equal pronuclei. Equal number and size of nucleoli, scattered in both pronuclei. The absolute number of nucleoli ranges between three and seven.

Z3 Equal pronuclei. Equal number and even or (and) uneven size of nucleoli, aligned in one pronucleus at the pronuclear junction. The other pronucleus with randomly scattered nucleoli. The absolute number of nucleoli ranges between three and seven.

Z4 Unequal or separated pronuclei.

Table 6.2: ASEBIR distribution of NPB in 2PNs.

NPB type	Definition	Description
1	3–7 polarized NPB	
2	Everything that is not 1 or 3	
3	Only 1 or 2 NPB in at least one of the PN	

(ASEBIR: Association for the Study of Reproductive Biology; NPB: Nucleolar precursor body; PN: Pronuclear; PNs: Pronuclei).

Table 6.3: ASEBIR classification on the basis of PN size.

Symmetry	Definition	Description
1	Same PN size	
2	Similar PN size	
3	Different PN size	

(ASEBIR: Association for the Study of Reproductive Biology; PN: Pronuclear).

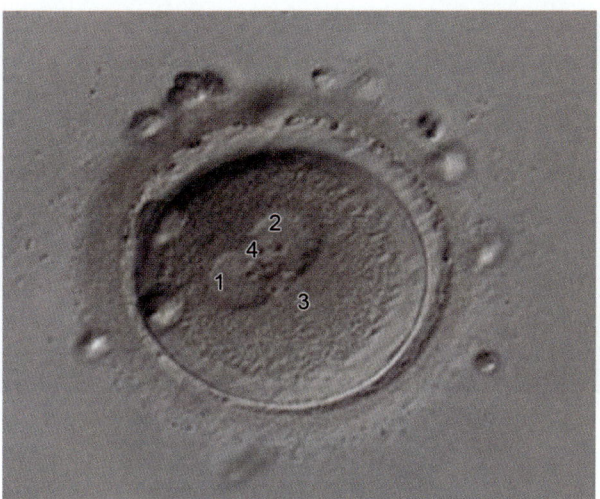

Fig. 6.3: Zygote showing more than 3 pronuclear (PN) on day 1.

blastomeres is assessed and each embryo is given a particular score based on the number and uniformity of blastomeres, fragmentation and presence of multinucleation. Number of blastomeres is known to have the highest predictive value.[9,10] Additionally, embryos must exhibit appropriate kinetics and synchrony of division. In normal developing embryos, cell division occurs every 18–20 hour.

Cell Number

The single cell zygote divides into 2–4 cells at 44–47 hours postinsemination (hpi) (day 2) and 7–10 cells after 67–71 hpi (day 3) (Figs. 6.4A to C).

Transferring a 4-cell embryo on day 2 has a higher implantation rate (IR) as compared to 2 or 5 cells, 3 or 6 cells, 1 cell or less than 6-cell embryo. Moreover, embryos on day 3 are evaluated on the basis of rate of cell division between day 2 and day 3. Thus, embryos can be categorized according to their implantation potential.

Embryos dividing either too slow or too fast may have metabolic and/or chromosomal defects.[11] Different morphological anomalies are often associated with each other, and uneven cleavage has shown to be related to multinucleation[12] and fragmentation.[13]

Size and Shape of the Blastomere

Cell regularity plays an important role in the cleavage stage embryos. Usually the blastomeres should be same or similar in size, to maximize the overall pregnancy outcome.[12,14] Irregular blastomeres may indicate cell division or a physiological alteration (Table 6.4).

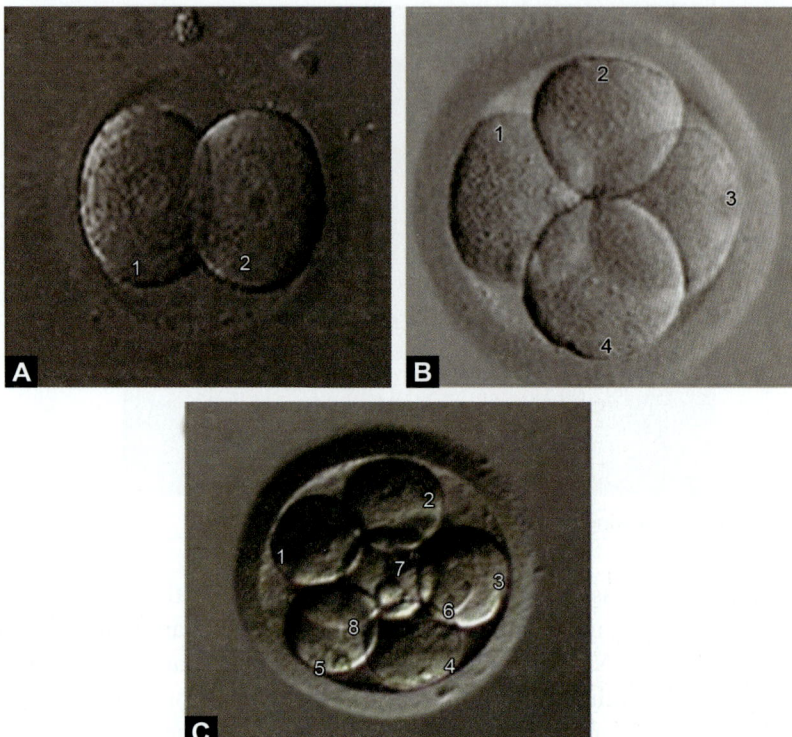

Figs. 6.4A to C: Embryos showing cell division. (A) 2-cell embryo at 45 hour; (B) 4-cell embryo at 47 hour; and (C) 8-celled embryo at 68 hour postinsemination.

Concordant observations were also reported wherein embryos with uneven sized blastomeres displayed a higher rate of multinucleation and aneuploidy, consequently lowering the IR.

When cell division is not synchronous, it corresponds to the fact that the cells from two different cell cycle coexist. As a result, embryos with 3, 5, 7, 9, etc. blastomeres have two different sizes of cells. Positive classification of embryos with odd number of cells is as follows:

- 3 cell: 1 large blastomere and 2 small blastomere
- 5 cell: 3 large blastomere and 2 small blastomere
- 7 cell: 1 large blastomere and 6 small blastomere
- 9 cell: 2 large blastomere and 7 small blastomere.

Table 6.4: Cell regularity in cleavage stage embryos.

Symmetry	Definition	Description
1	Same cell size	

Contd…

Contd…

Symmetry	Definition	Description
2	Similar cell size	
3	Different cell size	
4	One dominant cell	

Fragmentation

Fragmentation, also known as blebbing is portions of the embryo cell that has broken off and separated from the nucleated portion of the cell (Fig. 6.5). The degree of fragmentation, size of fragments and its distribution all contribute in evaluating the developmental potential of an embryo.

A good quality embryo should have no fragmentation or less fragmentation, i.e. less than or equal to 10%.[14] Numerous studies in literature have correlated a high degree of fragmentation with low IRs.[15] Moreover, fragmentation has also been related to aneuploidy.[16,17] In contrast, presence of low fragmentation has no negative or possibly even a positive impact on the developing embryo and the PRs.[18]

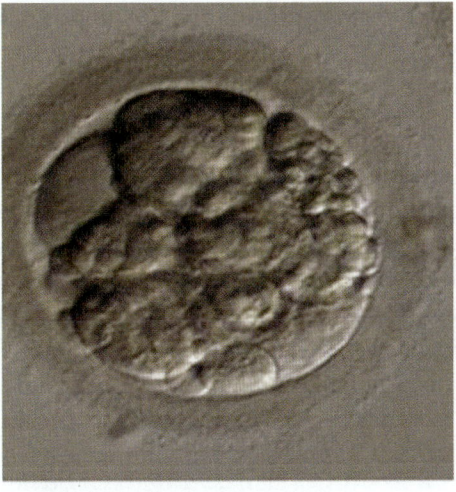

Fig. 6.5: Day 3 embryo exhibiting 20% of fragmentation.

Nucleation

Nucleation is defined as the presence of the nuclei in the blastomeres of the cleavage stage embryo. Ideally it should be one nucleus per blastomere, but no visible nuclei or multinucleation is often observed in cohort of embryos (Figs 6.6A and B).

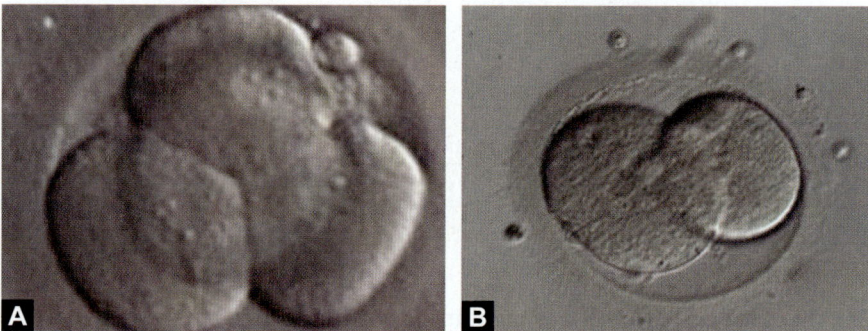

Figs. 6.6A and B: (A) 4-cell embryo showing distinct nuclei in each blastomere; and (B) 2-cell embryo showing multinucleation in one of the blastomere.

Multinucleation is the presence of more than one nucleus in each blastomere on day 2 or day 3 and has been associated with an increased rate of aneuploidy and chromosomal abnormalities.[12,19] It has been reported that multinucleated cells arise from a failure of cytokinesis, thereby leading to cleavage stage arrest *in vitro*.[12] Numerous other studies reported low IR and increased rate of abortions due to multinucleation in cleavage stage embryos.[20] Additionally, in extended culture systems, multinucleation was associated with a lower blastocyst formation rate.[9]

Cytoplasmic Pitting

Cytoplasmic pitting is characterized by the presence of numerous small pits on the surface of the cytoplasm (Fig. 6.7).[21] It indicates cytoplasmic activation on day 3 and should not be misjudged with extensive vacuolization.[22]

Acytoplasmic Ring

Acytoplasmic ring is formed during contraction of the cytoplasm leaving a large translucent ring without the organelles close to the edge of the blastomere (Fig. 6.8). The presence of an acytoplasmic ring relates to the cellular lysis[23] and thus is detrimental to the development of the embryo.

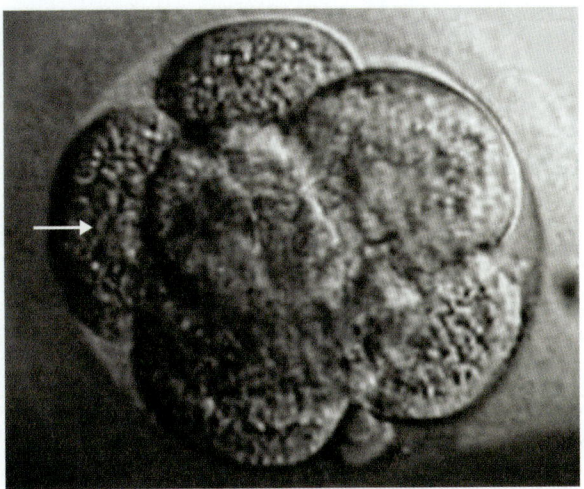

Fig. 6.7: Embryo showing pitting on day 3.

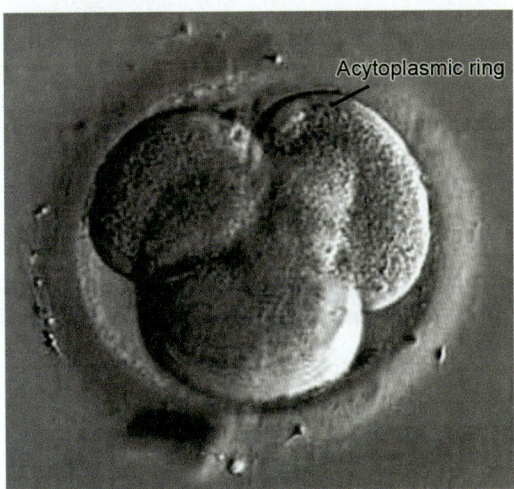

Fig. 6.8: Embryo showing acytoplasmic ring on day 2.

Cytoplasmic Anomalies

The cytoplasm of the cleaving embryos is normally pale in appearance and less granular.[24] Anomalies, such as cytoplasmic granularity and vacuoles can also be scored morphologically on day 2 or day 3 (Fig. 6.9). Extensive vacuolization is detrimental mainly to spatial development.[23]

According to the described parameters, embryos at 4-cell stage on day 2 and 7 or 8-cell stage on day 3 with minimum fragmentation, no multinucleation and with the absence of any cytoplasmic anomalies makes the most viable embryos.

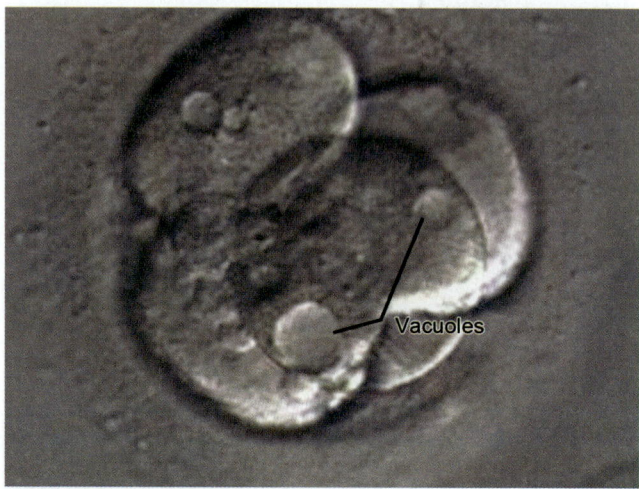

Fig. 6.9: 4-cell embryo exhibiting high number of small and medium vacuoles.

Morula Stage (Day 4)

On day 4 the embryos should be assessed 92 ± 2 hpi; is in that stage when embryos begin their transition from multiblastomeres to compacting or compacted embryo (Table 6.5). A good quality morula is composed of 16–32 blastomeres showing considerable compaction on day 4 (Fig. 6.10).[25]

Table 6.5: Classifying day 4 embryos according to degree compaction.

Compaction	Definition	Description
0	No compaction	
1	Loosing cell definition	
2	Starting compaction	
3	Very compacted	

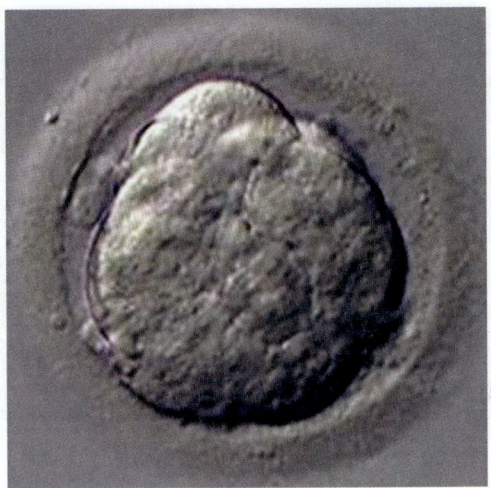

Fig. 6.10: A well-compacted morula on day 4.

Blastocyst Scoring (Day 5 and Day 6)

Usually, 5–6 days after fertilization, embryos develop to the blastocyst stage, consisting of two cell layers: (1) the outer cells of the blastocyst, forming the blastocyst structure itself are called the trophectoderm (TE) cells and (2) the cells located inside the blastocoel, often forming a cell clump at one pole of the blastocyst are called the inner cell mass (ICM) cells.

Generally, blastocysts are graded by evaluating three separate quality scores that include:

1. *Blastocoel cavity:* A defining moment in embryonic development is when fluid starts to accumulate between cells at the morulae stage of development. As the fluid's volume increases, a cavity appears gradually forming the blastocoel. As the development of blastocyst progresses, blastocoel increases resulting in thinning of the ZP. Finally, the blastocyst breaks free of the ZP through a process called hatching.

Depending on the degree of expansion and hatching status, there has been described different system for blastocysts grading but may be the most complete is the system presented by Hardarson et al. in 2012,[26] as it is a compilation between the Istanbul consensus document[27] and the system described by Gardner and Schoolcraft in 1999.[28] According to this system blastocyst can be classified as:

- Grade I (early blastocyst): It is the early stage of the blastocyst formation on D5 with a cavity occupying less than 50% of the volume of the embryo (Fig. 6.11)
- Grade II (cavitating blastocyst): The next stage of blastulation in which the cavity occupies half or more than half of the total volume of the embryo (Fig. 6.12)

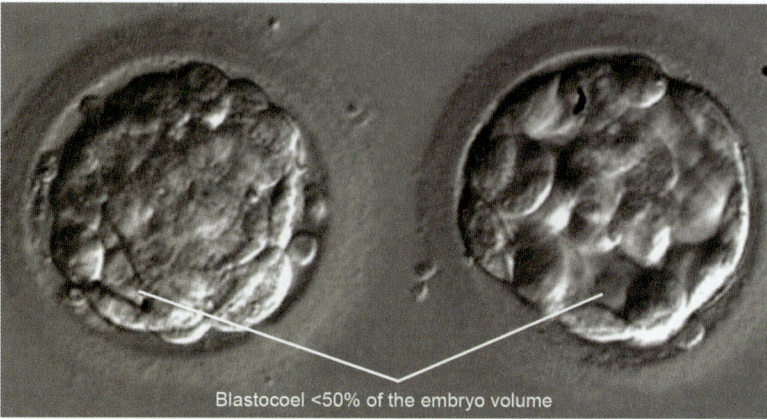

Blastocoel <50% of the embryo volume

Fig. 6.11: Early blastocyst with fluid-filled cavity occupying less than 50% of the volume of the embryo.

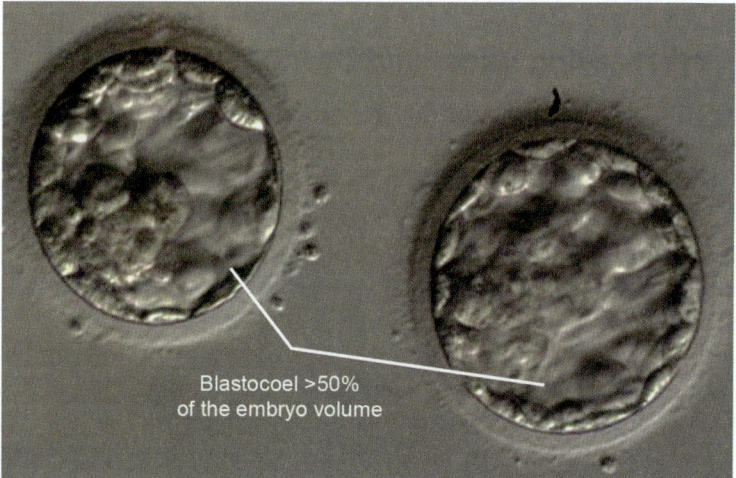

Blastocoel >50% of the embryo volume

Fig. 6.12: Cavitating blastocyst (left) and full blastocyst (right) and with fluid-filled cavity occupying more than 50% of the total volume of the embryo.

- Grade III (full blastocyst): These are those blastocysts in which the blastocoel cavity completely fills the embryo (Fig. 6.12)
- Grade IV (expanded blastocyst): It is the advance stage of the blastocyst in which the blastocoel cavity now is greater than the original volume of the embryo and it is characterized by zona thinning (Fig. 6.13)
- Grade V (hatching blastocyst): The blastocoel cavity is greater than the original volume of the embryo and the TE is herniating through a natural breach in the ZP (Fig. 6.14)
- Grade VI (hatched blastocyst): These are those in which the blastocyst has completely escaped from a natural breach in the ZP (Fig. 6.15).

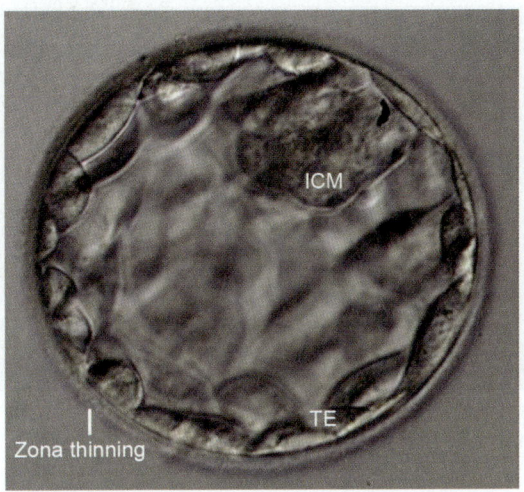

Fig. 6.13: Expanded blastocyst with well-compacted inner cell mass (ICM) and a cohesive trophectoderm.

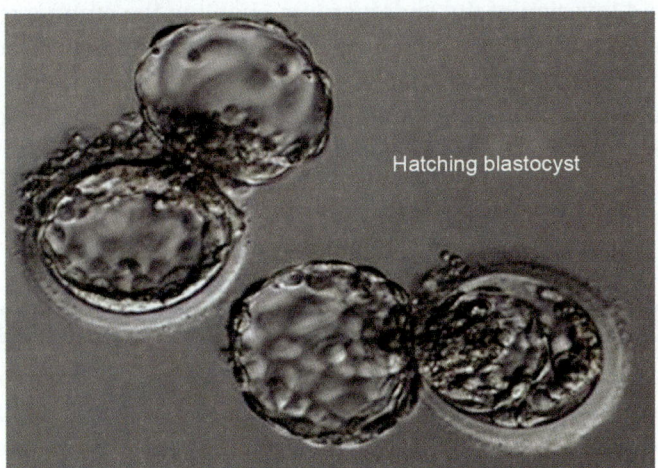

Fig. 6.14: Hatching blastocyst at 117 hour postinsemination.

2. *Inner cell mass*: Cells forming the ICM are compacted and oval in shape and its size varies between 1,900 µm² and 3,800 µm². ICM can range from tightly packed cells to loosely bound cells and thus are scored accordingly. They can be graded from A–D or 3 to 1, according to different grading systems, but basically the best ICM category (A or 1) contains many cells that are tightly packed together, the middle ICM category (B or 2) is composed of several cells that are loosely grouped and the worst category (C or 3) describes an ICM that contains very few cells that are loosely bound; category D would include those ICM that is degenerated or missing.[26]

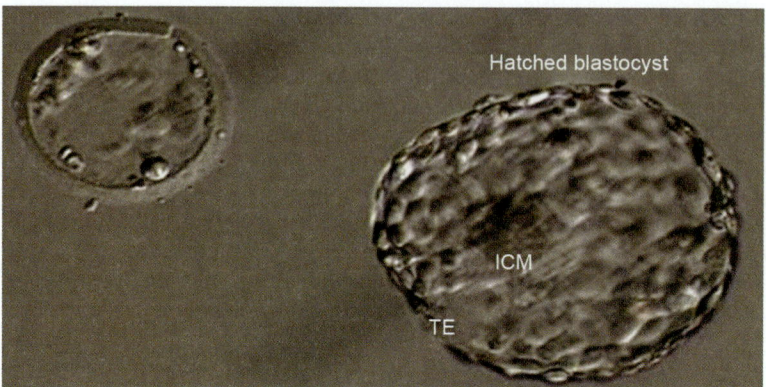

Fig. 6.15: Hatched blastocyst on day 6 of embryo culture.
(ICM: Inner cell mass; TE: Trophectoderm).

3. *Trophectoderm:* Trophectoderm is a single layer of cohesive cells forming the wall of the blastocyst cavity and it is scored on the basis of number and the cohesiveness of the cells. It plays an important role in the adhesion and invasion of the endometrium enabling the embryo to implant. Similar to ICM, TE are scored by their number and cohesiveness from A–D or 3 to 1. The best TE category (A or 1) contains many cells that form a cohesive epithelium, the middle TE category (B or 2) is composed of few cells forming a loose epithelium and the worst category (C or 3) describes a TE that contains very few, and large cells that struggle to form a cohesive epithelium; category D would include those TE that are degenerated.[26]

TIME-LAPSE MONITORING

Time-lapse monitoring (TLM) has made it easier for the embryologists to assess the embryo quality and development in real time instead of standardized time points, which only gives us a snapshot of the dynamic process. This enables us to evaluate abnormalities that may appear or disappear outside the set time range. Hence, continuous monitoring provides a complete picture of the embryo's developmental kinetics.

There are various TLM systems currently available: for instance, Embryo-Scope (FertiliTech) is an incubator with a built-in camera, whereas Primo Vision (Vitrolife) are small cameras that can be placed inside a regular incubator like Heracell. However in all these models, images are captured without removing the embryos from the incubator, thereby restricting exposure of embryos to suboptimal conditions. In addition, more detailed information on the timing of cell divisions, intervals between cell cycles and other important events including multinucleation, symmetry of blastomeres and dynamic PNs patterns can be annotated for analysis.

The aim of this technology is to maximize the chance of selecting the most viable embryo having a higher implantation potential based on morphokinetic parameters, thereby, encouraging elective single embryo transfer (eSET) and minimizing the risk of multiple pregnancies.

Numerous studies have demonstrated the predictive value of time-lapse system.[29-31] Moreover, studies have developed selection criteria and algorithms based on morphokinetic exclusion criteria to exclude morphologically normal embryos displaying aberrant cleavage patterns thus improving the PR and IR.[32]

EMBRYO TRANSFER

Embryo transfer (ET) is the final and one of the most critical procedures determining the success of an IVF cycle. Although tremendous progress has been made in the field of assisted reproduction, the IR has been maintained relatively low.[33] Multiple factors, such as poor embryo quality, compromised uterine receptivity and the ET technique itself has been documented to be responsible for the low IRs.[34]

Focusing on the ET technique, until recent years, ET was considered as a nondecisive factor as compared to the other procedures involved in IVF. However, numerous studies have highlighted the importance of a smooth ET to maximize the PRs.[35] ET technique can be divided into several components and we need to evaluate these components individually to optimize the technique and improve the success rates.

Various factors such as ultrasound guidance, choice of catheter, bacterial contamination of catheter, prolonged duration of ET, air bubble in the catheter, volume of media transferred, ease of the procedure and mock ET have an impact on the overall outcome (Box 6.2).

The ultimate aim of a successful ET is to deposit the embryos to a location in the uterus where chances of implantation increase. Disrupting the endometrium with the catheter, uterine contractions, damaging the embryo during the process of transfer or deposition of embryos in suboptimal locations are likely to cause a transfer failure.

Ease of Embryo Transfer

Numerous studies in literature have reported that difficult transfers often result in a lower PR and IR as compared to easy transfers, thereby correlating pregnancy outcomes with the overall ease of ET.[36] Despite its subjectivity, ease of transfer is considered an important determinant in successful implantation. In general, transfers that are more time consuming, because discomfort require a stiffer catheter or involve extra manipulations like using a tenaculum are described as difficult transfers. Presence of blood on the catheter after ET is also an indication of a difficult transfer, increasing the

---

Box 6.2: Factors contributing to a successful embryo transfer.

- Anatomical and physiological factors
  - Uterine contractions
  - Anatomy of cervix and uterus
  - Uterine fluid
  - Position of the uterus

- Technical factors
  - Catheter insertion and placement
  - Catheter withdrawal
  - Use of ultrasound guidance
  - Volume of transfer media transferred
  - Air or liquid combination
  - Viscosity of transferred media

- Catheter
  - Type
  - Tip shape
  - Diameter

- Embryo selection
  - Grading embryos

---

chances of retained embryos and significantly lowering the IR.[37] Additionally, several techniques like ultrasound guidance, trial transfers or using soft catheters during ET can enable easy transfers.

Trial or Mock Transfer

A mock transfer can be done either before ovarian stimulation or just before the ET. During the mock transfer, full length of the uterine cavity and the cervix is measured using a catheter. All findings are recorded for future reference and these notes enable clinicians to take further precautions during the actual ET.

There are studies correlating mock transfers with better PR and IR in comparison to no trial transfers.[38] Moreover, mock transfers have shown to decrease chances of difficult transfers during the actual ET.

Ultrasound Guidance or Clinical Touch

To facilitate easy insertion of catheter and to ensure the embryos are deposited in the optimal location, ultrasound-guided ET is of paramount importance. Sonographic guidance can help avoid touching the uterine fundus and ensure the catheter is directed properly. In clinical condition like, presence of fibroids in the uterus or in a severely flexed uterus, ultrasound guidance can be very helpful for the clinician. In addition, it is comforting for the patient to visualize the final step of their treatment. However, using an ultrasound during ET causes inconvenience of filling the patient's bladder is more time consuming and will require another operator. Some investigators have suggested performing transfers by clinical touch wherein clinicians move the catheter to visualize its location. In this method, patients discomfort is used to assess fundal contact.[39] Discomfort is often indicative of uterine contraction, which results in expulsion of embryos, consequently lowering the PR.[40] An alternate approach suggested was to transfer the embryos at a fixed distance from the external os (approximately 6 cm), however, this will vary according to the size of the uterus and the cervical length.[39]

Encouraging results from a 2010 Cochrane review suggests using ultrasound over clinical touch to improve clinical PR.[41] Several other meta-analysis has also supported this conclusion.[42,43] Some studies have also reported a decrease in the incidents of ectopic pregnancy using ultrasound guidance.[44,45]

Patient Preparation

Subclinical infection is one of the potential reasons of implantation failure. Positive culture from catheter tips and cervix has been associated with lower clinical PR.[46] To avoid this, it has been recommended to clean the vagina and cervix with saline. Cervical mucus is also known to plug the catheter tip thereby interfering with the ET. Embryos tend to adhere to mucus and thus get displaced when the catheter is withdrawn.

Types of Catheter

Several types of catheters are commercially available for ET. An ideal catheter should be malleable so that it can be advanced in the uterine cavity along its contour. Furthermore, catheters should be soft to avoid causing any kind of trauma to the endometrium or cervix. Although in difficult transfers, hard catheters may facilitate placement, they are associated with trauma, more bleeding and uterine contractions. The outer sheath of soft catheters can also be bent to align the catheter and the uterine axis.

With extensive use of ultrasound-guided ET, numerous echogenic catheters are commercially available now which enables us to visualize the entire catheter or only the tip on ultrasound. Studies have demonstrated higher PR where better using soft catheters such as Cook, and Frydman (Laboratoire CCD, France) and Wallace (Wallace Ltd., Colchester, England) were used in comparison to firm catheters like TDT (metal obturator), Tefcat (Cook Ob-Gyn, Spencer, IN, USA) and Tom Cat (Sherwood Medical, St. Louis, MO, USA).[47,48]

Embryo Loading

Among the aforementioned factors, less attention has been paid to embryo loading (EL). Different combinations of air and fluid volumes in the catheter

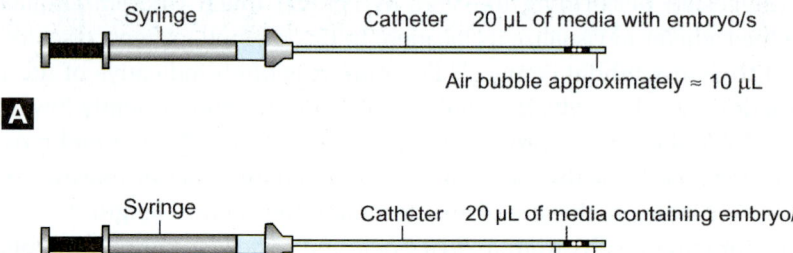

Figs. 6.16A and B: Embryo loading by (A) Fluid-only method; and (B) Air-fluid method.

are being used across different IVF centers. However, two catheter loading methods (air-fluid and fluid-only) have shown to improve the overall efficacy of ET (Figs. 6.16A and B).

General agreement in literature suggests improved clinical outcome by introducing air brackets around the embryo in the transfer media. Air column prevents premature expulsion of the embryo before transfer and also prevents embryo adhesion to the catheter during injection.[49] Furthermore, the air bubble is used as a marker to determine the embryo position in the uterus during ultrasound-guided ET.[50] On the contrary, studies supporting the fluid-only method postulate air as a nonphysiological factor having detrimental effect on the embryos, consequently affecting the IR.[51] Randomized controlled trials (RCTs) have reported no significant difference in the two loading techniques.[52]

Ideally, 20 µL of media surrounds the embryo in the catheter. Insufficient media (<10 µL) may interfere with embryo expulsion consequently affecting the IR.[53]

Embryos are vulnerable to environmental light, temperature or other agents in catheter and thus it is advised to decrease the time interval from loading the ET catheter to embryo deposition.[54]

Embryo Deposition

Randomized controlled trial has documented a higher PR when catheter tip was placed 15–20 mm from the fundus as compared to the traditional 10 mm. On the contrary, some investigators stress to take into account the length of the cavity (Table 6.6).[55] Despite the literature, the gold standard in the practice is transferring embryos in the mid to lower midportion of the uterus.

It is advisable to inject the embryos gently to avoid formation of bubbles and releasing excess media. However there is insufficient data to correlate the speed of injection with the PR.[56]

Table 6.6: Distance between the catheter tip and the fundus and its impact on the pregnancy rate and implantation rate.

Pregnancy outcome	Catheter tip (10 mm)	Catheter tip (15 mm)	Catheter tip (20 mm)
Pregnancy rate	39.3%	49.2%	60%
Implantation rate	20.6%	31.3%	33.3%

After injection, it is advisable to maintain the pressure on the plunger of the syringe to avoid retaining the embryos.[57] To minimize the negative pressure of the plunger, the catheter should be retracted slowly[58] and it is recommended to remove the outer sheath and the catheter simultaneously to prevent the plunger effect. Studies show no significant increase in PR when catheters were removed after an interval as compared to immediate withdrawal.

Postembryo Transfer

After ET, the catheter should be flushed and inspected for retained embryos by the embryologist. Any retained embryo should be loaded again for transfer. There is insufficient data to support the effect of reloading and transferring the retained embryo on the pregnancy outcome.[59] Prolonged bed rest (24 h) or brief bed rest (5–30 min) have shown no benefit over immediate ambulation.[56]

LIMITING THE NUMBER OF EMBRYOS TO TRANSFER

The mechanisms underlying the implantation phenomenon are unknown and after ET, the control of the transferred embryos will be lost and we cannot distinguish which embryos reach the endometrial cavity and whether all of them have the same chance of implantation. That assumption has lead during several years to transfer of two, three or even more embryos to increase the PRs.

Nevertheless, transferring two or three embryos increases the incidence of multiple gestations. The incidence of multiple gestations after IVF in United States has been relatively high (34%) as compared to Europe (24.5%). It is well established that high-order multiple pregnancy (HOMP) leads to increase risk of low-birth weight (< 2,500 g), preterm delivery (< 37 weeks gestation),[60] increased risk of neonatal morbidity and mortality, subsequently leading to long-term learning and developmental disabilities in infants.[61] Additionally, mothers are at a higher risk for pregnancy associated diabetes and hypertensive disorders, preeclampsia and postpartum hemorrhage.[62] The economic burden of multiple gestation further adds to the overall cost of the treatment.[63]

Although, multifetal reduction can be used to reduce the incidence of HOMP, the risk of pregnancy loss after fetal reduction is relatively high ranging between 4.5% and 15.4%. Moreover, the psychological, financial, ethical and religious factors can further make the whole process very stressful. To reduce the frequency of multiple gestations, there is a need to reduce the number of embryos being transferred by a better selection prior to the transfer.

Single Embryo Transfer versus Double Embryo Transfer

Several RCT have provided threshold values for the number of embryos transferred to achieve acceptable PRs and live birth rates. The most effective method to reduce occurrence of multiple pregnancy is to limit the number of embryos transferred.[64] However, it is difficult to generalize these prediction models and translate them into guidelines for every couple. Clinics that have shifted to double ET (DET) from high-order ET (three or more embryos) showed no difference in the PRs. However, a shift to single ET (SET) from DET can lower pregnancy and live birth rates.

In order to develop an effective ET policy that minimizes occurrence of multiple gestations, while maintaining the overall PRs and live birth rates, it is crucial for each IVF clinic to evaluate their own data. To determine the ideal number of embryos to be transferred, it is essential to customize the treatment according to the maternal age the quality of embryos and the number of cycles performed for the patient.

In general, consideration should be taken to carefully select patients for eSET. Independent of age, and good prognosis patient includes the following characteristics:
- Morphologically assessed good quality embryos
- First IVF cycle
- Surplus embryos to necessitate cryopreservation
- Patients with successful previous IVF cycle.

There is good evidence in literature to support the following recommendations determining the number of embryos to be transferred:[65]
- Women aged less than 35 years of age with good prognosis should be offered eSET.
- There are publications that defend the approach of combining eSET with a frozen ET (FET) to increase the cumulative live birth rates. The PR in such patients is equivalent to PR post-DET in young patients.[66,67] This is essential to minimize the chances of stimulating the patient again as surplus high quality embryos can be cryopreserved for subsequent attempt.
- Similarly, eSET should be strongly recommended in donor egg cycles, when the donor is less than 35 years of age.
- In women aged between 35 years and 37 years, not more than three embryos should be transferred in a fresh ET cycle. However, in patients

with good prognosis and having good quality embryos, no more than two cleavage embryos or blastocyst should be considered for transfer in the first or second cycle.

- In women aged between 38 years and 40 years, no more than three embryos should be transferred. Nevertheless, in case of extended culture only two blastocysts should be considered for transfer.
- In women aged more than 40 years, no more than three embryos or blastocyst should be transferred. There is insufficient data to recommend the number of embryos to be transferred in women aged more than 43 years.
- For FET, the number of good quality thawed embryos to be transferred should be similar in each of the above mentioned groups.

Anyway, couples should always be adequately counseled regarding chances of becoming pregnant in their particular situation and the risks involved in multifetal gestation.

Cleavage Stage Embryos versus Blastocyst Transfer

Culturing embryos to blastocyst stage is another method to promote single-ton gestation. Culturing embryos till D5 has inherent advantages in comparison to D3 embryos, in terms of better synchronization between the developing endometrium and the embryo, thereby improving the overall PRs.[68] Additionally, a blastocyst transfer ensures selection of only competent embryos that have undergone the genomic activation and thus have better developmental capability.[69] Studies in literature show that selecting embryos at the blastocyst stage have a lower risk of aneuploidies, thereby improving the implantation potential considerably.[70] RCT, have reported significant increase in the IR when embryos were transferred on D5 as compared to D3 of embryo culture.[70-73]

A significant increase in the live birth rates was also reported in a meta-analysis after blastocyst transfer.[74] Thus, transferring embryos on D5 may prove to be beneficial in selecting the most viable embryos from within a cohort. Consequently, transferring fewer blastocysts than cleavage stage embryos should be taken into consideration, especially in young patients with good prognosis.

A number of studies have demonstrated that the blastulation rate in patients with severe male infertility is significantly low. This can be attributed to the fact that paternal genes in the embryo are expressed from day 3 of embryo culture. Thus, recommending a blastocyst transfer in such clinical cases.[75]

Furthermore, extended culture plays an important role in patients with recurrent implantation failure. General agreement in literature suggests culturing embryos until D5 in patients with multiple failures to improve the IR, which in turn influences the live birth rates as well.[76,77]

Another advantage of blastocyst transfer is seen in patients who have to undergo preimplantation genetic diagnosis (PGD). In addition to the natural selection of potentially competent embryos, blastocyst stage biopsy enables availability of more genetic material, thereby preventing diagnostic errors.[78]

On the other side is fair mentioning that extended culture is associated with increased incidence of cycle cancelation, wherein no embryos are available for transfer due to embryo arrest at the cleavage stage.[79] Consequently, this affects the patient both financially as well as psychologically. To overcome this situation, embryos should be cultured till D5 only when good quality embryos are available on D3 of embryo culture. This will prevent the risk of not having any embryos for transfer on D5. In addition to this, increased cost and higher risk of monozygotic twinning are few more potential disadvantages of blastocyst transfer.[80]

CONCLUSION

In vitro fertilization is a multifaceted treatment comprising of various factors, each playing its role to achieve the desired endpoint of high live birth rates. Embryo selection and transfer is a crucial part of determining the success of an assisted reproductive technology (ART) cycle. One of the major concerns of ART is the occurrence of multiple gestations, which imposes considerable threat to both the maternal and fetal health. In order to minimize these risks, there is a need to limit the number of embryos transferred. Thus, it is essential to improve the current techniques of embryo selection by developing a more uniform and transferable grading system to assure selection of embryos with a higher implantation potential. In addition, optimizing the ET protocols would further help to contribute to clinical success.

REFERENCES

1. Zollner U, Zollner KP, Hartl G, et al. The use of a detailed zygote score after IVF/ICSI to obtain good quality blastocysts: the German experience. Hum Reprod. 2002;17(5):1327-33.
2. Balaban B, Urman B. Effect of oocyte morphology on embryo development and implantation. Reprod Biomed Online. 2006;12(5):608-15.
3. Tesarik J, Greco E. The probability of abnormal preimplantation development can be predicted by a single static observation on pronuclear stage morphology. Hum Reprod. 1999;14(5):1318-23.
4. Garello C, Baker H, Rai J, et al. Pronuclear orientation, polar body placement, and embryo quality after intracytoplasmic sperm injection and in-vitro fertilization: further evidence for polarity in human oocytes? Hum Reprod. 1999;14(10):2588-95.
5. Scott L, Alvero R, Leondires M, et al. The morpology of human pronuclear embryos is positively related to blastocyst development and implantation. Hum Reprod. 2000;15(11):2394-403.

6. Ardoy M, Calderón C, Arroyo G, et al. ASEBIR criteria for the morphological evaluation of human oocytes, early embryos and blastocysts. ASEBIR Clin Embryol Papers. 2008.

7. Staessen C, Van Steirteghem AC. The chromosomal constitution of embryos developing from abnormally fertilized oocytes after intracytoplasmic sperm injection and conventional in-vitro fertilization. Hum Reprod. 1997;12(2):321-7.

8. Sultan KM, Munné S, Palermo GD, et al. Chromosomal status of uni-pronuclear human zygotes following in-vitro fertilization and intracytoplasmic sperm injection. Hum Reprod. 1995;10(1):132-6.

9. Alikani M, Calderon G, Tomkin G, et al. Cleavage anomalies in early human embryos and survival after prolonged culture in-vitro. Hum Reprod. 2000;15 (12):2634-43.

10. Fisch JD, Rodriguez H, Ross R, et al. The Graduated Embryo Score (GES) predicts blastocyst formation and pregnancy rate from cleavage-stage embryos. Hum Reprod. 2001;16(9):1970-5.

11. Magli MC, Gianaroli L, Ferraretti AP, et al. Embryo morphology and development are dependent on the chromosomal complement. Fertil Steril. 2007;87(3): 534-41.

12. Hardarson T, Hanson C, Sjögren A, et al. Human embryos with unevenly sized blastomeres have lower pregnancy and implantation rates: indications for aneuploidy and multinucleation. Hum Reprod. 2001;16(2):313-8.

13. Hnida C, Engenheiro E, Ziebe S. Computer-controlled, multilevel, morphometric analysis of blastomere size as biomarker of fragmentation and multinuclearity in human embryos. Hum Reprod. 2004;19(2):288-93.

14. Holte J, Burglund L, Milton K, et al. Construction of an evidence-based integrated morphology cleavage embryo score for implantation potential of embryos scored and transferred on day 2 after oocyte retrieval. Hum Reprod. 2007;22(2):548-57.

15. Racowsky C, Jackson KV, Cekleniak NA, et al. The number of eight-cell embryos is a key determinant for selecting day 3 or day 5 transfer. Fertil Steril. 2000;73 (3):558-64.

16. Munné S. Chromosome abnormalities and their relationship to morphology and development of human embryos. Reprod Biomed Online. 2006;12(2): 234-53.

17. Ebner T, Yaman C, Moser M, et al. Embryo fragmentation in vitro and its impact on treatment and pregnancy outcome. Fertil Steril. 2001;76(2):281-5.

18. Alikani M, Cohen J, Tomkin G, et al. Human embryo fragmentation in vitro and its implications for pregnancy and implantation. Fertil Steril. 1999;71(5):836-42.

19. Kligman I, Benadiva C, Alikani M, et al. The presence of multinucleated blastomeres in human embryos is correlated with chromosomal abnormalities. Hum Reprod. 1996;11(7):1492-8.

20. Van Royen E, Mangelschots K, De Neubourg D, et al. Calculating the implantation potential of day 3 embryos in women younger than 38 years of age: a new model. Hum Reprod. 2001;16(2):326-32.

21. Biggers JD, Racowksy C. The development of fertilized human ova to the blastocyst stage in KSOM(AA) medium: is a two-step protocol necessary? Reprod Biomed Online. 2002;5(2):133-40.

22. Desai NN, Goldstein J, Rowland DY, et al. Morphological evaluation of human embryos and derivation of an embryo quality scoring system specific for day 3 embryos: a preliminary study. Hum Reprod. 2000;15(10):2190-6.

23. Veeck LL. Abnormal morphology of the human oocytes and conceptus. In: Veeck LL (Ed). An Atlas of Human Gametes and Conceptuses: An Illustrated Reference for Assisted Reproductive Technology. New York: The Parthenon Publishing group Inc.; 1999.

24. Hartshorne G. The embryo. Hum Reprod. 2000;15 Suppl 4:31-41.

25. Tao J, Tamis R, Fink K, et al. The neglected morula/compact stage embryo transfer. Hum Reprod. 2002;17(6):1513-8.

26. Hardarson T, Van Landuyt L, Jones G. The blastocyst. Hum Reprod. 2012;27 (1):i72-91.

27. Alpha Scientists in Reproductive Medicine and ESHRE Special Interest Group of Embryology. The Istanbul consensus workshop on embryo assessment: proceedings of an expert meeting. Hum Reprod. 2011;26(6):1270-83.

28. Gardner DK, Schoolcraft WB. In vitro culture of human blastocysts. In: Jansen R, Mortimer D (Eds). Towards Reproductive Certainty: Fertility and Genetics Beyond 1999: The Plenary Proceedings of the 11th World Congress. UK: Parthenon Publishing; 1999. pp. 378-88.

29. Campbell A, Fishel S, Bowman N, et al. Modelling a risk classification of aneuploidy in human embryos using non-invasive morphokinetics. Reprod Biomed Online. 2013;26(5):477-85.

30. Dal Canto M, Coticchio G, Mignini Renzini M, et al. Cleavage kinetics analysis of human embryos predicts development to blastocyst and implantation. Reprod Biomed Online. 2012;25(5):474-80.

31. Pribenszky C, Mátyás S, Kovács P, et al. Pregnancy achieved by transfer of a single blastocyst selected by time-lapse monitoring. Reprod Biomed Online. 2010;21(4):533-6.

32. Meseguer M, Herrero J, Tejera A, et al. The use of morphokinetics as a predictor of embryo implantation. Hum Reprod. 2011;26(10):2658-71.

33. Adamson GD, de Mouzon J, Lancaster P, et al. World collaborative report on in vitro fertilization, 2000. Fertil Steril. 2006;85(6):1586-622.

34. Schoolcraft WB, Surrey ES, Gardner DK. Embryo transfer: techniques and variables affecting success. Fertil Steril. 2001;76(5):863-70.

35. Mansour RT, Aboulghar MA. Optimizing the embryo transfer technique. Hum Reprod. 2002;17(5):1149-53.

36. Tomás C, Tikkinen K, Tuomivaara L, et al. The degree of difficulty of embryo transfer is an independent factor for predicting pregnancy. Hum Reprod. 2002; 17(10):2632-5.

37. Goudas VT, Hammitt DG, Damario MA, et al. Blood on the embryo transfer catheter is associated with decreased rates of embryo implantation and clinical pregnancy with the use of in vitro fertilization-embryo transfer. Fertil Steril. 1998;70(5):878-82.

38. Mansour R, Aboulghar M, Serour G. Dummy embryo transfer: a technique that minimizes the problems of embryo transfer and improves the pregnancy rate in human in vitro fertilization. Fertil Steril. 1990;54(4):678-81.

39. Lesny P, Killick SR, Tetlow RL, et al. Embryo transfer—can we learn anything new from the observation of junctional zone contractions? Hum Reprod. 1998; 13(6):1540-6.

40. Fanchin R, Righini C, Olivennes F, et al. Uterine contractions at the time of embryo transfer alter pregnancy rates after in-vitro fertilization. Hum Reprod. 1998;13(7):1968-74.

41. Brown J, Buckingham K, Abou-Setta AM, et al. Ultrasound versus 'clinical touch' for catheter guidance during embryo transfer in women. Cochrane Database Syst Rev. 2010;(1):CD006107.

42. Buckett WM. A meta-analysis of ultrasound-guided versus clinical touch embryo transfer. Fertil Steril. 2003;80(4):1037-41.

43. Abou-Setta AM, Mansour RT, Al-Inany HG, et al. Among women undergoing embryo transfer, is the probability of pregnancy and live birth improved with ultrasound guidance over clinical touch alone? A systemic review and meta-analysis of prospective randomized trials. Fertil Steril. 2007;88(2):333-41.

44. Tang OS, Ng EH, So WW, et al. Ultrasound-guided embryo transfer: a prospective randomized controlled trial. Hum Reprod. 2001;16(11):2310-5.

45. Sallam HN, Sadek SS. Ultrasound-guided embryo transfer: a meta-analysis of randomized controlled trials. Fertil Steril. 2003;80(4):1042-6.

46. Moore DE, Soules MR, Klein NA, et al. Bacteria in the transfer catheter tip influence the live-birth rate after in vitro fertilization. Fertil Steril. 2000;74(6): 1118-24.

47. Buckett WM. A review and meta-analysis of prospective trials comparing different catheters used for embryo transfer. Fertil Steril. 2006;85(3):728-34.

48. Abou-Setta AM, Al-Inany HG, Mansour RT, et al. Soft versus firm embryo transfer catheters for assisted reproduction: a systematic review and meta-analysis. Hum Reprod. 2005;20(11):3114-21.

49. Eytan O, Elad D, Zaretsky U, et al. A glance into the uterus during in vitro simulation of embryo transfer. Hum Reprod. 2004;19(3):562-9.

50. Lambers MJ, Dogan E, Lens JW, et al. The position of transferred air bubbles after embryo transfer is related to pregnancy rate. Fertil Steril. 2007;88(1):68-73.

51. Krampl E, Zegermacher G, Eichler C, et al. Air in the uterine cavity after embryo transfer. Fertil Steril. 1995;63(2):366-70.

52. Abou-Setta AM. Air fluid versus fluid-only models of embryo catheter loading: a systematic review and meta-analysis. Reprod Biomed Online. 2007;14(1):80-4.

53. Ebner T, Yaman C, Moser M, et al. The ineffective loading process of the embryo transfer catheter alters implantation and pregnancy rates. Fertil Steril. 2001; 76(3):630-2.

54. Matorras R, Mendoza R, Expósito A, et al. Influence of the time interval between embryo catheter loading and discharging on the success of IVF. Hum Reprod. 2004;19(9):2027-30.

55. Coroleu B, Barri PN, Carreras O, et al. The influence of the depth of embryo replacement into the uterine cavity on implantation rates after IVF: a controlled, ultrasound-guided study. Hum Reprod. 2002;17(2):341-6.

56. Bungum L, Bungum M. Embryo transfer. In: Gardner DK, Weissman A, Howles CM, Shoham Z (Eds). Texbook of Assisted Reproductive Technologies: Laboratory and Clinical Perspectives, 3rd edition. United Kingdom: Informa Healthcare; 2008.

57. Hearns-Stokes RM, Miller BT, Scott L, et al. Pregnancy rates after embryo transfer depend on the provide at embryo transfer. Fertil Steril. 2000;74(1):80-6.

58. Eytan O, Elad D, Jaffa AJ. Evaluation of the embryo transfer protocol by a laboratory model of the uterus. Fertil Steril. 2007;88(2):485-93.

59. Nabi A, Awonuga A, Birch H, et al. Multiple attempts at embryo transfer: does this affect in-vitro fertilization treatment outcome? Hum Reprod. 1997;12 (6):1188-90.

60. Tough SC, Greene CA, Svenson LW, et al. Effects of in vitro fertilization on low birth weight, preterm delivery, and multiple birth. J Pediatr. 2000;136(5):618-22.

61. Sunderam S, Chang J, Flowers L, et al. Assisted Reproductive Technology Surveillance—United States, 2006. MMWR Surveillance Summaries. 2009;58(SS05): 1-25.

62. Tallo CP, Vohr B, Oh W, et al. Maternal and neonatal morbidity associated with in vitro fertilization. J Pediatr. 1995;127(5):794-800.
63. Katz P, Nachtigall R, Showstack J. The economic impact of the assisted reproductive technologies. Nat Cell Biol. 2002;4 Suppl:s29-32.
64. Grifo JA, Flisser E, Adler A, et al. Programmatic implementation of blastocyst transfer in a university-based in vitro fertilization clinic: maximizing pregnancy rates and minimizing triplet rates. Fertil Steril. 2007;88(2):294-300.
65. Joint SOGC-CFAS. Guidelines for the number of embryos to transfer following in vitro fertilization No. 182, September 2006. Int J Gynaecol Obstet. 2008;102 (2):203-16.
66. Thurin A, Hausken J, Hillensjö T, et al. Elective single-embryo transfer versus double-embryo transfer in in vitro fertilization. N Engl J Med. 2004;351(23): 2392-402.
67. Heijnen EM, Eijkemans MJ, De Klerk C, et al. A mild treatment strategy for in-vitro fertilisation: a randomised non-inferiority trial. Lancet. 2007;369 (9563):743-9.
68. Gardner DK, Schoolcraft WB, Wagley L, et al. A prospective randomized trial of blastocyst culture and transfer in in-vitro fertilization. Hum Reprod. 1998;13 (12):3434-40.
69. Braude P, Bolton V, Moore S. Human gene expression first occurs between the four-and eight-cell stages of preimplantation development. Nature. 1988;332 (6163):459-61.
70. Karaki RZ, Samarraie SS, Younis NA, et al. Blastocyst culture and transfer: a step toward improved in vitro fertilization outcome. Fertil Steril. 2002;77(1):114-8.
71. Frattarelli JL, Leondires MP, McKeeby JL, et al. Blastocyst transfer decreases multiple pregnancy rates in in vitro fertilization cycles: a randomized controlled trial. Fertil Steril. 2003;79(1):228-30.
72. Margreiter M, Weghofer A, Kogosowski A, et al. A prospective randomized multicenter study to evaluate the best day for embryo transfer: does the outcome justify prolonged embryo culture? J Assist Reprod Genet. 2003;20(2):91-4.
73. Levron J, Shulman A, Bider D, et al. A prospective randomized study comparing day 3 with blastocyst-stage embryo transfer. Fertil Steril. 2002;77(6):1300-1.
74. Glujovsky D, Farquhar C, Quinteiro Retamar AM, et al. Cleavage stage versus blastocyst stage embryo transfer in assisted reproductive technology. Cochrane Database Syst Rev. 2016;(6):CD002118.
75. Shoukir Y, Chardonnens D, Campana A, et al. Blastocyst development from supernumerary embryos after intracytoplasmic sperm injection: a paternal influence? Hum Reprod. 1998;13(6):1632-7.
76. Blake DA, Farquhar C, Johnson N, et al. Cleavage stage versus blastocyst stage embryo transfer in assisted conception. Cochrane Database Syst Rev. 2007; (4):CD002118.
77. Guerif F, Bidault R, Gasnier O, et al. Efficacy of blastocyst transfer after implantation failure. Reprod Biomed Online. 2004;9(6):630-6.
78. Kahraman S, Beyazyürek C, Tac HA, et al. Recent advances in preimplantation genetic diagnosis. Adv Genom Genet. 2015;5(1):189-203.
79. Cutting R, Morroll D, Roberts SA, et al. Elective single embryo transfer: guidelines for practice British Fertility Society and Association of Clinical Embryologists. Hum Fertil (Camb). 2008;11(3):131-46.
80. Peramo B, Ricciarelli E, Cuadros-Fernández JM, et al. Blastocyst transfer and monozygotic twinning. Fertil Steril. 1999;72:1116-7.

Chapter 7

Oocyte and Embryo Vitrification

Ana Cobo, Aila Coello

INTRODUCTION

Vitrification is a cryopreservation procedure by which an aqueous solution is solidified into a glassy phase at low temperatures. This process is facilitated by applying high cooling rates and increasing viscosity using high concentration of cryoprotectants (CPAs).[1] These agents either permeate the cell membrane or create an osmotic gradient allowing reduce water content and, as a result, avoiding ice crystal formation. However, CPAs can be toxic at high concentration; thereby protocols have been modified in order to minimize damage. In this way, by significantly reducing the volume of the sample, the cooling rate is increased and the concentration of CPAs can be reduced while maintaining successful vitrification.

The essential role of cryopreservation in assisted reproductive technology (ART) has become obvious since the commencement of the infertility treatment, becoming a more flexible and efficient practice. Semen and embryo cryopreservation has been a successful strategy, routinely applied in *in vitro* fertilization (IVF) procedure for a long time. However, in spite of numerous studies conducted over the last 20 years, the reliability of oocyte cryopreservation is just being confirmed currently, thanks to vitrification.

METHODOLOGY: MEDIA AND DEVICES

The methodology used for oocyte and embryo vitrification may differ significantly between laboratories especially when different devices and solutions are used. Since the first vitrification solution was developed,[2] various CPAs have been proposed to be effective. Nowadays, a mixture of penetrating CPAs, such as ethylene glycol (EG) and dimethyl sulfoxide (DMSO) in combination with a nonpenetrating CPA, such as sucrose or trehalose, is the approach most commonly used.[3]

The basic procedure is simple and quick. Oocytes or embryos are exposed to a hypertonic solution composed of penetrating CPAs. At this point, water is removed from the cells to adjust osmolarity while CPAs begin to flow into them. The degree of permeability depends on the stage of embryo development and the type of CPA.[4] Then, oocytes or embryos are exposed briefly to a more concentrated solution composed of both penetrating and nonpenetrating CPAs which cause the proper cell dehydration. After this step, they are placed into a suitable container designed for vitrification and immediately submerged into liquid nitrogen (LN). The premise in the vitrification approach has been that the higher the cooling rate, the greater the likelihood that true vitrification can be achieved. However, high warming rate is also required as demonstrated recently.[5]

The cooling rate achieved will depend on the device and the volume of solution. Consequently, a variety of devices have been developed to facilitate rapid cooling; most of them are known as "open systems" because samples come into direct contact with LN during vitrification. Devices hermetically sealed before vitrification are known as "closed systems", which prevent samples from coming into direct contact with LN during vitrification. Obviously, the thermal isolation of samples in this way slows the cooling rate. The key to overcome this shortcoming is to find the optimal balance between the speed of cooling and warming and the necessary concentration of CPA for each step of exposure in order to reach the vitrified state without inducing osmotic swelling stress.[6]

The main drawback of using open system devices is the possibility of cross-contamination through direct contact of the vitrification sample with nonsterile LN. Although there are no documented cases of cross-contamination in the history of ART cryotransfers, it is vital that efforts be made to increase the safety of our cryopreservation methods. Hence, the design of devices that are able to prevent the risks associated with direct contact with LN during storage, while maintaining the advantages of open systems during the vitrification process, would be highly advisable. The sterilization of LN, either by filtering or by ultraviolet irradiation,[7] is also a good alternative, as is the use of vapor storage tanks, which are known to be safer than traditional ones and have proven to be very efficient in terms of preserving sample viability.[8]

OOCYTE VITRIFICATION

Nowadays the challenge of cryopreserve, storage for long time and successfully implant the female gamete is feasible thanks to vitrification. In spite of its great value, oocyte cryostorage has not been a valid option until relatively recently, due to the unavailability of successful methodologies. The reasons behind the long period of failures in the attempt to cryopreserve oocytes are currently well identified. Among them, the size and shape of the female gamete are two significant reasons. The female gamete is the largest cell of the human body, with a great content of water, which involves a higher probability of ice formation during the cryopreservation process. Chilling injury, defined as the irreversible damage to the cytoskeleton[9] and cell membranes[10] following exposure of cells to low temperatures (from +15°C to –5°C) before the nucleation of ice, is other major factor responsible for cell death during cryopreservation.[11] The ice crystal formation within the cytoplasm must be avoided, at all cost, in order to guarantee the survival and integrity of the oocytes when they are later thawed. Vitrification efficiently avoids chilling injury by the direct passage from room temperatures to −196°C and efficiently avoids ice formation.[12] As a result, these days we count on several efficient approaches able to provide successful outcomes comparable to those achieved with fresh oocytes.

There is a large population that is currently benefiting from oocyte vitrification technique, as cancer patients who need an option for fertility preservation (FP) before undergoing the potential sterilizing treatment,[13] or women who wish to delay their motherhood due to a variety of reasons.[14,15] Oocyte cryostorage brings additional advantages to ART programs being helpful to solve different clinical situations as in low-responder patients,[16] unpredictable unavailability of semen sample collection from the male partner, risk of suffering ovarian hyperstimulation syndrome,[17] or some other cases in which the embryo transfer is not advisable.[18] Undoubtedly, the ovum donation programs have also been major beneficiaries of egg banking.[19]

Ovum Donation Programs

Oocyte cryostorage results very useful to overcome the most common drawbacks involved with ovum donation as currently applied, such as synchronization between donors and recipients, long waiting lists subject to the availability of a suitable donor and the most important, the absence of a quarantine period. In our center, we have developed a consistent software tool that after entering parameters characteristic of the woman and her partner (as phenotypic traits, blood group, etc.) gives us a list of available donors and number of oocytes at that time on the bank, thus simplifying the process donor-recipient matching.

The first live birth after vitrification was obtained from a donated oocyte using an open system device (OPS) in 1999.[20] Since then, numerous publications using different types of devices corroborate the effectiveness of the technique (Table 7.1).

Our group, in 2008, published a study whose objective was to assess the impact of vitrification using donated oocytes, in terms of survival and development potential when compared to fresh oocytes.[21] To do this, a cohort of oocytes from a single donor was randomly divided into two groups: (1) in the first one, the oocytes were vitrified and (2) in the second one, the remaining oocytes were kept in the incubator (control fresh oocytes). Within an hour after vitrification we proceeded to devitrification and after two additional hours proceeded to simultaneous insemination of the two types of eggs, (1) fresh and (2) vitrified. The cryotop method employed for oocyte vitrification was that previously described by Kuwayama.[22] The study included 30 donors

Table 7.1: Key publications related to donated vitrified oocytes.

	Year	Device	Survival rate (%)	Pregnancy rate (%)
Kuleshova et al.	1999	OPS	64.7	33.3
Lacena et al.	2006	Cryotop	89.2	56.5
Cobo et al.	2008	Cryotop	96.9	65.2
Chang et al.	2008	Cryotop	85.4	83.3
Sher G et al.	2008	Cryotloop	96.1	81.2
Nagy et al.	2008	Cryotop	89.0	75.0
Cao et al.	2009	Cryoleaf	91.8	
Cobo et al.	2010	Cryotop	92.5	55.4
Noyes et al.	2010	Cryotip	87.0	63.0
Trokoudes et al.	2011	Cryotop	91.4	55.6
Garcia et al.	2011	Cryolock	89.4	61.8
Stoop et al.	2012	CBS high security	90.2	50.0
Papatheodorou et al.	2013	Vitrisafe	90.9	28.0
Sole et al.	2013	Cryotop	85.6	53.5
Figueira et al.	2014	Cryotop	77.1	37.7

and 30 recipients (509 oocytes; 231 vitrified oocytes and 219 fresh oocytes). After a survival rate of 96.9%, we found no differences in the rate of division in day 3 (77.6% vs 84.6% in vitrified in fresh) or the morphological quality of embryos (80.8% vs 80.5% of good quality embryos vitrified versus fresh). Likewise, both the blastocyst rate (48.7% vs 47.5%) and quality of embryos (81.1% vs 70%) were similar comparing fresh and vitrified.

We want to make special mention of the randomized, prospective, triple-blind, controlled clinical trial which included the largest sample size published to date, aimed to validate oocyte vitrification technique as a fundamental tool in running the bank of these gametes intended for programs ovo-donation.[19] The study included 600 donor or recipients (300 per each branch) and 3,039 vitrified versus 3,185 fresh oocytes. In this study, we demonstrated the noninferiority of vitrified oocytes regarding ongoing pregnancy rate by intention to treat [odds ratio (OR) = 0.921, 95% confidence interval (CI) 0.667–1.274]. The overall survival rate in this study was 92.5% and ongoing pregnancy rate by intention to treat was 43.7% in the case of patients who received vitrified oocytes compared to 41.7% obtained with fresh oocytes. This study definitively confirmed our previous observations about the nonalteration of vitrified oocytes potential to develop into embryos capable of generating competent ongoing pregnancies in a similar proportion to fresh oocytes.

Because of the great potential of vitrified oocytes, and similarly to what happens with fresh donations, after embryo transfer there are often surplus viable embryos, suitable to be vitrified for future transfers. In this case, we are talking about a double round of vitrification, first at oocyte stage and later at cleavage stage (day 3) or blastocyst stage. In a publication in 2013, we showed that the double vitrification has no effect on the delivery rate or live birth.[23] This study included 796 vitrified embryos generated from vitrified oocytes (N = 471 cycles) and 4,394 vitrified embryos generated from fresh oocytes (N = 2,629 cycles). The overall survival rate was 97.2% (95% CI 95.9–98.6) versus 95.7% (95% CI 94.9–96.4) for double vitrified versus once respectively (NS). The live birth rate per warming cycle was 33.8% versus 30.6% (NS). As showed, the OR of the delivery rate, the double vitrification had no effect on embryos regardless of whether they were in early stage development (day 3) or blastocyst stage (OR = 0.867, 95% CI 0.657–1.203).

We recently published an observational study in which our experience of 6 years with the egg banking program[24] was described. The analysis included 3,610 cycles of oocyte donation where 42,152 metaphase II (MII) were warmed with a survival rate of 92.6%. The impact of storage time on the survival rate and clinical outcome was calculated by establishing different time intervals from less than 6 months to over 5 years. In any case, the storage time did not affect survival or clinical outcomes. We believe that this is very reassuring information since success after long time storage guarantees the sustainability of the approach. The clinical, ongoing pregnancy and delivery rates were 55.0%, 45.3% and 37.6% respectively, thus confirming the consistency of the results as compared to our previous findings.[13,19] The likelihood of having surplus embryos available for additional cryotransfers was very high in this series due to the mean number of oocytes donated. The possibility of further cryotransfers increased cumulative outcomes, and thus maximized the yield of a single donation cycle, which is precisely what we show herein. The cumulative delivery rate per donation cycle increased to over 70% after three cryotransfers and rose to nearly 80% after five cryotransfers. These results render the donation cycle as highly efficient.

Kaplan-Meier analysis observed in Graph 7.1 provides interesting information about the number of vitrified oocytes consumed by a recipient (in either one or more cycles of ovum donation) necessary for a newborn. The analysis showed that the live-birth rate (LBR) increases exponentially, and the patient can achieve a baby with a probability of nearly 100% when about 3–4 cycles of egg donation (around 35–40 oocytes) are completed. This result confirms our previous findings while showing the excellent efficiency of egg banking.

Fertility Preservation

Vitrification of oocytes is currently being offered as an option for women who wish to preserve their gametes to allow them to have a chance to conceive in

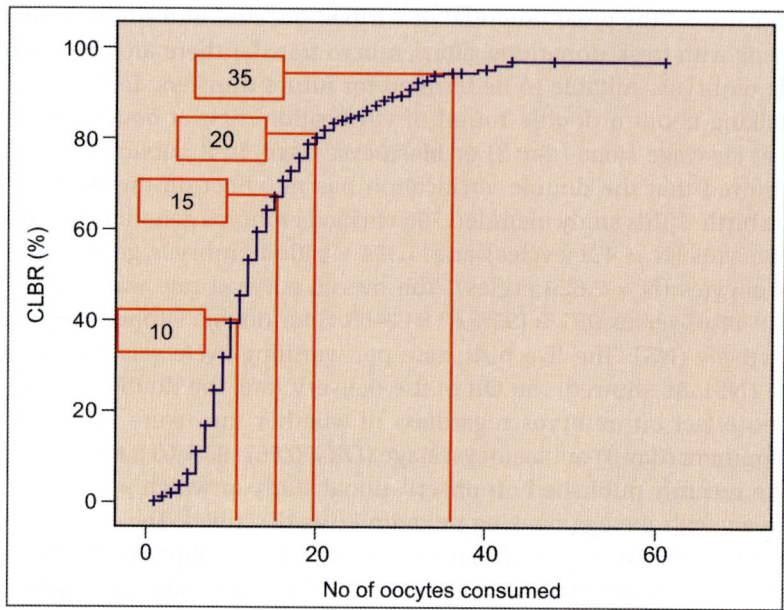

Graph 7.1: The Kaplan-Meier curve for the CDR of at least one baby, depending on the total number of oocytes consumed.
(CDR: Cumulative delivery rate; CLBR: Cumulative live birth rate).

the future and to have their own genetic offspring.[25] The main beneficiaries of this strategy are cancer patients who must undergo chemotherapy or radiotherapy and patients with other diseases who require potentially gonadotoxic treatments.

The first reported case in Europe of a pregnancy after FP using vitrification of oocytes was from our group in a patient, whose ovarian cortex was cryopreserved first, and after grafting, four stimulation cycles were performed to accumulate and vitrify mature oocytes; a later IVF cycle successfully ended in a twin pregnancy. Since then, various studies have reported clinical outcomes with cryopreserved oocytes for FP in cancer patients (Table 7.2).

Although FP may initially concern cancer patients, there are many other medical conditions that may compromise fertility, such as endometriosis or high-risk for early ovarian failure, where an intervention as safeguarding gametes for future use is required to uphold fertility potential. In addition, age-related decline of fertility is a very common condition in ART. Elective oocyte vitrification for nonmedical conditions is increasingly accepted as an option to postpone motherhood.[26] An updated data of FP for oncological and nononcological patients in IVI is showed in Table 7.3.

We have recently reported, in the largest series to date, our experience in FP in a population of women who electively decided to vitrify their gametes for future use. A clear, and expected, effect of female age was observed in

Table 7.2: Live birth reported after fertility preservation in cancer patients: slow freezing and vitrification of oocytes.

	Yang et al. 2007	Porcu et al. 2008	Sanchez Serrano et al. 2009	Kim et al. 2011	Garcia-Velasco et al. 2013	Alvarez et al. 2014	Da Motta et al. 2014
Type of malignancy	Hodgkin's lymphoma	Borderline ovarian tumor	Breast cancer	Chronic myeloid leukemia	Non-Hodgkin's lymphoma	Invasive ovarian carcinoma	Breast cancer
Cryopreservation technique	Slow freezing	Slow freezing	Combined OTC-SF + OV (Cryotop)	Vitrification (EMG)	Vitrification (Cryotop)	Vitrification (Cryotop)	Vitrification (Cryotip)
Age at FP	27	26	36	22	31	28	36
No. of cryopreserved oocytes	13	7	16	7	4	14	28
Storage time (years)	6	4	2	9	2	1	6
Pregnancy	Single*	Twin	Twin	Single	Single	Heterotopic	Triplet
Number of live births	1	2	2	1	1	1	1
Weeks of gestation	37	38	34	35 + 3 days	39	38	—
Weight of babies	3062	2100 and 2400	1650 and 1830	2410	3440	2651	2970
Sex of baby	Male	Females	Males	Male	Male	Male	—

*Gestational carrier

(EMG: Electron microscope grids; FP: Fertility preservation; OTC-SF: Ovarian tissue cryopreservation plus oocyte vitrification by cryotop).

Cause	No of patients	No of cycles	Clinical pregnancy (%)	Ongoing pregnancy (%)	LBR (%)
Table 7.3: Clinical outcome of oncological and nononcological FP patients.					
Oncological	289	395	46.05	32.89	68
Nononcological	50	69	37.93	29.31	14
Total	339	464	44.75	32.32	82

(FP: Fertility preservation; LBR: Live-birth rate).

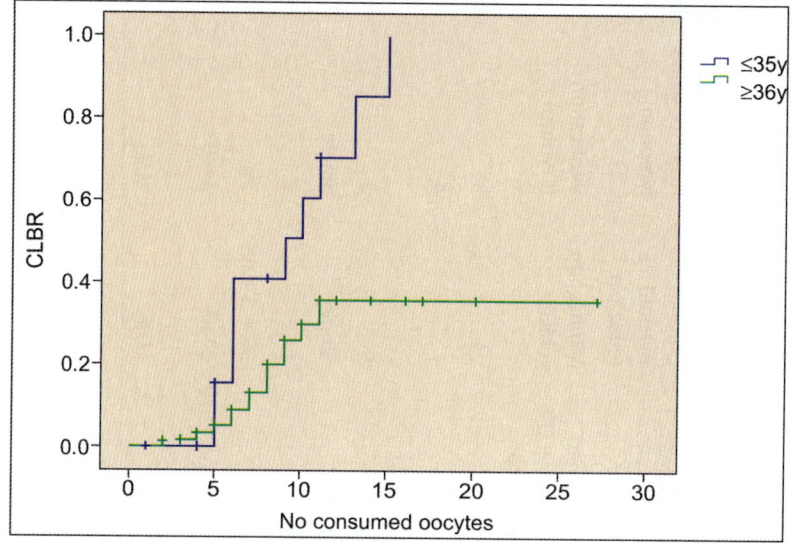

Graph 7.2: Kaplan-Meier plotting of the cumulative live-birth rate (CLBR) of at least one baby, depending on the total number of consumed oocytes and categorized by age. (CI: Confidence interval).

our data. Higher outcomes were achieved in women aged less than or equal to 35 years. In this group a larger number of oocytes were retrieved and finally vitrified, and the survival and clinical outcomes were equivalent to those achieved in our egg banking program for ovum donation, with the highest success rates in the youngest group of women (≤29 years). Otherwise, predictably fewer oocytes and worse outcomes were achieved as the age increased, resembling the results of the infertile population of similar age. There is a clear different probability of having a baby according to the number of oocytes consumed when the less than or equal to 35-year-old and more than 36-year-old groups are compared (P <0.05). Obviously, the more oocytes the higher the probability, but the relationship is not linear, as shown by the curves, and is strongly related to a powerful confounder, i.e. the age of the patient (Graph 7.2). When we looked at our data, we observed a huge difference in cumulative live-birth rate (CLBR) when using only five oocytes

(15.4%) compared with using eight (40.8%), which means an 8.4% increase in CLBR per additional oocyte, if women were less than or equal to 35 years old. If they were more than 36 years old using the same number of oocytes, the increase in CLBR was considerably more modest (from CLBR of 5.1% with the use of five oocytes to 19.9% when eight oocytes were consumed, meaning an increase in CLBR of 4.9% per additional oocyte). With 15 oocytes, the CLBR continued to increase in the less than 35-year-old group, whereas with the same number of oocytes the plateau was already reached in the group of women aged more than 36 years, meaning that at this point the success is independent from the number of oocytes used up. In light of this, we suggest that at least eight to ten MII oocytes should be vitrified to obtain a reasonable success rate.

Low-responder Patients

A potential alternative to the management of low responder (LR) is to create a large stock of oocytes by accumulating vitrified MII oocytes over several stimulation cycles and inseminating them all at the same time. Theoretically, this could help to increase the chances of success by endowing patients with a "normoresponder-like" status. We reported, in 2010, a study aimed to assess the efficiency of this new strategy for managing LR that takes advantage of vitrification as a way of creating larger cohorts of oocytes.[16] This study included 242 LR patients (594 cycles) whose mature oocytes were accumulated by vitrification and inseminated simultaneously (LR-Accu-Vit) and 482 patients (588 cycles) undergoing IVF or embryo transfer with fresh oocytes in each stimulation cycle (LR-fresh). The embryo transfer cancelation per patient was significantly lower in the LR-Accu-Vit group (9.1%) than the LR-fresh group (34.0%). This result showed that this strategy is useful to avoid patients abandoning treatment due to negative results that impair their ability to cope with the situation. Live-birth rate or patient was higher in the LR-Accu-Vit group (30.2%) than the LR-fresh group (22.4%) which confirmed the efficiency of this method for managing LR patients. The positive effects of this strategy are even more evident when cumulative outcome is considered, which endorses the treatment as a successful alternative for LR patients.

Other authors also reported the evaluation of this form of vitrification in the context of standard infertile patients. Rienzi et al.[27] conducted a prospective randomized sibling-oocyte study that included 120 fresh and 124 vitrified sibling oocytes from 40 infertile patients (mean age 35.5 ± 4.8 years). The survival rate was 97%, with a fertilization rate after intracytoplasmic sperm injection (ICSI) of 77% (95/124) per warmed oocyte and 79% (95/120) per warmed or inseminated oocyte. Moreover, the proportions of excellent quality embryos were the same in each group.

In another study, the cumulative outcome after the transfer of embryos derived from fresh and vitrified oocytes from a single ovarian stimulation cycle was calculated. The study included 182 ICSI cycles in which oocyte vitrification was also performed. The cumulative pregnancy rate (CPR) was calculated when after failing a fresh embryo transfer the patient underwent a second embryo transfer using embryos derived from the vitrified oocytes. Implantation rates in fresh and vitrification cycles were not significantly different for women less than or equal to 34 years.[28]

All these evidences suggest that vitrified oocytes are functionally similar to fresh oocytes in terms of fertilization, development and implantation potential.

EMBRYO VITRIFICATION

Vitrification was first applied in embryology with the use of mouse embryos almost 30 years ago,[2] with successfully vitrification in 1991 by Kono et al.[29] The first human pregnancy and delivery of a baby as a result of blastocyst vitrification was published in 2001.[30] Since these landmark publications, vitrification of human embryos has played an important role in assisted reproduction treatment. It allows increasing cumulative outcomes since several pregnancies can be achieved after only one ovum retrieval. Furthermore, it has been suggested that controlled ovarian stimulation with exogenous gonadotropins adversely affects endometrial receptivity in ART cycles.[31,32] Thus, there is a trend toward cryopreservation of all viable embryos in a fresh IVF cycle followed by transfer of frozen thawed embryos in a subsequent cycle. This policy leads to place embryos in a more physiologic environment resulting in a better embryo-endometrium synchrony.

In addition, cryopreservation programs are crucial for patients at risk of ovarian hyperstimulation syndrome as well as to allow time for the testing of embryos for genetic anomalies before transfer.[33]

Currently, vitrification is being increasingly applied to both early cleavage and blastocyst stage embryos. In 2013, we reported our experience with the application of vitrification with Cryotop system to our embryo cryopreservation program.[34] Based on 3,150 warming cycles (6,019 embryos), the overall survival rate was 95%, with 93% (95% CI 90.1–95.3) of day 2 and 95% (95% CI 94.3–95.7) of day 3 embryos fully intact upon warming. Figures 7.1A to D show cleavage stage embryos and blastocysts before and after vitrification. Similarly to what happened to early stages, our overall blastocyst survival rate involving almost 2,000 blastocysts was considerably high (Table 7.4).

Other authors have published similar outcomes using the Cryotop system.[35-37] In the past, other devices have been used for blastocyst vitrification. For example, Balaban et al. reported approximately 95% survival (234

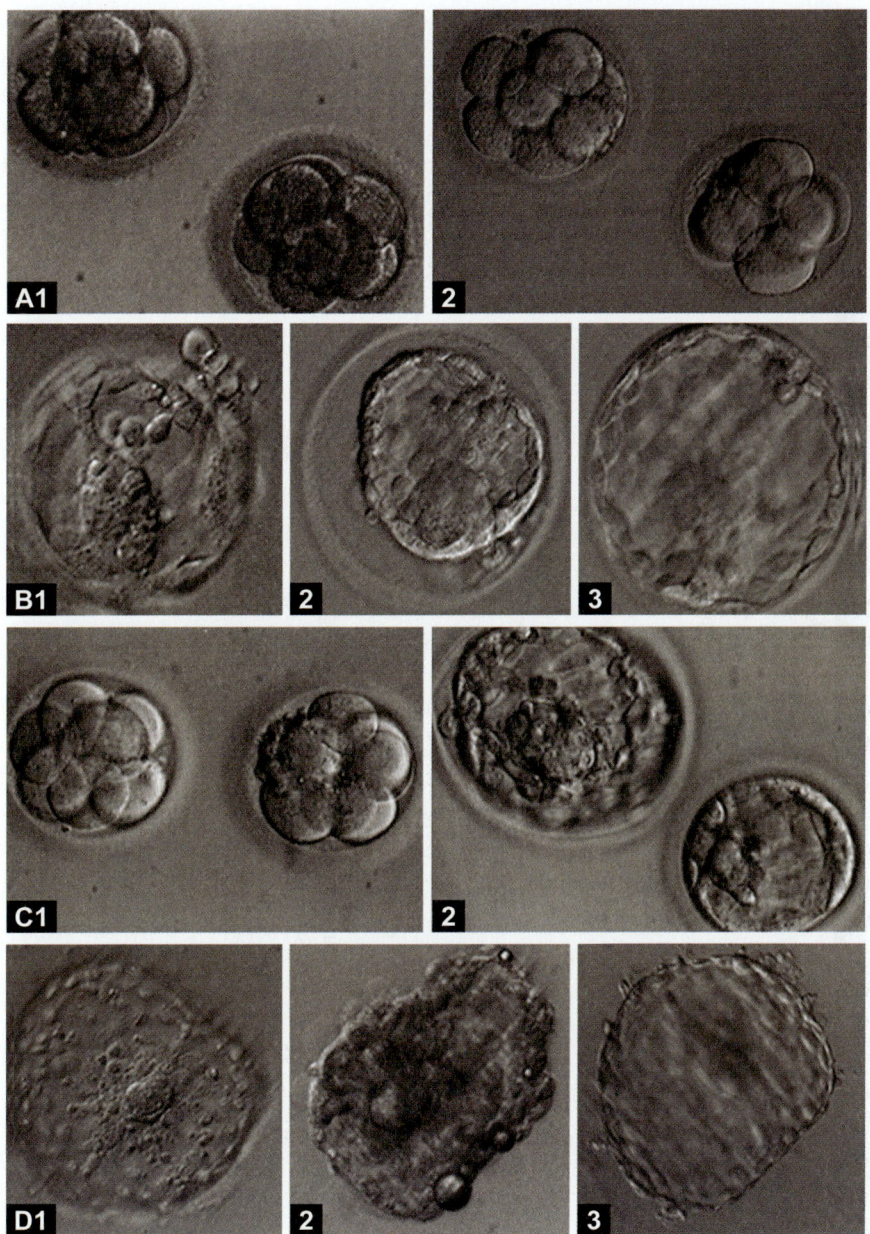

Figs. 7.1A to D: Cleavage stage embryos and blastocysts before and after vitrification. (A) Day 3 embryos [(1) Before vitrification, and (2) immediatly after warming], (B) [(1) Day 5 blastocyst [(1) Before vitrification, (2) 1 hour after vitrification (the reexpansion has not been completed), and (3) Fully reexpanded 3 hours after warming]; (C) [(1) Day 3 embryos before vitrification, and (2) Day 5 blastocyst developed from the day 3 warmed embryos]; and (D) Hatched day 6 blastocyst [(1) Before vitrification, (2) 1 hour after vitrification (the reexpansion has not been completed), and (3) Fully reexpanded blastocyst 5 hours after warming].

Table 7.4: Effect of blastocyst development on survival and live birth rates.

	Survival rate	95% CI (%)	P value	LBR/warming cycle	95% CI (%)	P value
Days 5 blastocysts (n = 1,079 warned embryos)						
Early blastocyst	432/458 (94.3%)	(91.7–96.7)	0.039	92/285 (32.3%)	(26.7–37.7)	0.21
Expanded blastocyst	537/549 (97.9%)	(96.7–99.0)[a]		155/349 (44.4%)	(39.2–49.6)[a]	
Hatching-hatched blastocyst	64/72 (88.8%)	(81.5–96.6)		14/41 (34.1%)	(19.6–48.6)	
Day 6 blastocyst (n = 952 warmed embryos)						
Early blastocyst	46/47 (97.9%)	(93.8–100)	0.107	6/35 (17.1%)	(4.6–29.6)[b]	0.201
Hatching-hatched blastocyst	328/335 (95.5%)	(95.8–98.8)		100/292 (34.2%)	(28.8–39.6)	
Expanded blastocyst	556/570 (97.5%)	(93.0–96.9)		96/276 (34.7%)	(29.1–40.3)	

[a,b]Different superscripts in the same column indicate statistical difference (P < 0.05)
(CI: Confidence interval; LBR: Live-birth rate).
Source: Cobo A, de los Santos MJ, Castelló D, et al. Outcomes of vitrified early cleavage-stage and blastocyst-stage embryos in a cryopreservation program: evaluation of 3,150 warming cycles. Fertil Steril. 2012;98(5):1138–46.

blastocysts warmed) with the use of the cryoloop, and a larger study of 1,129 vitrified blastocysts reported a 85.7% survival rate.[38] Similar outcomes were published by others involving 250–700 embryos.[30,39,40] Studies of the use of electron microscope (EM) grid, reporting data from 90–300 warmed blastocysts, have shown survival rates of approximately 50%.[41,42]

According to our data, expanded blastocysts on day 5 or day 6 achieved the highest survival rate. This finding contrasts with reports by other groups[43,44] suggesting that the likelihood of ice formation is higher in expanded blastocysts than in early blastocysts, in which the volume of the blastocoel cavity is much smaller. In fact, this is the rationale for provoking an artificial collapse of blastocysts before vitrification in some cases.[43,45,46] This is not a strategy we apply routinely, except in isolated cases of hatching blastocysts. It is possible that the high survival rate of our expanded blastocysts was due to the open system we use (Cryotop), because it ensures a very high cooling rate and, most importantly, an extremely high warming rate, which impedes the formation of ice (recrystallization) during warming.[5,47-52]

The delivery rate or warming cycle we obtained was 32.5% (95% CI 30.9–34.2). Overall implantation, clinical pregnancy, ongoing pregnancy, and LBRs per warming cycle were 35.5% (95% CI 33.5%–38.5%), 41.7% (95% CI 39.9%–43.4%), 32.6% (95% CI 31.0%–34.2%), and 38.1% (95% CI 36.4%–39.8%) respectively.

Other important aspect, it was the absence of variability in the before and after morphologic evaluation of early cleavage stages, thus confirming the safety of the cryopreservation method we employed.[53,54] These data confirmed that an efficient embryo cryopreservation program could be carried out with the help of the vitrification technique.[55]

REFERENCES

1. Yavin S, Arav A. Measurement of essential physical properties of vitrification solutions. Theriogenology. 2007;67(1):81-9.
2. Rall WF, Fahy GM. Ice-free cryopreservation of mouse embryos at -196 degrees C by vitrification. Nature. 1985;313(6003):573-5.
3. Coello A, Campos P, Remohi J, et al. A combination of hydroxypropyl cellulose and trehalose as supplementation for vitrification of human oocytes: a retrospective cohort study. J Assist Reprod Genet. 2016;33(3):413-21.
4. Alpha Scientists In Reproductive Medicine. The Alpha consensus meeting on cryopreservation key performance indicators and benchmarks: proceedings of an expert meeting. Reprod Biomed Online. 2012;25(2):146-67.
5. Seki S, Mazur P. The dominance of warming rate over cooling rate in the survival of mouse oocytes subjected to a vitrification procedure. Cryobiology. 2009;59(1):75-82.
6. Papatheodorou A, Vanderzwalmen P, Panagiotidis Y, et al. Open versus closed oocyte vitrification system: a prospective randomized sibling-oocyte study. Reprod Biomed Online. 2013;26(6):595-602.

7. Parmegiani L, Cognigni GE, Filicori M. Efficacy of ultraviolet sterilization of liquid nitrogen. Reprod Biomed Online. 2011;22(5):501.
8. Cobo A, Romero JL, Pérez S, et al. Storage of human oocytes in the vapor phase of nitrogen. Fertil Steril. 2010;94(5):1903-7.
9. Pickering SJ, Braude PR, Johnson MH, et al. Transient cooling to room temperature can cause irreversible disruption of the meiotic spindle in the human oocyte. Fertil Steril. 1990;54(1):102-8.
10. Ghetler Y, Yavin S, Shalgi R, et al. The effect of chilling on membrane lipid phase transition in human oocytes and zygotes. Hum Reprod. 2005;20(12):3385-9.
11. Watson PF, Morris GJ. Cold shock injury in animal cells. Symp Soc Exp Biol. 1987;41:311-40.
12. Liebermann J, Dietl J, Vanderzwalmen P, et al. Recent developments in human oocyte, embryo and blastocyst vitrification: where are we now? Reprod Biomed Online. 2003;7(6):623-33.
13. Cobo A, Domingo J, Pérez S, et al. Vitrification: an effective new approach to oocyte banking and preserving fertility in cancer patients. Clin Transl Oncol. 2008;10(5):268-73.
14. Dondorp WJ, De Wert GM. Fertility preservation for healthy women: ethical aspects. Hum Reprod. 2009;24(8):1779-85.
15. Garcia-Velasco JA, Domingo J, Cobo A, et al. Five years' experience using oocyte vitrification to preserve fertility for medical and nonmedical indications. Fertil Steril. 2013;99(7):1994-9.
16. Cobo A, Garrido N, Crespo J, et al. Accumulation of oocytes: a new strategy for managing low-responder patients. Reprod Biomed Online. 2012;24(4):424-32.
17. Herrero L, Pareja S, Losada C, et al. Avoiding the use of human chorionic gonadotropin combined with oocyte vitrification and GnRH agonist triggering versus coasting: a new strategy to avoid ovarian hyperstimulation syndrome. Fertil Steril. 2011;95(3):1137-40.
18. Herrero L, Pareja S, Aragonés M, et al. Oocyte versus embryo vitrification for delayed embryo transfer: an observational study. Reprod Biomed Online. 2014;29(5):567-72.
19. Cobo A, Meseguer M, Remohi J, et al. Use of cryo-banked oocytes in an ovum donation programme: a prospective, randomized, controlled, clinical trial. Hum Reprod. 2010;25(9):2239-46.
20. Kuleshova L, Gianaroli L, Magli C, et al. Birth following vitrification of a small number of human oocytes: case report. Hum Reprod. 1999;14(12):3077-9.
21. Cobo A, Kuwayama M, Pérez S, et al. Comparison of concomitant outcome achieved with fresh and cryopreserved donor oocytes vitrified by the Cryotop method. Fertil Steril. 2008;89(6):1657-64.
22. Kuwayama M, Vajta G, Kato O, et al. Highly efficient vitrification method for cryopreservation of human oocytes. Reprod Biomed Online. 2005;11(3):300-8.
23. Cobo A, Castellò D, Vallejo B, et al. Outcome of cryotransfer of embryos developed from vitrified oocytes: double vitrification has no impact on delivery rates. Fertil Steril. 2013;99(6):1623-30.
24. Cobo A, Garrido N, Pellicer A, et al. Six years' experience in ovum donation using vitrified oocytes: report of cumulative outcomes, impact of storage time, and development of a predictive model for oocyte survival rate. Fertil Steril. 2015;104(6):1426-34.
25. Cobo A, Garcia-Velasco JA, Domingo J, et al. Is vitrification of oocytes useful for fertility preservation for age-related fertility decline and in cancer patients? Fertil Steril. 2013;99(6):1485-95.

26. Cobo A, Garcia-Velasco JA, Coello A, et al. Oocyte vitrification as an efficient option for elective fertility preservation. Fertil Steril. 2016;105(3):755-64.

27. Rienzi L, Romano S, Albricci L, et al. Embryo development of fresh 'versus' vitrified metaphase II oocytes after ICSI: a prospective randomized sibling-oocyte study. Hum Reprod. 2010;25(1):66-73.

28. Ubaldi F, Anniballo R, Romano S, et al. Cumulative ongoing pregnancy rate achieved with oocyte vitrification and cleavage stage transfer without embryo selection in a standard infertility program. Hum Reprod. 2010;25(5):1199-205.

29. Kono T, Kwon OY, Nakahara T. Development of vitrified mouse oocytes after in vitro fertilization. Cryobiology. 1991;28(1):50-4.

30. Mukaida T, Nakamura S, Tomiyama T, et al. Successful birth after transfer of vitrified human blastocysts with use of a cryoloop containerless technique. Fertil Steril. 2001;76(3):618-20.

31. Bourgain C, Devroey P. The endometrium in stimulated cycles for IVF. Hum Reprod Update. 2003;9(6):515-22.

32. Kolibianakis E, Bourgain C, Albano C, et al. Effect of ovarian stimulation with recombinant follicle-stimulating hormone, gonadotropin releasing hormone antagonists, and human chorionic gonadotropin on endometrial maturation on the day of oocyte pick-up. Fertil Steril. 2002;78(5):1025-9.

33. Roy TK, Bradley CK, Bowman MC, et al. Single-embryo transfer of vitrified-warmed blastocysts yields equivalent live-birth rates and improved neonatal outcomes compared with fresh transfers. Fertil Steril. 2014;101(5):1294-301.

34. Cobo A, de los Santos MJ, Castelló D, et al. Outcomes of vitrified early cleavage-stage and blastocyst-stage embryos in a cryopreservation program: evaluation of 3,150 warming cycles. Fertil Steril. 2012;98(5):1138-46.

35. Hiraoka K, Hiraoka K, Kinutani M, et al. Blastocoele collapse by micropipetting prior to vitrification gives excellent survival and pregnancy outcomes for human day 5 and 6 expanded blastocysts. Hum Reprod. 2004;19(12):2884-8.

36. Stehlik E, Stehlik J, Katayama KP, et al. Vitrification demonstrates significant improvement versus slow freezing of human blastocysts. Reprod Biomed Online. 2005;11(1):53-7.

37. Kuwayama M, Vajta G, Ieda S, et al. Comparison of open and closed methods for vitrification of human embryos and the elimination of potential contamination. Reprod Biomed Online. 2005;11(5):608-14.

38. Takahashi K, Mukaida T, Goto T, et al. Perinatal outcome of blastocyst transfer with vitrification using cryoloop: a 4-year follow-up study. Fertil Steril. 2005;84(1):88-92.

39. Mukaida T, Nakamura S, Tomiyama T, et al. Vitrification of human blastocysts using cryoloops: clinical outcome of 223 cycles. Hum Reprod. 2003;18(2):384-91.

40. Huang CC, Lee TH, Chen SU, et al. Successful pregnancy following blastocyst cryopreservation using super-cooling ultra-rapid vitrification. Hum Reprod. 2005;20(1):122-8.

41. Cho HJ, Son WY, Yoon SH, et al. An improved protocol for dilution of cryoprotectants from vitrified human blastocysts. Hum Reprod. 2002;17(9):2419-22.

42. Choi DH, Chung HM, Lim JM, et al. Pregnancy and delivery of healthy infants developed from vitrified blastocysts in an IVF-ET program. Fertil Steril. 2000; 74(4):838-9.

43. Vanderzwalmen P, Bertin G, Debauche Ch, et al. Births after vitrification at morula and blastocyst stages: effect of artificial reduction of the blastocoelic cavity before vitrification. Hum Reprod. 2002;17(3):744-51.

44. Van Landuyt L, Stoop D, Verheyen G, et al. Outcome of closed blastocyst vitrification in relation to blastocyst quality: evaluation of 759 warming cycles in a single-embryo transfer policy. Hum Reprod. 2011;26(3):527-34.
45. Lucena E, Bernal DP, Lucena C, et al. Successful ongoing pregnancies after vitrification of oocytes. Fertil Steril. 2006;85(1):108-11.
46. Chang CC, Shapiro DB, Bernal DP, et al. Two successful pregnancies obtained following oocyte vitrification and embryo re-vitrification. Reprod Biomed Online. 2008;16(3):346-9.
47. Sher G, Keskintepe L, Mukaida T, et al. Selective vitrification of euploid oocytes markedly improves survival, fertilization and pregnancy-generating potential. Reprod Biomed Online. 2008;17(4):524-9.
48. Nagy ZP, Chang CC, Shapiro DB, et al. The efficacy and safety of human oocyte vitrification. Semin Reprod Med. 2009;27(6):450-5.
49. Cao YX, Xing Q, Li L, et al. Comparison of survival and embryonic development in human oocytes cryopreserved by slow-freezing and vitrification. Fertil Steril. 2009;92(4):1306-11.
50. Noyes N, Knopman J, Labella P, et al. Oocyte cryopreservation outcomes including pre-cryopreservation and post-thaw meiotic spindle evaluation following slow cooling and vitrification of human oocytes. Fertil Steril. 2010;94(6): 2078-82.
51. Trokoudes KM, Pavlides C, Zhang X. Comparison outcome of fresh and vitrified donor oocytes in an egg-sharing donation program. Fertil Steril. 2011;95 (6):1996-2000.
52. Garcia JI, Noriega-Portella L, Noriega-Hoces L. Efficacy of oocyte vitrification combined with blastocyst stage transfer in an egg donation program. Hum Reprod. 2011;26(4):782-90.
53. Stoop D, De Munck N, Jansen E, et al. Clinical validation of a closed vitrification system in an oocyte-donation programme. Reprod Biomed Online. 2012;24 (2):180-5.
54. Solé M, Santaló J, Boada M, et al. How does vitrification affect oocyte viability in oocyte donation cycles? A prospective study to compare outcomes achieved with fresh versus vitrified sibling oocytes. Hum Reprod. 2013;28(8):2087-92.
55. Figueira Rde C, Setti AS, Braga DP, et al. The efficiency of a donor-recipient program using infertile donors' egg cryo-banking: a Brazilian reality. J Assist Reprod Genet. 2014;31(8):1053-7.

Chapter 8

Embryo Biopsy and Tubing

Rishina Bansal, Shridutt Gaitonde, Navin Desai

INTRODUCTION

Preimplantation genetic diagnosis (PGD) in humans was developed in late 1980s in the United Kingdom. Initially, PGD revolved around determination of gender as an indirect means of avoiding an X-linked disorder. In 1989 in London, Handyside and Scott reported the first unaffected child born following PGD performed for an X-linked disorder.[1,2]

It is an increasingly common adjunct to *in vitro* fertilization (IVF) and it is used to identify genetic defects in embryos created through IVF before pregnancy. To undergo a PGD cycle, the patients have to start an IVF cycle in order to retrieve oocytes that will be fertilized and result into zygotes; those zygotes will develop into embryos progressing across different stages until being transferred to the patient's uterus. It is during this procedure when the biopsy has to be done in order to obtain cells and analyze the chromosomal status. That will allow the embryologist to discriminate those embryos considered as candidates to be transferred into the patient.

The PGD along with the polymerase chain reaction (PCR) allow us to identify inheritable diseases in the embryos as this technique amplifies a fragment of deoxyribonucleic acid (DNA) and facilitates the screening to identify monogenic diseases. Therefore, we can distinguish between:

- *Preimplantation genetic diagnosis:* It refers specifically to when one or both genetic parents has a known genetic abnormality and testing is performed on an embryo to determine, if it also carries a genetic abnormality
- *Preimplantation genetic screening (PGS):* It refers to techniques where embryos from presumed chromosomally normal genetic parents are screened for aneuploidy.

Preimplantation genetic diagnosis and PGS are presently the only options available for avoiding a high-risk of having a child affected with a genetic disease prior to implantation. Preimplantation genetic testing provides an alternative to current postconception diagnostic procedures, which are frequently followed by the difficult decision of pregnancy termination, if results are unfavorable.

In order to perform preimplantation genetic testing, it can be done at different stages of the embryo development, from the first polar body (PB1) of the oocyte, in which it is still not fertilized, the second PB (PB2), that appears after the fertilization, one or two blastomeres on day 3 of development to several cells from the blastocyst's trophectoderm (TE). The technique will imply in any of the cases the breaching of the zona pellucida (ZP) to create an artificial orifice and the extraction of the sample [polar body (PB)/blastomere/TE] for further analysis. In this chapter it will be detailed the available techniques for each of those procedures.

BREACHING OF THE ZONA PELLUCIDA

The ZP of mammalian oocytes and embryos is an acellular matrix composed of sulfated glycoproteins with different roles during fertilization and embryo development, and its main function of is the protection of the embryo and the maintenance of its integrity.[3]

Sampling of genetic material from oocytes and embryos relies on creating a hole in the ZP large enough for polar bodies (PBs) or blastomeres to be extruded, or TE cells to herniate out.[4] The hole size is critical, if too large several blastomeres can be dragged out with the one biopsied. If the hole is too small, stress on the blastomere may be excessive, leading to cell lysis.[5] The suggested opening diameter should be around 20–30 μm.[6]

Several methods can be used to rupture the ZP:
- Mechanical
- Chemical
- Laser
- Piezo-mediated devices.

Mechanical

This approach is simple and efficient but requires correct positioning of oocyte or embryo. Embryos denuded of corona cells are micromanipulated in microdrops of 4-(2-hydroxyethyl)-1-piperazineethanesulfonic acid (HEPES) buffered medium under paraffin oil. The procedure is performed at 37°C, under an inverted microscope. The embryo is held with a holding pipette, and the ZP is tangentially pierced with a microneedle from the 1- to the 11-o'clock position. The embryo is released from the holding pipette, and the part of the ZP between the two points is rubbed against the holding pipette until this area is completely dislodged from the rest of the oocyte or embryo.[3,7] Groups performing PBB favor this method.[4]

Chemical

The human ZP can be dissolved using a controlled, directed stream of a low pH solution as the acid Tyrode's (AT) solution (pH of AT = 2.2–2.6).[3] One advantage of AT drilling compared with the mechanical rupture is the possibility of increasing the size of the hole in the ZP.

In order to perform chemical zona drilling, the embryo is held with a holding pipette in such a way that the micropipette containing AT (internal diameter 3–5 mm) and located at the 3-o'clock position faces a large perivitelline space to avoid damaging the blastomeres. The acid solution is gently delivered with the help of a microinjector over a small area of the ZP, with the tip of the pipette positioned very close to the zona and gently scratching it. The hole should be between 15–20 μm, never more than 30 μm. As soon as a hole in the ZP is created, suction is applied to avoid excess AT entering the perivitelline space. If the inner region of the ZP is difficult to breach, creation of the hole can be facilitated by pushing the AT micropipette against the ZP. It is necessary to rinse the embryo several times in fresh culture medium immediately after the assisted hatching (AH) and biopsy procedure, prior to returning it back into the culture dish, to avoid detrimental effects of the acid solution on the blastomeres.

This was the preferred choice for cleavage stage biopsy.[8,9] It has advantages over mechanical zona dissection in terms of speed of safety. However, the safety and the ideal size of the hole is difficult to standardize and depends on the amount of acid used and skill of the personnel (Figs 8.1A to D).[4]

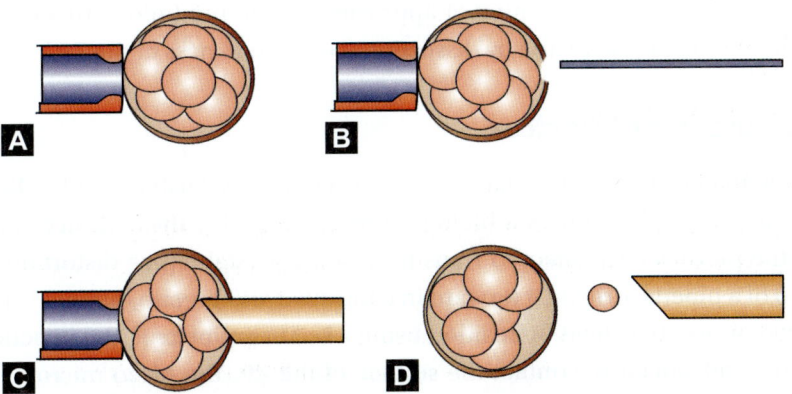

Figs. 8.1A to D: Schematic representation of zona drilling using acid Tyrode's.

Laser

The application of a laser on the ZP for AH results in photoablation of the ZP. The drilling mechanism is explained by a thermal effect induced at the focal point by absorption of the laser energy by water and/or ZP macromolecules, leading to thermolysis of the ZP. The effect on the ZP is greatly localized, and the holes obtained are cylindrical and precise.[3]

The preferred model of laser is the near-infrared (NIR) solid-state compact diode 1.48 mm laser. The advantage of using light as a cutting tool is that it removes the need for a double tool holder and either disposable or reusable cutting tools. It is extremely precise and, if used appropriately, provides consistent, reproducible, and rapid results.[10] Furthermore, the likelihood of introducing contamination or pH changes in the medium surrounding the embryo is greatly reduced as neither microtools nor reagents are required to dissect the zona.[11] The 1.48 mm diode laser is small but, at the appropriate pulse duration, can emit light at power levels sufficient to cause selective thermal disruption of the ZP glycoproteins and is not absorbed by water.[11] This noncontact laser can be inserted into the body of the microscope on which the manipulations take place or be integrated in a special objective and the beam delivered to the target through the dish.[12]

A culture dish with several 10 μL drops of HEPES buffered culture medium and overlaid with prewarmed mineral oil has to be prepared shortly before the procedure. Embryos selected for transfer are placed individually in separate drops, and the dish is placed on the heated stage of the inverted microscope equipped with the laser technology. It is recommended to stabilize the embryo with a holding micropipette. An area between two blastomeres with a large perivitelline space has to be chosen for laser drilling. Routinely, a single opening of approximately 30 μm (about 10% of the ZP circumference) is created by dissecting the full thickness of the ZP.[3]

Piezo-mediated Devices

Piezo-actuated micromanipulation was developed by Yoshida and colleagues, and its application as a biological research tool.[13] These devices harness the piezoelectric effect to transmit a small crystal lattice distortion to the tip of a pipette, driving it forward in controlled and precise manner.[14] The embryo or oocyte is held in position using a holding pipette.[15] The injection pipette is advanced to contact the surface of the ZP. The piezo micromanipulator (PMM) is activated with foot switch as pipette is pushed through the zona. It introduce a small negative pressure within the microinjection pipette and apply piezo pulses (start with intensity = 3, frequency = 6) while gently pushing the microinjection pipette toward the holding pipette. The tip should rapidly pass through the zona, emerging into the perivitelline space. Stop pushing as soon as you see this. Failure to control the tip risks subjecting the plasma membrane to high-intensity piezo, resulting in rapid cell lysis. The piezo impact force is applied until the ZP is almost penetrated (Table 8.1).[13]

Table 8.1: Cleavage stage embryo biopsy methods: benefits, limitations and critical factors to success.

Method	Benefits	Limitations	Critical factors
Mechanical	Less invasive to embryo Improved survival after freezing-thawing Inexpensive	Difficult to learn Operator dependent Time-consuming	Operator skill essential Appropriate tools needed
Chemical	Relatively inexpensive Widespread clinical experience	Operator dependent Difficult to limit aperture size Effect on cryopreservation Double tool holder optimal	Acidified Tyrode's pH Sensitive control of acid Rinse acid from embryos
Laser	Rapid and reproducible Simple to use Software	Capital cost Not all systems portable Invisible thermal damage or stress	Laser alignment and calibration Pulse duration and number Distance between laser and zona pellucida (ZP)
Piezo	Precise movement Minimize damage to oocytes	Operator dependent Delicate technique Piezo pulse displaces Microinjection needle tip	Additional tools required Pressure to open zona Operator skill essential

BIOPSY PROCEDURES

Theoretically, PGD can be accomplished at any developmental stage between the mature oocyte and blastocyst, but to date, only three discrete stages have been proposed: (1) PB, (2) cleavage stage, and (3) blastocyst.

Polar Body Biopsy

Polar bodies are by-products of meiotic division of the oocyte. PB1 is the by-product of the first meiotic division and contains the counterpart of the oocyte chromosomes, which are diploid at this stage. This is why it is an indirect approach to infer the genetic or chromosomal status of the oocyte without losing its reproductive capability.[16] As the information obtained through this PB1 refers only to the mother inheritance, it is not possible to detect the chromosomal abnormalities that occur after fertilization. The PB2 is extruded after fertilization, so by extruding the extra 23 chromosome set the number of chromosomes in the oocyte is reduced by half.[17] This can be also biopsied and analyzed.

Polar body biopsy was first proposed in 1990s by Verlinsky and collaborators.[18] Since then, several groups have applied PBB to a variety of diagnostic applications like detection of single gene disorders, translocation analysis, human leukocyte antigen (HLA) typing and detection of X-linked disorders.[12] However, most cases of PB diagnosis are performed for aneuploidy screening, but PBs provide information only on the female part, which is critical in the case of certain monogenetic diseases. In a recessive disease, PB analysis will only distinguish whether the oocyte carries the normal or the affected allele but the state of the corresponding embryo will be determined by the paternal allele and can be normal, unaffected (carrier), or affected.[16] There is ongoing discussion on the need to biopsy and analyze both PBs. A recent study showed that in younger women, PB1 is more prone than PB2 to meiotic errors causing aneuploidies, whereas the opposite holds true in older women.[19,20]

Technical Aspects of Polar Body Biopsy

Recent investigations using polarization microscopy have shown that some oocytes presenting a PB1 may still be in telophase I owing to the presence of a connective spindle strand between the PB1 and the oocyte.[18] Such a spindle bridge is a remnant of the meiotic division and occurs during formation of PB1 as well as at the completion of the second meiotic division after extrusion of the PB2. The spindle bridge is present for only a limited time period, which is usually 1–2 hours after extrusion of the PB1 or PB2. In view of this, PBB should not be performed within too short time after their formation. As long as chromosomal material from the oocyte is still attached to these spindle fibers there is a risk of pulling this material out during biopsy, which may result in enucleating the oocyte.[16,17]

Chronology

- *Day 0:* Follicle retrieval, oocyte denudation and biopsy of the PB1 of the metaphase II (MII) oocytes after 2–4 hours. Perform the intracytoplasmic sperm injection (ICSI) 1–4 hours after the biopsy
- *Day 1:* Fertilization assessment after 17–20 hours and biopsy of the PB2 before 24 hours from the ICSI.

The removal of the PB1 and PB2 can be done at separate times (sequential approach) or at the same time (simultaneous approach). Simultaneous biopsy of the PB1 and PB2 requires only one manipulation and helps to reduce stress to the oocyte. It is best accomplished in a time window of

8–14 hours after fertilization. Too early biopsy bears the risk of spindle remnants in the PB2, and too late biopsy may result in a PB1 that already started disintegration or degeneration. The latter problem is especially important, if the analysis is based on fluorescence *in situ* hybridization (FISH), because it may contribute to diagnostic failures.[21,22] For simultaneous biopsy it can sometimes be difficult to distinguish PB1 and PB2 or to accurately separate PB1 and PB2 in case of fragmentation. Using single-nucleotide polymorphism (SNP)-based analysis of heterozygosity could help to identify and distinguish them.[18] Otherwise, sequential biopsy may be preferred, if a fragmented PB1 is already present at the time of injection.

Steps to Follow

Zona opening to remove the PBs can be done by any one of the abovementioned techniques (mechanical, chemical, laser or piezo-mediated devices).

A 60 mm petridish with three 50 µL drops of HEPES buffered culture medium to wash the oocytes and purgue the biopsy pipette, one 25 µL drop to place the oocyte and another 25 µL drop on its side to release the PB once biopsied, and overlaid with prewarmed mineral oil, has to be prepared shortly before the procedure. Prepare one dish per oocyte to be analyzed. Once the selected oocytes are placed in the drops, place the dish on the heated stage of the inverted microscope equipped with the laser technology. The PBB is best accomplished when the oocyte is affixed to the holding capillary with the PB1 at the 6- or 12-o'clock position and the PB2 located right of the first one but in the same focal plane. An opening of 15–18 µm of diameter is drilled at 2–3-o'clock, and by pushing the biopsy capillary into the perivitelline space, both PBs can be removed simultaneously and be deposited in the clean drop for further analysis by PCR or FISH. The positioning of the PB2 next to the aspiration capillary allows pushing the PB2 far to the left side toward the holding capillary, and this stretching movement usually is enough to break the cytoplasmic bridge between the PB2 and the oocyte. Due to the use of a blunt-ended capillary, even manipulation in direct vicinity to the oolemma does not damage the oocyte (Figs. 8.2A to D).

The gold standard is the use of laser for the AH, as the main benefit is that laser drilling and subsequent biopsy can be performed without changing the culture dish or the pipettes (in contrast to using AT for example) and thereby preventing contamination during diagnosing the sample with PCR.[23,24]

Genetic Screening

- *Analysis by fluorescence in situ hybridization (FISH):* Immediately after the biopsy of an oocyte, the corresponding PBs are placed in a neighboring droplet of HEPES medium until all oocytes are biopsied. For FISH, it

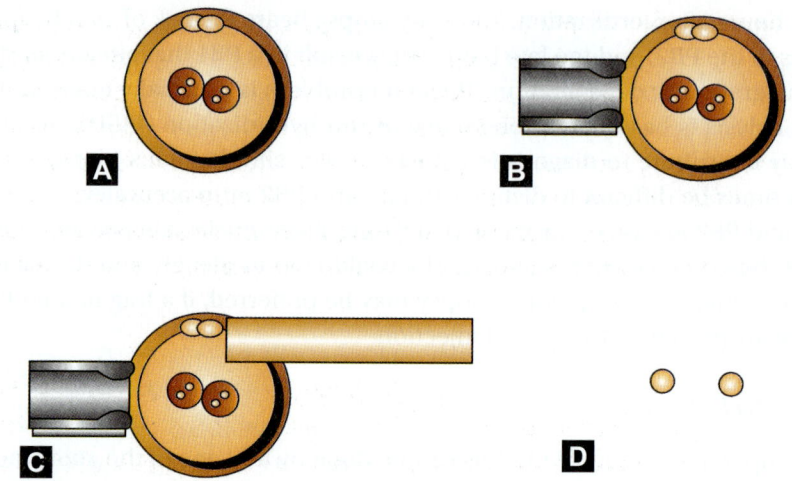

Figs. 8.2A to D: Schematic representation of polar body biopsy.

is not essential to place the PB1 and PB2 in different droplets, as they can be visually distinguished during fluorescence evaluation. Due to the small cytoplasmic content of PBs, a special pretreatment like hypoosmotic swelling or proteinase/pronase treatment prior FISH is not necessary. For transfer onto the glass slide, PBs of one oocyte are removed from their drop and transferred into a tiny drop (0.2 mL) of water placed on a clean glass slide. The small volume guarantees that the PB will attach to the slide within a small area and that the fluid will dry out very fast, which reduces the risk of a dislocation of the PB on the slide. It is recommended to use for this transfer the biopsy capillary and to perform the complete procedure under visual control at the microscope. Placing the PBs directly at the bottom of the slide will prevent floating and rupture of the PBs. The drying process must be observed under a stereomicroscope, and the final location of the PB after air-drying should be marked on top of the slide by encircling with a diamond marker. With some experience, PBs from 6 oocytes to 10 oocytes can be placed within a round area of 10 mm, each encircled with the marker. Subsequent fixation can be performed with 2–3 drops of 10 mL methanol or acetic acid (3:1, ice-cold –20°C) followed by another fixation after air-drying using methanol at room temperature for 5 minute.[25]

- *Analysis by polymerase chain reaction or array comparative genomic hybridization (array CGH):* In contrast to the isolation for FISH, the differentiation of the PB1 and PB2 is crucial for any PCR-based evaluation, either for monogenetic diseases or for array CGH. Therefore, the PB1 and PB2 are released after biopsy in different droplets with medium in a dish covered with mineral oil. These droplets should be rather large (approximately 10 mL) as this will facilitate to aspirate the PBs without sucking up some mineral oil. For PCR, the PBs need to be transferred into a PCR tube. This can be easily done by preloading the PCR tube with 1.6 mL buffer [phosphate buffered saline (PBS) or cell extraction buffer]. Using a low-volume pipette (0.2–2.0 mL), one PB is aspirated in a total of 0.4 mL medium and released into the buffer in the PCR tube by pipetting several times up and down. This process must be done in a laminar air flow in order to avoid any contamination with other cells or genetic material.[12]

Pitfalls

A major problem of the PB approach apart from just accounting for maternal genome is the interpretation of the results with FISH, especially for PB1. Whereas PB2 formation and aging can be precisely controlled because the time point of injection initiates the course of PB2 extrusion, the situation is different for PB1. At the time of ovum pickup the majority of oocytes are already in MII, but it is unknown at what time PB1 has been extruded and how long the chromatin of PB1 is already prone to an aging process. This aging process affects the quality of the DNA, the coherence of the chromatids, its dispersion after isolation on a slide, and, therefore, hybridization efficiency. In contrast, isolation and amplification of PB1 DNA for array CGH can be accomplished with more than 90% success rates, even from PBs that show signs of degeneration.[16]

In view of the costs of array CGH, the economic impact of PBB has to be considered as well. Because both PBs need to be separately analyzed, costs are doubled. Bearing in mind the fact that not all oocytes develop into viable embryos is another drawback of PBB.[16]

If the biopsy of both PBs is done at different time points, one should avoid drilling another opening. If PBs were retrieved through separate openings, problems may arise at the time of hatching because the embryo could hatch through both openings simultaneously and therefore may get trapped within the zona.[12]

Blastomere Biopsy

Cleavage stage or blastomere biopsy has remained the most widely practiced form of embryo biopsy worldwide according to the European Society of Human Reproduction and Embryology (ESHRE) PGD Consortium, accounting for approximately 90% of all reported PGD cycles to date.[26] Currently, this embryo biopsy strategy requires the removal of one or more cells from each embryo on day 3 of development.

The biopsy is performed when the embryo is typically composed of 6–8 blastomere cells to avoid compromising its development. Despite this, there is currently no consensus between clinics as to how many blastomeres should be removed for the genetic analysis. Some groups advocate the removal of a single blastomere, while others recommend that two blastomeres be biopsied in order to obtain a conclusive PGD result.[26]

Technical Aspects of Blastomere Biopsy

Intracytoplasmic sperm injection is the recommended technique for all PGD cases involving DNA amplification to reduce the chance of paternal contamination from extraneous sperm attached to the ZP or nondecondensed sperm within blastomeres. Similarly, as far as is practically and safely possible, all cumulus cells should be removed before biopsy as these cells can contaminate both FISH, array CGH and PCR-based diagnoses.

The use of standard IVF culture medium during biopsy is acceptable but its effectiveness may be highly dependent upon the developmental stage of the embryo biopsied with compacting 8-cell embryos proving more difficult to biopsy. Thereby, it is better to use commercially produced calcium- and magnesium-free (Ca^{2+}- or Mg^{2+}-free) medium which temporarily reverses calcium-dependent cell-cell adhesion, it is widely available and is used by many centers for routine clinical biopsy with the benefit of reducing the frequency of cell lysis[27] combined with a shorter time needed to perform the biopsy procedure.

Embryos are graded and selected for biopsy, however, it is "acceptable" to exclude very poor quality embryos from the embryo biopsy procedure.[28] Biopsy at cleavage stages is based on the principle that at these stages, the blastomeres remain totipotent and equivalent, such that the removal of a single blastomere will (a) provide a representative sample of the entire embryo and (b) compromise the embryo only to the extent of one-eighth of the embryo mass rather than removal of a developmentally crucial blastomere. The importance of selecting a blastomere with a single visible interphase nucleus cannot be stressed enough. Aside from the increased diagnostic efficiency observed in mononucleated blastomeres,[29] mononucleation is a marker for and directly correlates with implantation potential. Nevertheless, embryos containing blastomeres, all of which have no visible nucleus, should still be considered for biopsy as nuclear material is likely to be present and should yield results in molecular tests.[29] Time spent in careful examination of the embryo and orientation to selectively remove specific blastomeres is essential to attain the high diagnostic efficiencies required for clinical effectiveness. The following criteria can be used to select embryos for biopsy:[30,31]

- *Cell number:* More than 5 cells
- *Fragmentation:* Less than 20%
- *Multinucleate:* Less than 50%
- *Nucleus:* Present.

Chronology

- *Day 0:* Follicle retrieval, oocyte denudation and ICSI 3–5 hours after the ovum pickup
- *Day 1:* Fertilization assessment after 16–19 hours
- *Day 2:* Embryo development assessment after 44–47 hours
- *Day 3:* Embryo development assessment after 72 hours and cell biopsy and genetic analysis by array CGH or PCR
- *Day 5:* Selection of the normal or nonaffected embryos available for transfer.

Day 3 biopsy provides the diagnostic laboratory 2–3 days to run the test. Given that most IVF programs do not have their own genetic laboratories, this would still allow time for the biopsied samples to be shipped to a reference laboratory, the analysis to be done, and the result reported back to the clinical program in time for a fresh transfer.[32]

Steps to Follow

Zona opening to remove the PBs can be done by any one of the abovementioned techniques (mechanical, chemical, laser or piezo-mediated devices). Once done the opening of the ZP, there are three different approaches to retrieve the blastomeres: (1) aspiration, (2) fluid displacement and (3) mechanical displacement, but the most widely used method of removal of cells is aspiration. The advantage with the aspiration method is the capability to select the cell to be removed and with an appropriate training, the risk of cell lysis is very low.

The aspiration pipette is approximated to the hole and then introduced very carefully; once it is in the same focal plane than the desired blastomere it is gently aspirated while avoiding contact or disruption of the remaining cells of the embryo (under 40x magnification). Remove the aspiration pipette with the blastomere attached and leave the cell close by the embryo. If it is required to biopsy a second cell, the aspiration pipette has to be entered again into the embryo through the same hole to repeat the operation. Release the embryo from the holding pipette carefully to avoid it aspirating the biopsied cells (under 20x magnification) (Figs. 8.3A to D). Push up the pipettes and place them into the next biopsy drop. Once the biopsy is concluded, the biopsied embryos should be thoroughly rinsed postbiopsy to remove traces of biopsy medium and shifted to the culture dishes. The biopsied blastomeres will remain in the biopsy dishes till further processing for the genetic analysis. Biopsied embryos must be cultured singly in individual wells or dishes with a clear identification system to ensure tracking of blastomeres removed and easy identification of embryos postdiagnosis.[27]

Genetic Screening

- *Analysis by fluorescence in situ hybridization:* For a successful FISH, the blastomeres fixation is crucial. The purpose of the process is not only to fix

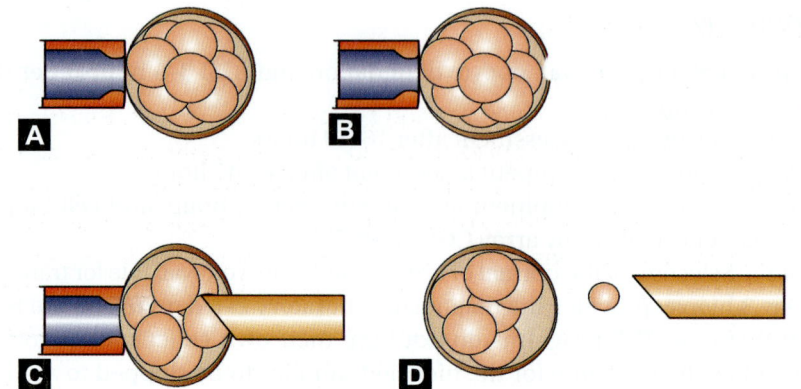

Figs. 8.3A to D: Schematic representation of blastomere biopsy.

the nuclei of each single cell eliminating the remaining cytoplasm but also to do it in a way in which the nuclei integrity and its characteristics remain preserved.

There are different methods to fix the blastomeres, being the most common Tarkowski method that uses a hypotonic solution and Carnoy fixative.[33]

Embryos are considered normal or balanced for the autosomal chromosomes when two signals are present for each of the probes used. Embryos are considered normal or balanced for the sex chromosomes when two signals are present for X chromosome probes and no signals are present for Y chromosome probes, or when one signal was present for each of the X and Y chromosome probes. Extra or missing signals are considered to represent an unbalanced chromosome complement, which renders the embryo not suitable for transfer. Signals are considered split, if the signals are less than two domains apart and hence counted as one signal. For embryos that underwent biopsy of two blastomeres, the embryo is considered mosaic, if one blastomere is defined as normal or balanced and the other blastomere as unbalanced. The overall result for these embryos is recorded as unbalanced and not suitable for transfer. Two blastomeres are considered to be concordant if both blastomeres gave the same result of either normal or balanced or unbalanced.[26] FISH is no longer used as the preferred method and has been replaced by array CGH.

- *Analysis by polymerase chain reaction or array CGH:* Blastomere or TE cells are placed inside PCR tubes containing PBS solution with the help of glass capillaries (new capillary to be used for each individual cell). After releasing the cell the remaining fluid is released in a separate PCR tube to create a blank. The PCR tube is closed and shipped to the genetics laboratory for analysis.

Trophectoderm Biopsy

On day 5 and 6 of development the embryo has until 300 cells distributed between an inner cell mass (ICM) and the TE or outer cell mass. The main advantage is that the amount of genetic material available for analysis increases because instead of having a single blastomere (maximum two) as with the day 3 biopsy, it is possible to obtain several blastomeres from the TE. The general recommendation is to obtain 4–5 nuclei.[34] Moreover, it is considered a less invasive technique, as the ICM remains intact. Another advantage is that, as mentioned, only the embryos that reach the blastocyst stage are biopsied, so there is a prior developmental selection.

Technical Aspects of Trophectoderm Biopsy

Before undergoing the TE biopsy on day 5 it is advisable to do AH for ZP breaking on day 3 to facilitate the controlled extrusion of TE.

Chronology

- *Day 0:* Follicle retrieval, oocyte denudation and ICSI 3–5 hours after the ovum pickup
- *Day 1:* Fertilization assessment after 16–19 hours
- *Day 2:* Embryo development assessment after 44–47 hours
- *Day 3:* Embryo development assessment after 72 hours and AH
- *Day 5:* Embryo assessment, TE biopsy and genetic analysis by array CGH, vitrification of the analyzed embryos
- *Day 6:* Embryo assessment, TE biopsy and genetic analysis by array CGH, vitrification of the analyzed embryos.

  In a further cycle with endometrial preparation, selection of the normal or nonaffected embryos available, thawing and transfer.

Steps to Follow

Usually, the ZP breaking is done on day 3 of development. On days 5 and 6 (and on rare occasions day 7), the embryos have to be assessed and in case of having any fully differentiated good quality blastocyst will be biopsied. Once the blastocyst is placed in the biopsy dish, attached it to the holding pipette with the suction, identifying the ICM and keeping it at 12- or 6-o'clock. The aspiration pipette is approximated to the hole, where the TE cells extruding from the expanded blastocyst are gently pulled (around 5–7 cells are enough). To change from the 40x objective to the laser objective and then make a few pulses of the laser at cell junctions in order to safely remove the cells without disrupting the ICM. Release the blastocyst from the holding pipette and move quickly the biopsy pipette over the holding to separate the blastocyst from the TE cells by friction. Release the blastocyst and the biopsied TE cells and pull up the pipettes to avoid aspirating any of them by mistake. Once finished the biopsy, shift the blastocyst to the culture dish after gently washing. The TE biopsied remains on the biopsy dish until their further processing for either array CGH or PCR. Following TE biopsy, the blastocysts will be vitrified using vitrification kits according to the manufacturer's instructions (Figs. 8.4A to C).[35,36]

Genetic Screening

- *Analysis by fluorescence in situ hybridization:* Trophectoderm samples are spread onto microscope slides, using a modified version of the methanol or acetic acid fixation method.[37] The isolated cells are individually washed once in 1% sodium citrate and transferred onto a glass slide and fixed using 3:1 methanol:acetic acid solution. The preparations is air dried, washed in PBS for 5 minute and dehydrated in 70, 85 and 100% ethanol. Fixed nuclei are then viewed using a phase contrast microscope and their location is marked with a diamond pen. Standard two round 9 chromosomes FISH (MultiVysion PB probe panel and the 4CC custom probe panel) are performed using a commercial ready-to-use probe mix.[38]
- *Trophectoderm cell analysis using array CGH:* Biopsied samples obtained during the study are washed in sterile PBS solution in a laminar flow cabinet to avoid any contamination of the sample, placed in microcentrifuge tubes containing 2 µL of PBS and then processed for array CGH analysis according to the protocol using a commercial genetic laboratory.[38]

Clearly, each of these stages is biologically different, and thus, the strategic considerations have both advantages and disadvantages (Table 8.2).[1]

Looking at the various technical aspects, day 5 biopsy looks like a better choice for biopsy: (I) extended culture enables selection of embryos with a greater chance of implantation and live delivery, (II) embryos reaching

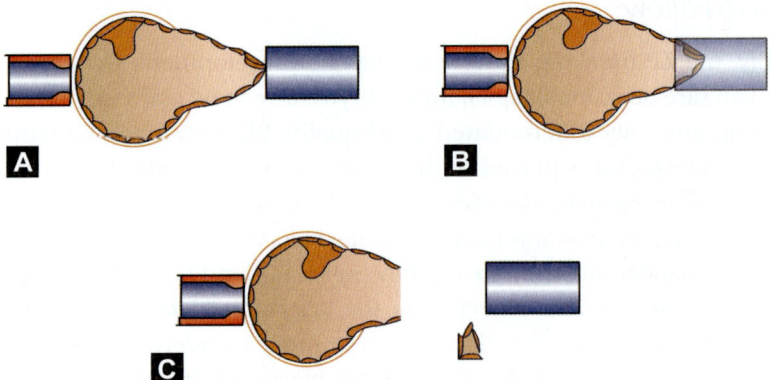

Figs. 8.4A to C: Schematic representation of trophectoderm biopsy.

Table 8.2: Comparison between different types of biopsies and their indication.

Method	Day performed	Type of cells removed	Indications	Zona drilling	Cell removal	Limitations
Polar body	1st PB D0 2nd PB D1 or simultaneously both on D1	1st and 2nd PB	PGS monogenics carried by mother	Laser Mechanical Beveled pipette	Aspiration	Only maternal chromosomes
Cleavage stage	D3	Blastomeres	PGS monogenics, sexing, chromosome abnormalities	Laser Mechanical Tyrode's acid	Aspiration Displacement	Postzygotic mosaicism
Blastocyst	D5	Trophectoderm	PGS monogenics, sexing, chromosome abnormalities	Laser Mechanical Tyrode's acid	Herniation	Postzygotic mosaicism Arrest prior to biopsy Vitrification program

(PB: Polar body; PGS: Preimplantation genetic screening).

blastocyst stage enriches for euploid embryos, and (III) extended culture does not lead to a significant loss of euploid embryos capable of implantation.

However, we need to apply powerful study design and come up with more evidence.[19,22,26,28,39-42]

SAFETY OF EMBRYOS

As with any micromanipulation procedure involving human gametes or embryo, every reasonable precaution should be taken to minimize cellular damage and stress during the procedure. General precautions include correct installation, calibration and maintenance of all micromanipulation equipment (particularly the laser). Biopsy and cell preparation should be performed by a suitably qualified and trained person.[1] Utmost care should be taken to ensure that no harm is done to the human embryo. One must be careful not to violate the principle percept of medical science—"primum non nocere"—"first do no harm".

VITRIFICATION

A major challenge at present is to develop an effective standardized method for cryopreservation of biopsied embryos. With the high rate of multiple pregnancies reported after PGD, it is imperative to develop effective methods of cryopreservation that will:

- It allow storage of unaffected embryos for later transfer, so that the numbers transferred can be limited to two or even single embryo transfer.
- It provides additional time to perform more diagnostic tests.[1,25]

CONCLUSION

Preimplantation genetic screening is a testing tool which gives us more information about the embryo apart from morphology assessment. It would help in selecting genetically normal embryos for transfer enabling higher pregnancy and implantation rates. Looking at the comparison and various technical aspects, day 5 biopsy looks like a better choice for biopsy as it gives us more information and rules out mosaicism.

REFERENCES

1. Harper JC. Introduction. Harper JC, Delhanty JDA, Handyside AH (Eds). Preimplantation Genetic Diagnosis. London, UK: John Wiley & Sons; 2001, pp. 3-12.
2. Scott RT, Upham KM, Forman EJ, et al. Cleavage-stage biopsy significantly impairs human embryonic implantation potential while blastocyst biopsy does not: a randomized and paired clinical trial. Fertil Steril. 2013;100(3):624-30.
3. Nagy ZP, Varghese AC, Agarwal A. Practical Manual of In Vitro Fertilization: Advanced Methods and Novel Devices, 1st edition. New York: Springer-Verlag; 2012. p. 703.

4. Griffiths T. Embryo biopsy. In: Coward K, Wells D (Eds). Textbook of Clinical Embryology. Cambridge: Cambridge University Press; 2013. pp. 286-99.

5. Cohen J, Feldberg D. Effects of the size and number of zona pellucida openings on hatching and trophoblast outgrowth in the mouse embryo. Mol Reprod Dev. 1991;30(1):70-8.

6. Montag M. A Practical Guide to Selecting Gametes and Embryos. New York: CRC Press; 2014. p. 328.

7. Selva J. Assisted hatching. Hum Reprod. 2000;15(Suppl 4):65-7.

8. El-Toukhy T, Braude P. Preimplantation Genetic Diagnosis in Clinical Practice, 1st edition. London: Springer-Verlag; 2014. p. 228.

9. Geber S, Bossi R, Lisboa CB, et al. Laser confers less embryo exposure than acid tyrode for embryo biopsy in preimplantation genetic diagnosis cycles: a randomized study. Reprod Biol Endocrinol. 2011;9:58.

10. Modern Times Group (MTG). Octax laser and software. [online] Available from www.mtg.com. [Accessed March, 2017].

11. Han TS, Sagoskin AW, Graham JR, et al. Laser-assisted human embryo biopsy on the third day of development for preimplantation genetic diagnosis: two successful case reports. Fertil Steril. 2003;80(2):453-5.

12. Montag M, Köster M, van der Ven K, et al. Polar body biopsy. In: Nagy ZP, Varghese AC, Agarwal A (Eds). Practical Manual of In Vitro Fertilization: Advanced Methods and Novel Devices, 1st edition. New York: Springer-Verlag; 2012. pp. 455-9.

13. Yoshida N, Perry AC. Piezo-actuated mouse intracytoplasmic sperm injection (ICSI). Nat Protoc. 2007;2(2):296-304.

14. Huang T, Kimura Y, Yanagimachi R. The use of piezo micromanipulation for intracytoplasmic sperm injection of human oocytes. J Assist Reprod Genet. 1996;13 (4):320-8.

15. Prime Tech Ltd. Prime Tech Piezo PMM4G and ICSI. [online] Available from www.primetech-jp.com/en/03support/images/p-icsi.pdf. [Accessed March, 2017].

16. Montag M, Köster M, Strowitzki T, et al. Polar body biopsy. Fertil Steril. 2013;100 (3):603-7.

17. Vayena E, Rowe PJ, Griffin PD. Current Practices and Controversies in Assisted Reproduction: Report of a meeting on "Medical, Ethical and Social Aspects of Assisted Reproduction" held at WHO Headquarters in Geneva, Switzerland 17-21 September 2001. Geneva: World Health Organization; 2002. p. 381.

18. Verlinsky Y, Ginsberg N, Lifchez A, et al. Analysis of the first polar body: preconception genetic diagnosis. Hum Reprod. 1990;5(7):826-9.

19. Fragouli E, Alfarawati S, Goodall NN, et al. The cytogenetics of polar bodies: insights into female meiosis and the diagnosis of aneuploidy. Mol Hum Reprod. 2011;17(5):286-95.

20. van der Ven K, Montag M, van der Ven H. Polar body diagnosis - a step in the right direction? Dtsch Arztebl Int. 2008;105(11):190-6.

21. Munné S, Dailey T, Sultan KM, et al. The use of first polar bodies for preimplantation diagnosis of aneuploidy. Hum Reprod. 1995;10(4):1014-20.

22. Magli MC, Montag M, Köster M, et al. Implementing polar body biopsy and chromosome copy number analysis by array comparative genomic hybridisation: technical experiences from the ESHRE PGS Task Force pilot study. Hum Reprod. 2011;26(1):3181-4.

23. Montag M, van der Ven K, van der Ven H. Erste klinische Erfahrungen mit der Polkörperdiagnostik in Deutschland. J Fertil Reprod. 2002;4(1):7-12.

24. Montag M, Schimming T, van der Ven H. Spindle imaging in human oocytes: the impact of the meiotic cell cycle. Reprod Biomed Online. 2006;12(4):442-6.

25. Montag M, van der Ven K, van der Ven H. Polar body biopsy. In: Gardner DK, Weissman A, Howles CM, Shoham Z (Eds). Textbook of Assisted Reproductive Techniques: Laboratory and Clinical Perspectives, 3rd edition. New York: Informa Healthcare; 2008. pp. 357-70.

26. Brodie D, Beyer CE, Osborne E, et al. Preimplantation genetic diagnosis for chromosome rearrangements - one blastomere biopsy versus two blastomere biopsy. J Assist Reprod Genet. 2012;29(8):821-7.

27. Harton GL, Magli MC, Lundin K, et al. ESHRE PGD Consortium/Embryology Special Interest Group—best practice guidelines for polar body and embryo biopsy for preimplantation genetic diagnosis/screening (PGD/PGS). Hum Reprod. 2011;26(1):41-6.

28. Magli MC, Gianaroli L, Ferraretti AP, et al. Embryo morphology and development are dependent on the chromosomal complement. Fertil Steril. 2007;87(1): 534-40.

29. Cui KH, Matthews CD. Nuclear structural conditions and PCR amplification in human preimplantation diagnosis. Mol Hum Reprod. 1996;2(1):63-71.

30. Igenomix: Pioneers in reproductive genetics. Advanced Reproductive Genetic Testing Services. [online] Available from www.igenomix.us. [Accessed March, 2017].

31. McArthur SJ, Leigh D, Marshall JT, et al. Pregnancies and live births after trophectoderm biopsy and preimplantation genetic testing of human blastocysts. Fertil Steril. 2005;84(6):1628-36.

32. Scott KL, Hong KH, Scott RT. Selecting the optimal time to perform biopsy for preimplantation genetic testing. Fertil Steril. 2013;100(3):608-14.

33. Tarkowski AK. An air-drying method for chromosome preparations from mouse eggs. Cytogenetics. 1966;5(6):394-400.

34. De Boer KA, Catt JW, Jansen RP, et al. Moving to blastocyst biopsy for preimplantation genetic diagnosis and single embryo transfer at Sydney IVF. Fertil Steril. 2004;82(2):295-8.

35. Lathi RB, Massie JA, Gilani M, et al. Outcomes of trophectoderm biopsy on cryopreserved blastocysts: a case series. Reprod Biomed Online. 2012;25(5): 504-7.

36. Adler A, Lee HL, McCulloh DH, et al. Blastocyst culture selects for euploid embryos: comparison of blastomere and trophectoderm biopsies. Reprod Biomed Online. 2014;28(4):485-91.

37. Velilla E, Escudero T, Munné S. Blastomere fixation techniques and risk of misdiagnosis for preimplantation genetic diagnosis of aneuploidy. Reprod Biomed Online. 2002;4(1):210-7.

38. Capalbo A, Wright G, Elliott T, et al. FISH reanalysis of inner cell mass and trophectoderm samples of previously array-CGH screened blastocysts shows high accuracy of diagnosis and no major diagnostic impact of mosaicism at the blastocyst stage. Hum Reprod. 2013;28(8):2298-307.

39. Braude P, Pickering S, Flinter F, et al. Preimplantation genetic diagnosis. Nat Rev Genet. 2002;3(12):941-53.

40. Verlinsky Y, Cohen J, Munne S, et al. Over a decade of experience with preimplantation genetic diagnosis: a multicenter report. Fertil Steril. 2004;82(2): 292-4.

41. Harper JC, Sengupta SB. Preimplantation genetic diagnosis: state of the art 2011. Hum Genet. 2012;131(2):175-86.

42. Yan L, Wei Y, Huang J, et al. Advances in preimplantation genetic diagnosis/screening. Sci China Life Sci. 2014;57(7):665-71.

Chapter 9

Time-lapse Imaging: A New Technology for Embryo Development

Carmela Albert, Pilar Gámiz, Natalia Basile, Marcos Meseguer

INTRODUCTION

In classical *in vitro* fertilization (IVF), embryo assessment is based on time-point evaluation during embryo development, and a clear correlation between embryo morphology and viability has been well established. The final decision for embryo transfer is based primarily on developmental stage, blastomere symmetry and the quality of the inner cell mass (ICM) and trophectoderm (TE) at the day of transfer.

Even though great knowledge has been achieved through this approach it has been demonstrated that embryo status can markedly change within a few hours.[1-4] In addition, inter and intraobserver variability is a commonly described problem[5] probably due to the subjective nature surrounding traditional morphological assessment.[3,6-10] In theory, increasing the number of observations could provide better information of the development of the embryo and therefore improve its assessment.[3,11,12] However, increased handling and higher evaluation frequency will expose the embryo to undesirable changes in temperature, humidity and gas composition.[11-13]

Time-lapse systems (TMSs) represent a solution to this problem. In 1997, Payne et al.[14] developed time-lapse cinematography to manage an intermittent observation of the process of oocyte fertilization. Later on, the observation period was augmented while maintaining optimal culture conditions[2] and nowadays TMSs increases the number of morphologic observation for assess embryo quality and allow the complete observation of the entire process of embryo development in the IVF laboratory. In addition to that, the TMS reduce the handling of samples and hence the human risk, implies a minimization of culture media, mineral oil and gas consumption, facilitates the detection of abnormal events that would normally occur between observations, reduce inter and intraobserver variations and decrease the number of hours needed by the embryologist in the laboratory.[15]

Morphokinetics, defined as the combination of the embryo appearance (morphology) and the timing in which cellular events occur, has been introduced as a new concept to improve embryo selection. TMS allows the precise determinations of the onset, and duration of an interval between cell divisions. The use of this strategy could allow single embryo transfers (SETs) without jeopardizing the overall IVF success,[16] becoming very attractive especially in European countries in which legislation is stricter about the number of embryo transferred.[15]

MODELS IN MARKET

There are different available options of TMS in the market. Some of them present all the items integrated in one single equipment, e.g. EmbryoScope® (Vitrolife), Geri (Genea Biomedx) and Miri® TL (Esco Medical). Others offer the option of introducing a microscope inside an available incubator, e.g. Primo Vision® (Vitrolife) and the Eeva™ Test (Merck Serono). Tables 9.1 and 9.2 describe the clinical and technical features of all the TMS available in the market.

Table 9.1: Technical features compared between the time-lapse systems available in the market.

Technical features	EmbryoScope®	Primo Vision®	Eeva™ test	Geri	Miri® TL
Microscopy	Phase contrast	Phase contrast	Dark field	Phase contrast	Phase contrast
Image capture frequency	Each 10 minutes	Each 10 minutes	Each 5 minutes	Each 5 minutes	Each 5 minutes
Focusing levels	7	Several	1	Several	Several
Patients per system	6	1	1	6	6
Embryos per dish	12	16	12	16	14
Integrated incubator	Yes	No	No	Yes	Yes
Data analysis	Manual	Manual	Manual	Manual	Manual

Table 9.2: Clinical features compared between the time-lapse systems available in the market.

Clinical features	EmbryoScope®	Primo Vision™	Eeva™ test	Geri	Miri® TL
Automatic assessment	No	No	Yes	No	No
Worker dependent	Yes	Yes	No	Yes	Yes
Time consuming	Yes	Yes	No/ Automatic	Yes	Yes
Selection algorithm	Set by the user	Set by the user	Present	Set by the user	Set by the user

Contd…

Contd...

Clinical features	EmbryoScope®	Primo Vision™	Eeva™ test	Geri	Miri® TL
Blastocyst formation prediction by day 3	No	No	Yes	No	No
Implantation prediction by day 3	Yes	Yes	Yes	No	No
Prospective validated	Yes	No	Yes	No	No

KINETIC PARAMETERS (INDIVIDUAL + CALCULATED)

As described at the proposed guidelines on the nomenclature and annotation of dynamic human embryo monitoring by a time-lapse user group, we can define the following morphokinetic individual variables:[17]

- *t0:* Time of IVF or midtime of microinjection [intracytoplasmic sperm injection (ICSI) or intracytoplasmic morphologically selected sperm injection (IMSI)]
- *tPB2:* The second polar body completely detached from the oolemma
- *tPN:* Fertilization is confirmed
- *tPNa:* Appearance of individual pronuclei (PN); tPN1a, tPN2a, and tPN3a
- *tPNf:* Time of PN disappearance; tPN1f, and tPN2f
- *tZ:* Time of PN scoring
- *t2 to t9:* Time to two to nine discrete cells
- *tSC:* First evidence of compaction
- *tMf/p:* End of compaction
    "f" corresponds to fully compacted
    "p" corresponds to partial compaction
- *tSB:* Initiation of blastulation
- *tByz:* Full blastocyst
    "y" corresponds to morphology of ICM
    "z" corresponds to morphology of TE cells
- *tEyz:* Initiation of expansion; first frame of zona thinning
- *tHNyz:* Herniation; end of expansion phase and initiation of hatching
- *tHDyz:* Fully hatched blastocyst.

Additionally we can define calculated variables that represent a certain cell stage or cycle duration (Fig. 9.1):

Pronuclei duration	$VP = tPNf - tPNa$
Duration of first cell cycle	$ECC1 = t2 - tPB2$
Duration of second cell cycle	$ECC2 = t4 - t2$

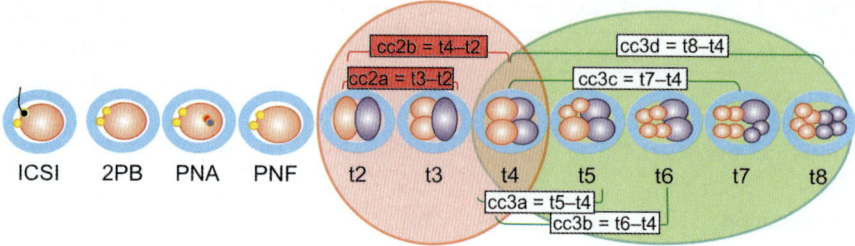

Fig. 9.1: Graphical representation of kinetic variables up to the 8-cell stage. (ICSI: Intracytoplasmic sperm injection; PB: Polar body).

Duration of single blastomere cell cycle	$cc2a = t3-t2$
	$cc2b = t4-t2$
Duration of third cell cycle	$ECC3 = t8-t4$
Duration of single blastomere cell cycle	$cc3a = t5-t4$
	$cc3b = t6-t4$
	$cc3c = t7-t4$
	$cc3d = t8-t4$
Synchronization of cell divisions	$s2 = t4-t3$
Synchronization of cleavage pattern	$s3 = t8-t5$
Duration of compaction (dcom)	tMf–tSC (full compaction)
	tMp–tSC (partial compaction)
Duration of blastulation (dB)	tB–tSB
Duration of blastocyst expansion (dexp)	tHN–tE
Duration of blastocyst collapse (dcol)	tBCend(n)–tBCi(n)
"n" is number of episodes of collapse and reexpansion	
Duration of reexpansion (dreexp)	treexpend(n)–treexpi(n)
Duration of herniation (8dHN)	tHN–tHD

BLASTOCYST DEVELOPMENT STUDIES

Kinetic markers have been associated to good quality embryos and to the prediction of blastocyst formation (Table 9.3).

In 2010, Wong et al.[18] analyzed kinetic parameters of 100 embryos that were cultured up to day 5 or 6 of development.[18] Three parameters were founded as predictors of blastocyst formation: (1) P1: duration of the first cytokinesis (14.3 ± 6.0 min), (2) P2: interval between the end of the first mitosis and the initiation of the second mitosis (11.1 ± 2.2 h) and (3) P3: the synchrony between the second and third mitosis (1.0 ± 1.6 h). The authors concluded that embryo development to the blastocyst stage could be predicted with 94% of sensitivity and 93% of specificity after using those parameters. Embryos with one or more values outside these ranges were expected to arrest. The time of completion of the second and third mitosis was also analyzed by

Table 9.3: Kinetic markers associated to the prediction of blastocyst formation.

Author	Study design	N embr-yos	Embryo origin	Time-lapse system	Predictive marker identified
Wong et al. 2010	Retrospective Study	100	Super-numerary frozen 2PN	Modified Olympus IX-70/71; CKK-40/41	1st cytokinesis, P2 and P3
Hashimoto et al. 2012	Experimetal study	80	Donated human embryos for research	Biostation CT	Duration of 2nd (t4–t3) and 3rd mitotic division (t8–t5)
Hlinka et al. 2012	Retrospective study	180	Clinical IVF routine	Primovision	c2, c3 and c4; i2, i3, and i4
Cruz et al. 2012	Retrospective cohort study	834	Oocyte donation cycles	Embryoscope	t4, s2, DC 3 Sells, tM; UN 2 cells
Chamayou et al. 2013	Retrospective study	224	Fresh oocyte ICSI treatments	Embryoscope	t1, t2, t4, t7, t8, tC–tF and s3
Kirkegaard et al. 2013	Prospective multicenter cohort	571	Fresh oocyte ICSI treatments	Embryoscope	1st cyto-kinesis, t3, DC 3 cells
Conhagan et al. 2013	Prospective multicenter cohort study	233	Fresh oocyte ICSI treatments	Eeva	P2 and P3
Kirkegaard et al. 2014	Retrospective multicenter study	1519	Fresh oocyte ICSI treatments	Embryoscope	P2 and P3
Cetinkaya et al. 2014	Retrospective observational cohort study	3354	Clinical IVF routine	Embryoscope	CS2
Yang et al. 2015	Prospective observational study	345	Metaphase I donated for research	Primovision	Cleavage patterns
Milewsky et al. 2015	Retrospective observational study	432	Fresh oocyte ICSI treatments	Embryoscope	t2, t5, cc2, SC
Storr et al. 2015	Prospective cohort study	380	Fresh oocyte ICSI treatment	Embryoscope	s3, t8, tEB
Motato et al. 2016	Retrospective study	7483	Clinical IVF routine	Embryoscope	tM; t8–t5

(DC: Direct cleavage; ICSI: Intracytoplasmic sperm injection; IVF: *In vitro* fertilization; PN: Pronuclei).

Hashimoto et al.,[19] who observed that high-scoring blastocysts took significantly shorter times for these divisions.

Hlinka et al.[20] analyzed 180 embryos that resulted in 28 pregnancies. After calculating the average duration of the interphases and cleavages of a subset of implanting embryos, the author established a uniform time patterning of cleavage clusters (c) and interphases (i); most specifically: $i2 = 11 \pm 1$, $i3 = 15 \pm 1$, $i4 = 23 \pm 1$ h/$c2 = 15 \pm 5$, $c3 = 40 \pm 10$, $c4 = 55 \pm 15$. Embryos falling within these values showed a higher rate of blastocyst development than those falling outside this range (88.2% vs 13.3%). In addition, higher morphological abnormality rates were observed in embryos falling outside the optimal ranges.

In a retrospective cohort study, Cruz et al.[21] monitored 834 embryos. Mean timings for the variables t2, t3, t4, t5, tM, cc2 and s2 were calculated for embryos that developed to blastocyst and for those that did not. Quartiles were defined for each parameter in association with the proportion of good and poor morphology blastocysts. Finally, optimal ranges were proposed as follows: t2, 24.3–27.9 hour; t3, 35.4–40.3 hour; t5, 48.8–56.6 hour; s2, less than 0.76 hour; and cc2, less than 11.9 hour. The following deselection criteria were also recorded: uneven blastomere size at the 2-cell stage and abrupt division from zygote to 3-blastomere embryo. In general, it was observed that embryos performing earlier cleavages had significantly higher developmental potential to day 5. Therefore, the capability to reach blastocyst stage seemed to be related to early embryo division kinetics.

In 2013, Chamayou et al.,[22] reported time intervals of morphokinetic parameters identified as predictors of embryo competence. In this retrospective study, embryos were divided into three groups: (1) implanted (72), (2) nonimplanted (106) and (3) arrested (66). Each kinetic parameter for every single embryo was compared and significant differences were found. The authors concluded that day 3 embryos develop into viable blastocysts when their kinetic parameters met the following ranges: t1 [18.4–30.9 hours postinsemination (hpi)], t2 (21.4–34.8 hpi), t4 (33.1–57.2 hpi), t7 (46.1–82.5 hpi), t8 (46.4–97.8 hpi), tC – tF (7.7–22.9 hpi) and s3 (0.7–30.8 hpi).

A couple of prospective studies were performed in 2013; Kirkegaard et al.,[23] analyzed 571 embryos from good prognosis patients and reported three markers linked to high-quality blastocysts: duration of the first cytokinesis, duration of 3-cell stage and direct cleavage to 3-cell, all of them with comparable predictive value but with no connection to implantation results. Conaghan et al.,[24] accomplished a two phase multicenter study to develop and validate an algorithm to predict blastocyst formation. A total of 1,727 embryos were monitored by an automatic cell tracking software. The time between cytokinesis 1 and 2 (P2) and the time between cytokinesis 2 and 3 (P3) turned out to be the strongest parameters in the prediction model. The results indicated a higher probability of usable blastocyst formation when both P2 and P3 were within specific cell division timing ranges (P2, 9.33–11.45 hours;

and P3, 0–1.73 hours) and a low probability when either P2 or P3 were outside the specific cell timing ranges. Through this model, the authors observed that usable blastocysts could be predicted with a specificity of 84.2% [95% confidence interval (CI) = 78.7%–88.5%], sensitivity of 58.8% (95% CI = 47.0%–69.7%), positive predictive value (PPV) of 54.1% (95% CI = 42.8%–64.9%), and negative predictive value (NPV) of 86.6% (95% CI = 81.3%–90.6%). By comparison, the same prediction based on morphology alone was achieved with a specificity of 52.1% (95% CI = 39.7%–64.6%), sensitivity of 81.8% (95% CI = 70.6%–92.9%), PPV of 34.5% (95% CI = 31.5%–37.5%), and NPV of 90.9% (95% CI = 87.3%–94.5%). The authors concluded that the use of this algorithm significantly improved the specificity (84.2% vs 52.1%; P<0.0001) and PPV (54.1% vs 34.5%; P<0.01) of usable blastocyst predictions enabling embryologists to better discriminate which embryos would be unlikely to develop to blastocyst. Therefore, they recommend the adjunctive use of this algorithm to improved embryo selection.

The Conaghan model was tested retrospectively by a different group using a set of 1,519 transferred embryos with known clinical outcome.[25] According to the algorithm, embryos were classified into usable and nonusable. The difference in implantation rate (IR) between the usable group and the whole cohort was 30% indicating that IRs could increase using this model. In addition, the percentage of nonusable embryos that resulted in implantation was 50.6% causing alert regarding the discard of viable embryos. Even though the Conaghan model was developed for blastocyst formation and the endpoint of this study was clinical outcome, the authors expressed that implanted embryos should derive from the usable embryo group and not from the nonusable group (or at least not in such high proportion). The possible explanation, according to the authors, could be that the model is based on narrow time intervals.

In 2015, Cetinkaya et al.[26] studied 17 kinetic markers on 3,354 embryos cultured up to day 5. The parameters: t8–t5, cleavage synchronicity from 4 to 8 cells (CS4–8) and cleavage synchronicity from 2 to 8 cells (CS2–8) were found as good indicators. In particular, CS2-8 defined as: CS2-8 = [(t3–t2) + (t5–t4)]/(t8–t2) was selected as the best predictor on day 3 for blastocyst formation and quality [area under the curve (AUC): 0.786]. The authors concluded that relative timings (time intervals and relative ratios) were better indicators of development than absolute time points that cannot be standardized for general applicability in different laboratories.

Yang et al.[27] took a different approach and developed a study to describe different types of abnormal divisions and how they may affect the developmental potential of the embryo. Seven types of divisions within two categories were defined according to the impact caused on blastocyst development. Category 1 included divisions with low impact on the development potential—normal division, uneven blastomere formation and appearance of big fragments.

Category 2 included divisions with high impact on embryo development—direct cleavage, fragmentation, developmental arrest and disordered division. Taking this in consideration a hierarchical classification model was developed based on the division patterns during the three initial embryo cleavages rather than on morphokinetic parameters as in previous studies. Day 3 embryos were then classified into six categories "A" to "F" according to the number and category of the abnormal cleavages they had presented. More specifically: (A) embryos that had normal cleavage in the initial three cleavages, (B) embryos that had category 1 behaviors in all three cleavages, (C) embryos undergoing category 1 behaviors in the initial two cleavages and category 2 behaviors in the third cleavage, (D) embryos that showed category 1 behaviors in the first cleavage and one of the two blastomeres (partial) showed category 2 behaviors in the second cleavage, (E) embryos that showed category 1 behaviors in the first cleavage and two blastomeres (all) showed category 2 behaviors in the second cleavage, and (F) embryos that showed category 2 behaviors in the first cleavage. The model was validated in a prospective observational study in which images from 345 embryos were acquired. The study revealed that 72.2% of the embryos presented at least one abnormal division. According to the model, blastocyst formation rate decreases from 94.8% to 21.2%, good quality blastocyst formation rate decreases from 70.8% to 3.8% and IR (for those that were transferred) decreases from 67% to 0% as we move on from "A" to "F".

In a study by Milewski et al. the parameters t2, t3, t4, t5, cc2 and s2 were measured and differences were observed between embryos that reached the blastocyst stage and embryos that arrested. A total of 432 embryos were analyzed. The resultant data for each parameter was divided in 4 intervals (C1–C4) and score values were assigned in order to find out which parameter values corresponded to the highest blastocyst development rate. The highest ones generally belonged to compartments C3 and C2. The extreme compartments, C1 and C4, had the lowest rates. The univariate logistic regression analysis concluded that all the studied parameters were significantly associated to blastocyst development. However, after multivariate logistic regression only t2, t5 and cc2 parameters were taken into account and combined into a new parameter (SC) defined as predictor of development to blastocyst.[28]

Storr et al. recorded the timings of 380 blastocysts and found eight significant prediction markers of top-quality blastocyst: s3, t6, t7, t8, tM, tSB, tB and tEB. Out of these potential predictors, s3 was identified as the one with the best individual discriminatory capacity before compaction (area under the curve—AUC 0.585, 95% CI 0.534–0.635), and tEB was identified as the best predictor regardless of embryo stage (AUC 0.727, 95% CI 0.675–0.775). By combining ts3, tEB and t8, a model with higher discriminatory capacity for predicting top-quality embryos was proposed.[29]

Diamond et al.[30] found that, adjunctive use of Eeva test is highly informative and allow embryologist to consistently improve the selection of embryos with high developmental potential.

Motato et al. in 2016[31] published a three-phase observational, retrospective, single-center clinical study, in which the author described the events associated with blastocyst formation and implantation based on the largest sample size ever described with time-lapse monitoring:

- *Phase 1:* Embryo scoring based on a classification tree to select embryos with higher blastocyst formation probabilities. The observed correlations between morphokinetic parameters and blastocyst formation are the basis for a proposed hierarchical classification procedure to select viable embryos with a high blastocyst formation potential. A detailed retrospective analysis of cleavage times was made for 7,483 zygotes. A total of 17 parameters were studied and several were significantly correlated with blastocyst formation and implantation. The most predictive parameters for blastocyst formation were: time of morula formation, tM (81.28–96.0 hours after ICSI), and t8–t5 (≤8.78 hours) or time of transition of 5-blastomere embryos to 8-blastomere embryos with a receiver operating characteristic (ROC) curve value = 0.849 (95% CI, 0.835–0.854). These parameters were less predictive of implantation, with a ROC value = 0.546 (95% CI, 0.507–0.585).

- *Phase 2:* Blastocyst transferred and IR. Owing to the lack of a relationship between the previously described variables with implantation potential, the authors identified new variables by comparing transferred blastocysts (n = 383) that implanted with those that did not implant (n = 449). Once again they analyzed 17 morphokinetic parameters and identified the variables: time for expansion blastocyst, tEB (107.9–112.9 hours after ICSI), and t8–t5 (5.67 hours after ICSI) to predict blastocyst implantation, with a ROC curve value = 0.591 (95% CI, 0.552–0.630). Using these data, a hierarchical model representing a classification tree was proposed. The model subdivided blastocysts into four categories from A to D with higher or lower IR (i.e. from 72.2% in category A to 39.7% in category D).

- *Phase 3:* Validation of the implantation model. After the conclusion of phase 2, the created model was validated on an independent data set composed of 257 embryos and 123 blastocysts with known implantation data (KID) embryos, giving a ROC of 0.596 (95% CI, 0.526–0.666; P = 0.008).

The authors concluded that the inclusion of kinetic parameters into score evaluation could improve blastocyst selection criteria as well as predict blastocyst formation with high accuracy. In addition, the proposed models classify embryos according to their probabilities of blastocyst stage and implantation.

The most recent study on blastocyst prediction was published by Aparicio et al.[32] in 2016 the authors founded that there is a direct correlation between blastocyst rate and percentage of optimal blastocyst according to each of the categories: high, medium and low. A total of 3,002 embryos were automatically classified by means of the Eeva system according to the timing of P2 and P3. These embryos were also classified with the use of Association for the Study of Reproductive Biology (ASEBIR) morphology classification. The results suggest that the automated embryo diagnostic test provided extra information to the embryologist to select the best embryos, independently from clinical features of the patient or day of transfer.

IMPLANTATION STUDIES

In addition to blastocyst formation, the scientific community has also correlated kinetic markers to embryo implantation as an endpoint (Table 9.4).

Starting in 2008, Lemmen et al.,[33] retrospectively compared time lapse recordings of a small group of embryos transferred at the 4-cell stage that resulted in eight pregnancies. In this case, the author observed that nuclei appearance in the first blastomere following the first cleavage was faster in embryos that implanted versus those that did not, and that the nuclei appearance in the first two blastomeres was significantly more synchronous ($P<0.05$).

Three years later, Meseguer et al.[1] published a study were explaining several parameters were correlated with embryo implantation. The study was based on 247 KID embryos and it developed a hierarchical model that subdivided embryos into six categories from A to F. Four of these categories (A–D) were further subdivided into two subcategories (+) or (–) (Flowchart 9.1). The hierarchical classification procedure starts with a morphological screening of all embryos in a cohort to eliminate those embryos that are clearly not viable (i.e. highly abnormal, atresia or clearly arrested embryos). Those embryos that are clearly not viable are discarded and not considered for transfer (category F). Next step in the model is to exclude embryos that fulfill any of the three exclusion criteria: (1) uneven blastomere size at the 2-cell stage, (2) abrupt division from one to three or more cells or (3) multinucleation at the 4-cell stage (category E). The subsequent levels in the model follow a strict hierarchy based on the binary timing variables t5, s2 and cc2. First, if the value of t5 falls inside the optimal range (48.8–56.6 h), the embryo is categorized as A or B. If the value of t5 falls outside the optimal range (or if t5 has not yet been observed at 64 h), the embryo is categorized as C or D. If the value of s2 falls inside the optimal range (≤ 0.76 h) the embryo is categorized as A or C depending on t5; similarly, if the value of s2 falls outside the optimal range, the embryo is categorized as B or D depending on t5. Finally, the embryo is categorized with the extra plus (+), if the value for cc2 is inside the optimal range (≤ 11.9 h) (A+/B+/C+/D+) and is categorized with a minus (–) as (A–/B–/C–/D–), if the value for cc2 is outside the optimal range.

Table 9.4: Kinetic markers associated to the embryo implantation as an endpoint.

Author	Study design	Total number of embryos	Embryo origin	Time-lapse system	Predictive marker identified/utilized
Lemen et al. 2008	Retrospective study	19	IVF/ICSI cycles	Nikon Diaphot 300 microscope with camera in a closed system	Nuclei apperance in the first blastomere
Meseguer et al. 2011	Retrospective study	247	ICSI cycles	EmbryoScope	t5, s2, cc2, UN 2 cell, MN 4 cell, DC 1–3 cells
Arazello et al. 2012	Prospective study	159	ICSI cycles	EmbryoScope	PN breakdown
Hlinka et al. 2012	Retrospective study	114	ICSI cycles	Primovision	c2, c3 and c4; i2, i3 and i4
Rubio et al. 2012	Multicenter retrospective study	5225 (1659 transferred)	IVF cycles from donated and autologous oocytes	EmbryoScope	DC 2–3 cells
Freour et al. 2013	Retrospective analysis and prospectively collected database	191	ICSI cycles	EmbryoScope	t4 and s3
Chamayou et al.	Retrospective study	178	ICSI cycles	EmbryoScope	cc3
Kirkgaard et al. 2013a	Prospective cohort study	84	ICSI cycles	EmbryoScope	None
Rubio et al. 2014	Prospective randomized control trial	2638	ICSI cycles from donated oocytes	EmbryoScope	T5; s2; cc2; UN 2 cell; MN 4 cell; DC 1–3 cells

Contd...

Contd...

Author	Study design	Total number of embtyos	Embryo origin	Time-lapse system	Predicative marker identified/utilized
Aguilar et al. 2012	Retrospective cohort study	1448	ICSI cycles from donated oocytes	EmbryoScope	Time to 2PB; PF; length of S-phase
Basile et al. 2012	Retrospective multicentric study	1122	ICSI cycles from donated and autologous oocytes	EmbryoScope	Cc2, t3, t5, UN 2 cell, MN 4 cell, DC 1–3 cells
Vermilea et al. 2014	Retrospective multicentric study	331	IVF/ICSI cycles	Evea	P2 and P3
Freour et al. 2015	Retrospective study	528	ICSI cycles	EmbryoScope	t5, s2, cc2, UN 2 cell, MN 4 cell, DC 1–3 cells
Dominguez et al. 2015	Retrospective cohort study	28	ICSI cycles from donated oocytes	EmbryoScope	Cc2
Adamson et al. 2016	Prospective concurrent cohort study		ICSI and IVF cycles from autologous oocytes	Eeva	P2 and P3
Goodman et al. 2016	Prospective randomized controlled trial	2092	ICSI and IVF cycles from autologous oocytes	EmbryoScope	Cc2, s2, t5, s3, tSB, MN, irregular division

(DC: Direct cleavage; ICSI: Intracytoplasmic sperm injection; IVF: *In vitro* fertilization; MN: Multinucleation; PB: Polar body; PN: Pronuclei).

Flowchart 9.1: Algorithm by Meseguer et al. (2011)

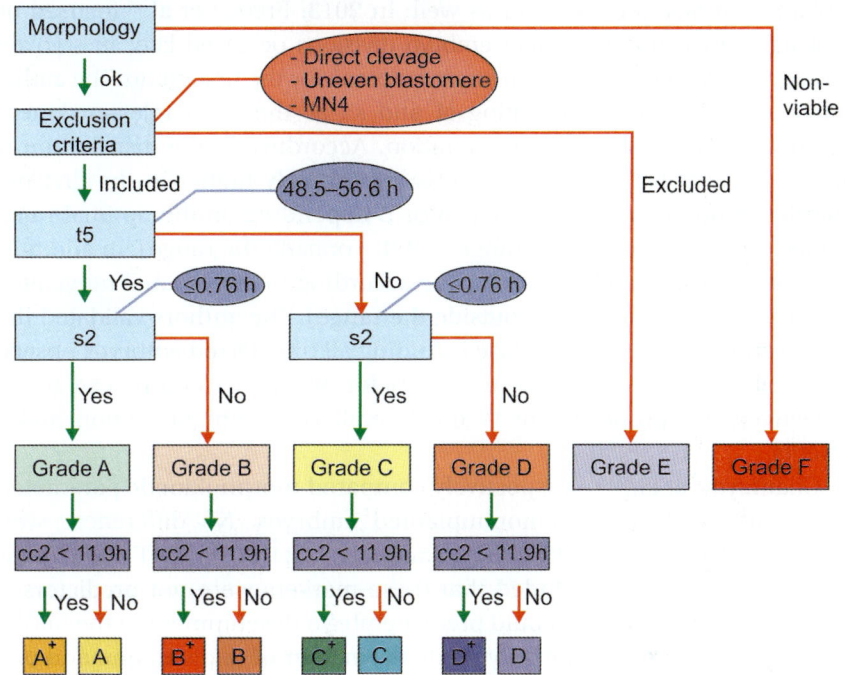

In 2012, Azzarello et al.[34] performed a prospective study transferring 159 embryos and proposed the variable 'time of pronuclear breakdown' as a predictor of pregnancy. In this study, the pronuclear breakdown of embryos resulting in live birth occurred significantly later than those that did not. In fact, the author proposed the limit of 20 hour 45 minutes and recommended to avoid transferring embryos presenting pronuclear breakdowns at earlier times.

The same year, Hlinka et al.,[20] proposed a novel method to predict implantation. The model relied on cleavage ratings of the embryos; more specifically time pattering of cleavage clusters and interphases were used to select the highest quality embryos. Diagnostic relation between blastocyst implantation and cleavage success was 100% specific for all the embryos analyzed (180) and all the pregnancies resulted from timely cleaved embryos.

Direct cleavage is another parameter that has been correlated with implantation. Meseguer et al.[1] initially observed this phenomenon based on 247 KID embryos. Later on, these findings were confirmed by a multicenter retrospective study performed by Rubio et al.[35] In this case the number of embryos analyzed was much higher (5225) and embryo implantation for embryos presenting direct cleavage from two to three cells (DC 2 to 3 <5 hours) was statistically lower than for those with normal cleavage pattern. Only 1 out of 109 embryos with DC 2–3 cells resulted in clinical pregnancy.

The impact of extrinsic factors on embryo kinetics and its relation with implantation has been studied as well. In 2013, Freour et al.[36] focused on smoking women observing that embryo divisions occurred later in smokers than in nonsmokers, resulting in worst outcome for the first group. The author analyzed 191 embryos indicating t4 and s3 as the most relevant kinetic parameters with respect to implantation. According to the distribution of these two variables, implantation was significantly higher in the first two quartiles. Embryos were graded as A or B depending on the optimal range defined for t4 (A = inside the range and B = outside the range). In addition, embryos were given a "+" or "−" value according to the optimal range of s3 (+ = inside the range and − = outside the range). The authors validated this classification model in a database including all transferred embryos observing IRs of 38.7%, 33.3%, 30.7% and 15.3% for A+, A−, B+ and B− categories, respectively. The proportion of A+ and A− embryos was higher in nonsmoker patients.

Chamayou et al.,[22] retrospectively compared morphokinetic parameters of 72 implanted and 106 nonimplanted embryos. No differences were found for PN appearance, PN disappearance, t1, t2, t4, t7, t8, tC–tF and s3 parameters. The authors concluded that these markers were not predictors of implantation but that they could predict embryo development to the blastocyst stage. In this study, the only predictor marker of implantation and production of a viable pregnancy was cc3. Embryos with cc3 between 9.7 and 21 hours seemed to have the highest probability of implantation and clinical pregnancy.

As opposed to many authors, Kirkegaard et al.,[23] showed no differences in the timings of cellular division or embryonic stage between implanted and nonimplanted embryos. The study was based on the observation of 84 SETs. The author defined the duration of first cytokinesis, duration of the 3-cell stage and direct cleavage to three cells as predictors of high quality embryo development but not of implantation or pregnancy. Therefore, this group concluded that a universal algorithm for optimal timing might not be feasible.

Validation of Meseguer's algorithm from 2001[1] came along with a triple-blind randomized prospective controlled trial published by Rubio et al. in 2014.[37] In this study, 405 patients were included in the control group in which embryos were selected based purely on morphology and 438 patients were included in the study group in which embryos were selected based on the algorithm. IRs were significantly higher in the study group (44.9%; 95% CI, 41.4–48.4) versus the control group (37.1%; 95% CI, 33.6–40.7). In addition, the ongoing pregnancy rate was also higher in the study group versus the control group (54.5%; 95% CI, 49.6–59.2 vs 45.3%; 95 CI, 40.3–50.4). The authors concluded that morphokinetic variables allow us to reject embryos with lower implantation while distinguishing those with higher implantation probabilities. Selecting embryos through kinetic markers may therefore improve reproductive outcomes.[37]

A second randomized controlled trial published by a different group reached similar results although they were not able to achieve statistical significance.[38] As opposed to Rubio's study, in which both study groups had different culture conditions (standard incubator vs EmbryoScope), one of the strengths of this study was that it was the first one to evaluate all embryos cultured within identical culture conditions and to demonstrate whether the addition of continuously monitored morphokinetic parameters improve clinical outcomes compared with conventional once daily morphologic assessment. The study anticipated a 10% increase and although it did not reach statistical significance, there were increased clinical pregnancy and IRs with the use of the additional parameters. In addition, the time of the start of blastulation, the absence of multinucleation, and the use of a score based on morphology and kinetics were significant predictors of implantation. The authors concluded that in this dynamic and evolving field, larger studies were needed to confirm their findings.

In 2014, Aguilar et al.[39] studied the human's first cell cycle and its impact on implantation based on morphokinetics. For this aim the author did a retrospective analysis of 1,448 transferred embryos and compared the timings of second polar extrusion, first and second pronuclear appearance, pronuclear abuttal, pronuclear fading and length of S-phase between implanted and nonimplanted embryos. The time ranges successfully linked to implantation were: 3.3–10.6-hour for second polar body extrusion, 22.2–25.9-hour for pronuclear fading and 5.7–13.8-hour for the length of S-phase.

The same year, Basile et al.[40] continued the study by Meseguer et al.[1] and published an improved version of the algorithm by studying a larger data set of embryos from four different IVF clinics (Flowchart 9.2). For that aim a sequential approach was adopted by the author. During phase 1 of the study, an algorithm was developed taking in consideration morphokinetic data of 754 KID embryos that were selected for transfer based only on conventional morphological criteria. The new algorithm included the variables t3, cc2 and t5 in combination with morphology and exclusion criteria [direct cleavage (DC), uneven blastomere size (UBS) and multinucleation (MN)] and classified embryos from A to E according to their implantation potential. Subsequently, during phase 2 of the study, the predictive ability of this new algorithm was tested by applying it for embryo classification in a different group of IVF patients (885 cycles). Considering only cycles with known implantation (100% or 0% implantation, n = 1,137), a significant decrease in IR was observed as embryo categories decreased from A to E. More specifically: "A" 32%, "B" 28%, "C" 26.25%, "D" 20.19% and "E" the lowest 17% P< 0.001.

Another study by VerMilyea et al.[41] established the relationship between implantation and three embryo categories derived from a computer automated TMS. The system classified embryos into the categories: high, medium or low based on the variables P2 and P3. According to this multicenter study

Flowchart 9.2: Algorithm by Basile et al. (2015).

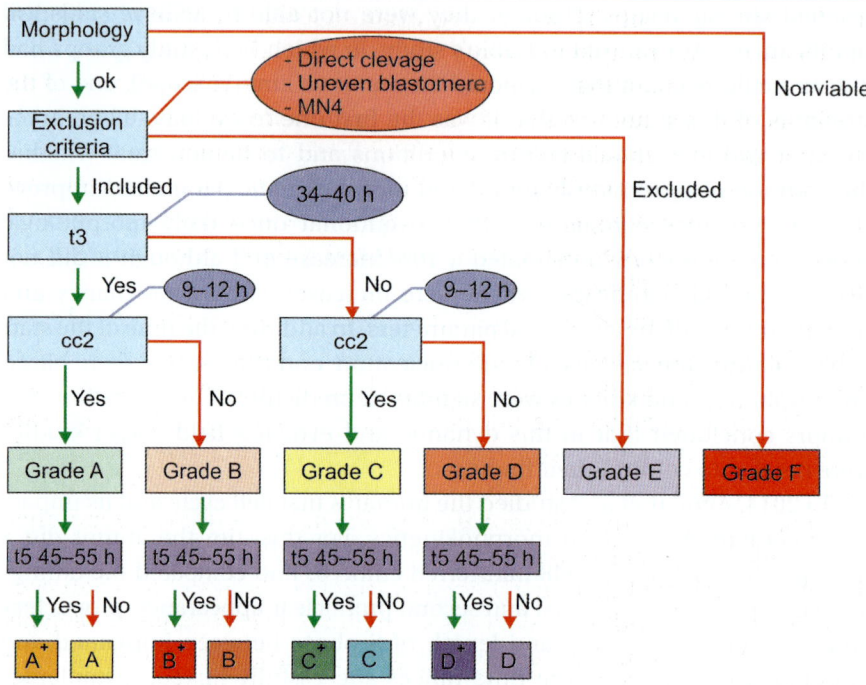

(205 patients) IRs were significantly linked to the three categories; more specifically: 37%, 35% and 15% for high, medium and low respectively. In addition, clinical pregnancy rate for patients that had one or more "high" embryos transferred embryos was significantly higher (51% vs 34%; P = 0.02).

A most recent study published by Adamson et al. in 2016,[42] tested the same technology in a prospective way. The aim of the study was to prove if an automatic time-lapse test (TL-test) combined with traditional morphology improves day 3 IRs compared with morphology alone. Two concurrently collected groups of patients were compared: those who received a day 3 transfer with the use of the TL test together with morphology (test group), and those who received a day 3 transfer with the use of morphology alone (control group). To further assess the impact of the automated TL-test score, the authors evaluated the implantation potential of embryos assigned by the TL-test as category TL-high versus TL-low among all transferred embryos (TL-high: duration of 2-cell stage within 9.33–11.45 hours and duration of 3-cell stage within 0–1.73 hours; TL-low: outside the TL-high ranges) and among those with only good morphology. Analysis of the study's primary endpoint, IR showed a significantly higher IR for day 3 transfer among the test group (30.2%, 58/192) than the control group (19.0%, 84/442; P = 0.003); clinical pregnancy rate was also significantly higher among the test group (46.0%, 45/98) than the control group (32.1%, 71/221; P = 0.02). Within the test group, patients receiving at least one TL-high embryo had significantly higher IRs than patients receiving only TL-low embryos (36.8% vs 20.6%). TL-high compared with TL-low embryos had significantly higher IRs (44.7% vs 20.5%). Among morphologically good embryos, TL-high embryos were more likely to implant than TL-low embryos (44.1% vs 20.6%). The authors concluded that the noninvasive TL-test adds valuable information to traditional morphologic grading and that it should be used to increase clinician's confidence in recommending elective SET (eSET) with day 3 transfer, and that we would expect higher IRs and higher clinical pregnancy rates, as well as reduced multiple pregnancy rates, compared with patients with embryos not assessed by the TL-test.

Limitations on the external performance and the universal use of published algorithms have been addressed.[43] In a study published by Freour et al.,[36] an external validation of Meseguer's algorithm[1] was performed in an unselected patient population. The model was applied showing a heterogeneous distribution of IRs in the resultant categories. In addition, correlation coefficients were significantly lower than the ones in the original study. However, a simplified version from the model (in which only the two main morphokinetic variables, t5 and s2, were consider and not cc2) performed acceptably. The author explained that the differences could be the result of differences in oxygen culture conditions, oocyte source (donor cycles versus autologous cycles), restrictions in the studied population and/or the stimulation protocols used. The conclusion was that a hierarchical prediction model should not be used universally in an unselected population; it should be center specific.

Flowchart 9.3: Algorithm by Dominguez et al. (2015).

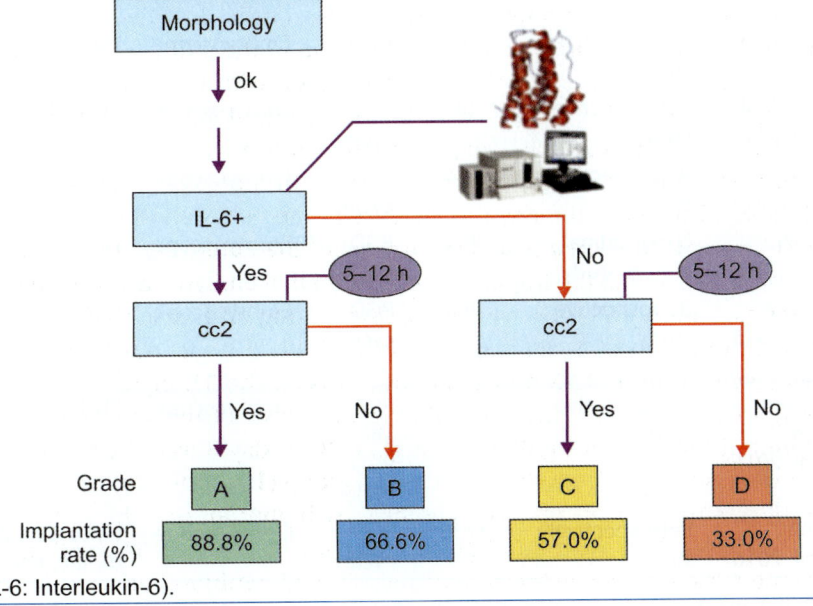

(IL-6: Interleukin-6).

The combination of technologies may be the key for improving results in the future. Dominguez et al.,[44] combined proteomics and time-lapse analysis of implanted[16] and nonimplanted[12] embryos. After logistic regression analysis the model identified the presence or absence of protein interleukin-6 (IL-6) and the duration of cc2 as the most relevant embryo features. Based on these results, the author developed a hierarchical model (*see* Flowchart 9.3) based on these two variables classifying embryos in four categories "A–D". IRs are expected to decrease as we move on from A to D as observed in this study (A = 88.8%, B = 66.6%, C = 57% and D = 33%).[40]

ANEUPLOIDY STUDIES

The correlation between euploidy and embryo kinetics has been studied as well (Table 9.5).

In 2010 Wong et al.,[18] collected single embryos for gene expression analysis and revealed that embryos with P1, P2, and P3 outside of the optimal ranges exhibited abnormal ribonucleic acid (RNA) patterns for embryo cytokinesis, microRNA (miRNA) biogenesis, and maternal messenger RNA

Table 9.5: Studies analyzing the correlation between euploidy and embryo kinetics.

Author	Study design	N^{er} embryos	Embryo origin	Time-lapse system	Predictive marker identified
Chavez et al. 2012	Research study	75	Freezed zygotes	Custom-built miniature microscope system	4 cells stage
Campbell et al. 2013	Retrospective study	98	PGD cycles	Embryoscope	tSB, tB
Campbell et al. 2013	Retrospective study	88	PGD cycles	Embryoscope	FHB, LB
Basile et al. 2014	Retrospective study	504	PGD cycles	Embryoscope	t5–t2, cc3
Rienzi et al. 2015	Longitudinal cohort study	455	PGD cycles	Embryoscope	No correlation
Chawla et al. 2015	Retrospective study	460	PGD cycles	Embryoscope	tPNf, t2, t5, cc2, cc3 and t5–t2
Vera-Rodri-guez et al. 2015	Retrospective study	85	PCR and PGD cycles	Embryoscope	PNd
Minasi et al. 2016	Retrospectively study	1730	PGD cycles	Embryoscope	t4, t4–t3, tSB, tB, tEB, tHB

(PCR: Polymerase chain reaction; PGD: Preimplantation genetic diagnosis).

(mRNA) reserve, suggesting that embryo fate may be predetermined and inherited very early in development (by the 4-cell stage).

Chavez et al.[45] subsequently observed that euploid embryos clustered tightly in the P1, P2, or P3 window that was predictive of blastocyst formation according to Wong's study. Performing further molecular analysis, the authors discovered that fragmentation dynamics, together with P1, P2 and P3, could potentially distinguish euploid from aneuploid embryos at the 4-cell stage considering that the fragments contained nuclear deoxyribonucleic acid (DNA), kinetochore proteins, and whole chromosomes as detected by fluorescence *in situ* hybridization (FISH).

In 2013, Campbell et al.[46] elaborated an aneuploidy risk model based on the differences of tSB and tB between euploid and aneuploid embryos that had undergone TE biopsy. The model includes three categories: (1) low-risk, tB less than 122.9 hpi and tSB less than 96.2 hpi, (2) medium-risk, tB less than 122.9 hpi and tSB 96.2 hpi, and (3) high-risk, tB 122.9 hpi.[36] The same group in a different study[47] applied this model to evaluate its effectiveness and potential clinical impact for unselected IVF patients without undergoing preimplantation genetic screening (PGS) after analyzing KID embryos. The study revealed significant differences in fetal heart rate (72.7; 25.5; 0) and live-birth rate (61.1; 19.2; 0) between the three categories low, medium and high respectively. This demonstrates that time-lapse imaging using defined morphokinetic data can be used to classify human preimplantation embryos according to their risk of aneuploidy, without performing biopsy and PGS, and that this correlates well with clinical outcomes.

The following year Basile et al.[48] also correlated morphokinetics with embryo aneuploidy based on 77 patients undergoing genetic screening due to recurrent miscarriage or implantation failure. In this case embryo biopsy was performed on day 3 of development and the total number of embryos analyzed was 504. A logistic regression analysis was used to select and organize which observed timing events (expressed as binary variables inside or outside the optimal range) were most relevant to select embryos with higher probability of being chromosomally normal. The model identified t5–t2 odds ratio (OR) = 2.853 (95% CI 1.763–4.616) followed by cc3 OR = 2.095 (95% CI 1.356–3.238) as the most relevant variables related to normal chromosomal content. An algorithm for embryo selection based on these two variables classifies embryos from A to D (Flowchart 9.4) with significant differences in the percentage of normal embryos as we move on from A to D. More specifically: A: 35.9%, B: 26.4%, C: 12.1%, and D: 9.8% (p< 0.001).

As opposed to the previous studies, Rienzi et al.[49] reported no correlation at all between 16 commonly detected morphokinetic parameters and embryo ploidy. This was a longitudinal cohort study conducted using 455 blastocysts from 138 patients at increased risk of aneuploidy because of advance maternal age, history of unsuccessful IVF treatments or both. The analyzed parameters included: t2, t3, t4, t5, t8, cc1, cc2, s2, s3, cc3, cc3 or cc2, t5–t2, syngamy, tSB, tSC and tB.

Flowchart 9.4: Algorithm by Basile et al. (2014).

In 2015 two studies observed correlations between embryo kinetics and euploidy. The first one, reported by Chawla et al.,[50] identified tPNf, t2, t5, cc2, cc3 and t5–t2 as parameters that significantly differed between chromosomally normal and abnormal embryos. The second one by Vera-Rodriguez et al.[51] combined chromosomal assessment and single cell quantitative reverse transcription polymerase chain reaction (RT-qPCR) to simultaneously obtain information from all the blastomeres of human embryos until approximately the 8-cell stage (n = 85). According to their results, the chromosomal status of aneuploid embryos (n = 26) correlates with significant differences in the duration of the first mitotic phase when compared with euploid embryos (n = 28). Moreover, gene expression profiling in this study suggested that a subset of genes is differentially expressed in aneuploid embryos during the first 30-hour of development.

In 2016 Minasi et al.,[52] in a retrospective study analyzed the morphology and morphokinetic of 1,730 blastocysts, obtained in 530 preimplantation genetic diagnosis (PGD) cycle. They found that the euploid blastocyst started to form, reached the full stage, expanded and hatched significantly faster, compared to aneuploid ones. Although there seems to be a relationship between the ploidy status and blastocyst morphology or development dynamic, the evaluation of morphological and morphokinetic parameters cannot currently be improved upon, and therefore replace, PGS.

However, time-lapse monitoring could be used in conjunction with PGS to choose, the blastocyst to analyzed or select that one that should be transferred.

RESEARCH STUDIES

We can use also kinetic markers and cleavage pattern to learn the behavior of the embryos until blastocyst stage.

Regarding ploidy, Grau et al.[53] described that half tripronucleated (TPN) ICSI-derived embryos became diploid during early *in vitro* development, whereas the other TPN embryos remained triploid. Regarding morphokinetics, Escrich et al.[54] reported that TPN embryos showed a delay at all the timings that cells cleaved at, except the cleavage timing to 5 cells, and significantly prolonged second and third cell cycles (cc2 and cc3, respectively) when compared to bipronucleated (BPN) embryos. However, once the ploidy of the TPN embryos was known, the TPN population was not homogeneous in most morphokinetic variables.

Taking this information into account, Grau et al.[55] showed that TPN embryos displayed different morphokinetic behavior according to ploidy; TPN self-corrected to diploidy were morphokinetically closer to correctly fertilized embryos, and morphokinetic variable t5 can predict their ploidy.

CONCLUSION

Static observations obtained from standard microscopes have contributed significantly to the knowledge of embryo development; however it is becoming more challenging to identify embryos with the highest implantation potential due to the static and notoriously subjective character of this type of morphological evaluation. The study of embryo kinetics through time-lapse technology has given rise to new markers for embryo selection representing a new and exciting powerful tool for viewing cellular activity and embryogenesis in a coherent and uninterrupted manner, otherwise not available through standard microscopy.

The present chapter presents an overview of the most recent studies that describe the use of this new technology in the IVF laboratory. It is our opinion that standard morphological assessment should remain the gold standard to initiate embryo evaluation; however, if possible, it should be complemented with the detection of kinetic markers known to improve clinical results. This new approach will allow the embryologist to perform a more accurate and objective embryo selection and therefore the goal of a SET slowly becomes more tangible.

REFERENCES

1. Meseguer M, Herrero J, Tejera A, et al. The use of morphokinetics as a predictor of embryo implantation. Hum Reprod. 2011;26(10):2658-71.
2. Mio Y, Maeda K. Time-lapse cinematography of dynamic changes occurring during in vitro development of human embryos. Am J Obstet Gynecol. 2008;199 (6):660.e1-5.
3. Gardner DK, Meseguer M, Rubio C, et al. Diagnosis of human preimplantation embryo viability. Hum Reprod Update. 2015;21(6):727-47.
4. Alpha Scientists in Reproductive Medicine and ESHRE Special Interest Group of Embryology. The Istanbul consensus workshop on embryo assessment: proceedings of an expert meeting. Hum Reprod. 2011;26(6):1270-83.

5. Baxter Bendus AE, Mayer JF, Shipley SK, et al. Interobserver and intraobserver variation in day 3 embryo grading. Fertil Steril. 2006;86(6):1608-15.

6. Kaser DJ, Racowsky C. Clinical outcomes following selection of human preimplantation embryos with time-lapse monitoring: a systematic review. Hum Reprod Update. 2014;20(5):617-31.

7. Paternot G, Wetzels AM, Thonon F, et al. Intra- and interobserver analysis in the morphological assessment of early stage embryos during an IVF procedure: a multicentre study. Reprod Biol Endocrinol. 2011;9:127.

8. Sundvall L, Ingerslev HJ, Breth Knudsen U, et al. Inter- and intra-observer variability of time-lapse annotations. Hum Reprod. 2013;28(12):3215-21.

9. Arce JC, Ziebe S, Lundin K, et al Interobserver agreement and intraobserver reproducibility of embryo quality assessments. Hum Reprod. 2006;21(8):2141-8.

10. Scott L. The biological basis of non-invasive strategies for selection of human oocytes and embryos. Hum Reprod Update. 2003;9(3):237-49.

11. Meseguer M, Rubio I, Cruz M, et al Embryo incubation and selection in a time-lapse monitoring system improves pregnancy outcome compared with a standard incubator: a retrospective cohort study. Fertil Steril. 2012;98(6):1481-9.e10.

12. Kirkegaard K, Ahlström A, Ingerslev HJ, et al. Choosing the best embryo by time lapse versus standard morphology. Fertil Steril. 2015;103(2):323-32.

13. Zhang JQ, Li XL, Peng Y, et al. Reduction in exposure of human embryos outside the incubator enhances embryo quality and blastulation rate. Reprod Biomed Online. 2010;20(4):510-5.

14. Payne D, Flaherty SP, Barry MF, et al. Preliminary observations on polar body extrusion and pronuclear formation in human oocytes using time-lapse video cinematography. Hum Reprod. 1997;12(3):532-41.

15. Basile N, Caiazzo M, Meseguer M. What does morphokinetics add to embryo selection and in-vitro fertilization outcomes? Curr Opin Obstet Gynecol. 2015;27(3):193-200.

16. Herrero J, Meseguer M. Selection of high potential embryos using time-lapse imaging: the era of morphokinetics. Fertil Steril. 2013;99(4):1030-4.

17. Ciray HN, Campbell A, Agerholm IE, et al. Proposed guidelines on the nomenclature and annotation of dynamic human embryo monitoring by a time-lapse user group. Hum Reprod. 2014;29(12):2650-60.

18. Wong CC, Loewke KE, Bossert NL, et al. Non-invasive imaging of human embryos before embryonic genome activation predicts development to the blastocyst stage. Nat Biotechnol. 2010;28(10):1115-21.

19. Hashimoto S, Kato N, Saeki K, et al. Selection of high-potential embryos by culture in poly(dimethylsiloxane) microwells and time-lapse imaging. Fertil Steril. 2012;97(2):332-7.

20. Hlinka D, Kalatová B, Uhrinová I, et al. Time-lapse cleavage rating predicts human embryo viability. Physiol Res. 2012;61(5):513-25.

21. Cruz M, Garrido N, Herrero J, et al. Timing of cell division in human cleavage-stage embryos is linked with blastocyst formation and quality. Reprod Biomed Online. 2012;25(4):371-81.

22. Chamayou S, Patrizio P, Storaci G, et al. The use of morphokinetic parameters to select all embryos with full capacity to implant. J Assist Reprod Genet. 2013;30(5):703-10.

23. Kirkegaard K, Kesmodel US, Hindkjaer JJ, et al. Time-lapse parameters as predictors of blastocyst development and pregnancy outcome in embryos from good prognosis patients: a prospective cohort study. Hum Reprod. 2013;28(10):2643-51.

24. Conaghan J, Chen AA, Willman SP, et al. Improving embryo selection using a computer-automated time-lapse image analysis test plus day 3 morphology: results from a prospective multicenter trial. Fertil Steril. 2013;100(2):412-9.e5.

25. Kirkegaard K, Campbell A, Agerholm I, et al. Limitations of a time-lapse blastocyst prediction model: a large multicentre outcome analysis. Reprod Biomed Online. 2014;29(2):156-8.

26. Cetinkaya M, Pirkevi C, Yelke H, et al. Relative kinetic expressions defining cleavage synchronicity are better predictors of blastocyst formation and quality than absolute time points. J Assist Reprod Genet. 2015;32(1):27-35.

27. Yang ST, Shi JX, Gong F, et al. Cleavage pattern predicts developmental potential of day 3 human embryos produced by IVF. Reprod Biomed Online. 2015;30(6):625-34.

28. Milewski R, Kuć P, Kuczyńska A, et al. A predictive model for blastocyst formation based on morphokinetic parameters in time-lapse monitoring of embryo development. J Assist Reprod Genet. 2015;32(4):571-9.

29. Storr A, Venetis CA, Cooke S, et al. Morphokinetic parameters using time-lapse technology and day 5 embryo quality: a prospective cohort study. J Assist Reprod Genet. 2015;32(7):1151-60.

30. Diamond MP, Suraj V, Behnke EJ, et al. Using the Eeva Test™ adjunctively to traditional day 3 morphology is informative for consistent embryo assessment within a panel of embryologists with diverse experience. J Assist Reprod Genet. 2015;32(1):61-8.

31. Motato Y, de los Santos MJ, Escriba MJ, et al. Morphokinetic analysis and embryonic prediction for blastocyst formation through an integrated time-lapse system. Fertil Steril. 2016;105(2):376-84.e9.

32. Aparicio-Ruiz B, Basile N, Pérez Albalá S, et al. Automatic time-lapse instrument is superior to single-point morphology observation for selecting viable embryos: retrospective study in oocyte donation. Fertil Steril. 2016;106(6):1379-85.e10.

33. Lemmen JG, Agerholm I, Ziebe S. Kinetic markers of human embryo quality using time-lapse recordings of IVF/ICSI-fertilized oocytes. Reprod Biomed Online. 2008;17(3):385-91.

34. Azzarello A, Hoest T, Mikkelsen AL. The impact of pronuclei morphology and dynamicity on live birth outcome after time-lapse culture. Hum Reprod. 2012; 27(9):2649-57.

35. Rubio I, Kuhlmann R, Agerholm I, et al. Limited implantation success of direct-cleaved human zygotes: a time-lapse study. Fertil Steril. 2012;98(6):1458-63.

36. Fréour T, Dessolle L, Lammers J, et al. Comparison of embryo morphokinetics after in vitro fertilization-intracytoplasmic sperm injection in smoking and nonsmoking women. Fertil Steril. 2013;99(7):1944-50.

37. Rubio I, Galán A, Larreategui Z, et al. Clinical validation of embryo culture and selection by morphokinetic analysis: a randomized, controlled trial of the EmbryoScope. Fertil Steril. 2014;102(5):1287-94.e5.

38. Goodman LR, Goldberg J, Falcone T, et al. Does the addition of time-lapse morphokinetics in the selection of embryos for transfer improve pregnancy rates? A randomized controlled trial. Fertil Steril. 2016;105(2):275-85.e10.

39. Aguilar J, Motato Y, Escribá MJ, et al. The human first cell cycle: impact on implantation. Reprod Biomed Online. 2014;28(4):475-84.

40. Basile N, Vime P, Florensa M, et al. The use of morphokinetics as a predictor of implantation: a multicentric study to define and validate an algorithm for embryo selection. Hum Reprod. 2015;30(2):276-83.

41. VerMilyea MD, Tan L, Anthony JT, et al. Computer-automated time-lapse analysis results correlate with embryo implantation and clinical pregnancy: a blinded, multi-centre study. Reprod Biomed Online. 2014;29(6):729-36.

42. Adamson GD, Abusief ME, Palao L, et al. Improved implantation rates of day 3 embryo transfers with the use of an automated time-lapse-enabled test to aid in embryo selection. Fertil Steril. 2016;105(2):369-75.e6.

43. Kirkegaard K, Ahlström A, Ingerslev HJ, et al. Choosing the best embryo by time lapse versus standard morphology. Fertil Steril. 2015;103(2):323-32.

44. Dominguez F, Meseguer M, Aparicio-Ruiz B, et al. New strategy for diagnosing embryo implantation potential by combining proteomics and time-lapse technologies. Fertil Steril. 2015;104(4):908-14.

45. Chavez SL, Loewke KE, Han J, et al. Dynamic blastomere behaviour reflects human embryo ploidy by the four-cell stage. Nat Commun. 2012;3:1251.

46. Campbell A, Fishel S, Bowman N, et al. Modelling a risk classification of aneuploidy in human embryos using non-invasive morphokinetics. Reprod Biomed Online. 2013;26(5):477-85.

47. Campbell A, Fishel S, Bowman N, et al. Retrospective analysis of outcomes after IVF using an aneuploidy risk model derived from time-lapse imaging without PGS. Reprod Biomed Online. 2013;27(2):140-6.

48. Basile N, Nogales Mdel C, Bronet F, et al. Increasing the probability of selecting chromosomally normal embryos by time-lapse morphokinetics analysis. Fertil Steril. 2014;101(3):699-704.

49. Rienzi L, Capalbo A, Stoppa M, et al. No evidence of association between blastocyst aneuploidy and morphokinetic assessment in a selected population of poor-prognosis patients: a longitudinal cohort study. Reprod Biomed Online. 2015;30(1):57-66.

50. Chawla M, Fakih M, Shunnar A, et al. Morphokinetic analysis of cleavage stage embryos and its relationship to aneuploidy in a retrospective time-lapse imaging study. J Assist Reprod Genet. 2015;32(1):69-75.

51. Vera-Rodriguez M, Chavez SL, Rubio C, et al. Prediction model for aneuploidy in early human embryo development revealed by single-cell analysis. Nat Commun. 2015;6:7601.

52. Minasi MG, Colasante A, Riccio T, et al. Correlation between aneuploidy, standard morphology evaluation and morphokinetic development in 1730 biopsied blastocysts: a consecutive case series study. Hum Reprod. 2016;31(10):2245-54.

53. Grau N, Escrich L, Martín J, et al. Self-correction in tripronucleated human embryos. Fertil Steril. 2011;96(4):951-6.

54. Escrich L, Grau N, Meseguer M, et al. Detailed kinetics and morphology analysis of human triplonucleated embryos: a comparison with correctly fertilized transferred embryos. Fertil Steril. 2013;28:171.

55. Grau N, Escrich L, Galiana Y, et al. Morphokinetics as a predictor of self-correction to diploidy in tripronucleated intracytoplasmic sperm injection-derived human embryos. Fertil Steril. 2015;104(3):728-35.

Chapter 10

Design, Equipment and Personnel Management

Irene Rubio Palacios, Javier Herrero Zapata

INTRODUCTION

The purpose of this chapter is to provide key aspects for the design of the ART unit, the necessary equipment and personnel management in terms of requirements and safety, based on the specific procedures that an ART unit can offer.

Designing an ART laboratory involves the consideration of many aspects, which can be encompassed into two groups. On the one hand, recommendations and obligations applicable at the time of designing the lab and providing proper facilities and equipment, on the other hand, the setting of specific objectives for the service being offered.[1] On the first group, laboratory set-up providing ART services would have to be setup as per the guidelines of the reproductive medicine societies of the respective nations.[9] Success of any ART unit mainly depends on the infrastructure of the laboratories and the formation of the personnel working. In this sense, a detailed layout and assessment of all laboratory furniture and equipment is essential prior to construction and can drastically improve the cost-benefit ratio. Regarding the personnel, authorized technical staff with a good theoretic background and proved experience and competence in the concerned specialty is critical for the well functioning of the unit.

LABORATORY

Laboratory Design

As described in the "European Society of Human Reproduction and Embryology (ESHRE) guidelines for good practice in *in vitro* fertilization (IVF) laboratories", a laboratory should have adequate space to follow good laboratory practice.[2] There are different key points that should be taken into account. The first step is to determine the estimated number of cycles the laboratory is expected to perform in a given time period. The second point to consider should be the design and organization of the laboratories, where the most recent developments in facilities, equipment and procedures should be considered. Immediately after, attention should be payed to embryologist or andrologist comfort in order to minimize risks to gametes by means of maximizing the efficiency and use of space.[3] To ensure an optimal handling of gametes during the treatment, there should be a dedicated andrology laboratory, an IVF laboratory with a different area dedicated to cryopreservation, and a separated area for the administrative work, such as record keeping and data entry. In those cases in which preimplantation genetic diagnosis (PGD) treatments are offered also, a separated laboratory should be included in the design.

Another important point is the location of each of the laboratories respect to the other areas. The semen collection room, if possible, adjacent to the andrology laboratory to facilitate the handling of the collected specimen. In fact, the ideal location of the andrology laboratory is between the semen collection room and the insemination room. The IVF laboratory must be adjacent to the operating room where the clinical procedures are performed. The cryopreservation area should be included in the core of the IVF but separated by walls to ensure proper isolation from the nitrogen sources and with visible access to the interior (via a window or camera). The cryostorage units should be continuously monitored and equipped with alarm systems detecting any out of range temperature and/or levels of liquid nitrogen (LN). All the staff dealing with LN should be trained in safety aspects of its use, and protection devices as glasses, cryogloves, etc. should be used during LN handling. The PGD laboratory, if any, should be also in a separated isolated room. It should be provided with a safety fume hood for analysis using fixatives and other toxic reagents. In addition, its isolation is crucial to prevent contamination during the tubing processes.

Regarding the laboratory building, the walls and ceiling should have absolute minimum number of penetrations. The materials used in laboratory construction, painting, flooring and furniture should be appropriate for clean room standards, minimizing volatile organic compounds (VOCs) release and embryo toxicity. The walls should reach the roof and be made of joint free stainless steel; covered with epoxy paint (no interior paint should contain materials like formaldehyde, acetaldehyde, benzene, etc.). Avoid false ceiling construction. Floor should be dust, crevices and crack free. It should be covered with large marble tiles, or granite tiles; alternately, with vitrified tiles. Bench surfaces should be resistant to acid, alkali, solvent and heat. Door will require seals and sweeps, and should be lockable. Another important issue is that electrical wearing should be concealed. Continuous power supply with power protection is essential. It is very important also to take into account that ducts and equipment must be laid out in such a way that routine and emergency maintenance and repair work can be performed outside the laboratory with minimum disruption.[4] Consideration should also be given to local health and safety requirements.

The location of storage areas and equipment, such as incubators, centrifuges and cryoequipment should be logically planned for efficiency and safety within each working area. It should have enough space to storage LN cylinders and tanks, disposables, media and other supplies. The laboratories design should ensure optimal workflow over minimal distances while handling reproductive cells during all treatment phases.

Laboratory designer must keep in mind that laboratory personnel has to work for long hours. It is essential to take into account aspects related to ergonomics, such as bench height, adjustable chairs, microscope eye height, efficient use of space and surfaces, sufficient air condition and the amount of daylight, all contribute to a working environment that minimizes distraction and fatigue.[3]

Laboratory Air Quality

During the *in vitro* culture of both gametes and embryos they are under a wide variety of artificial and stressful conditions as temperature and light variations, or changes in the percentage of oxygen (O_2) or carbon dioxide (CO_2) that could ultimately affect their viability. In addition to that, they are exposed also to substances that circumstantially will be present in their environment as dust particles, glass powder, plastic shavings, VOCs and disinfectants. All those conditions that potentially may affect the development of gametes and embryos can be minimized by the laboratories transformation into white rooms.

The maintenance of cleanliness is an uncompromising issue in a white room. Air should be clean, free of dust, smoke, gases and microbes. For that purpose, the clinic and hence the laboratories should be located away from traffic, dust and fumes. The air supply in the laboratory should be equipped with filters, preferably high efficiency particulate arrestance (HEPA) filters to minimize the airborne contamination, and VOC control.[3] To create a positive pressure is recommended also to minimize air contamination.

The access to the laboratories should be restricted to authorized personnel. All the individuals handling samples in the laboratory should change into clean clothes made up of cotton preferably, and wear slippers and non-powered gloves while working in the laboratory (and the rooms for changing clothes should be separate from the laboratory).[3]

A water source is also required for hand washing, ideally it should be located in a corner and deep enough to avoid splashing.[5]

As mentioned in the previous point, attention should be given to the operator comfort. In this sense, humidity and temperature should be completely controlled according to climate and seasonal variation. As a reference, the temperature of airflow within laboratory should be around 20–24°C and at less than 40% relative humidity.

EQUIPMENT

A detailed layout and assessment of all laboratory furniture is essential prior to construction in order to reach the best space achievement and create a distribution as more comfortable and functional as possible. Equipment should be suitably located in the laboratory to allow accessibility and sequential utilization, thus minimizing the need for frequent movement of specimens or reagents.

A detailed list of equipment should be prepared out and checked against the planned location of each item, and should be of adequate capacity to meet workload requirement and easy to disinfect and keep clean to avoid contamination. Also an automatic emergency backup power system must be in place for all critical equipment.

All the equipment must be validated as fit for its purpose, and the performance verified by calibrated instruments. Equipment should be in good working condition at all times; for this purpose, periodic inspection and cleaning should be done (the frequency will depend on the type of equipment); also a calibration check for all equipment using reference standards or reference material (Table 10.1). In fact, all the tasks related to equipment validation, calibration, maintenance and repair must be documented and records retained. Accepted ranges of use for all measured parameters should be determined and recorded. If measurements are out of range, corrections should be made and their effectiveness verified.[3]

For every item of equipment, the instruction manual and simplified instructions where needed, should be available. Laboratories should have necessary instructions for operation and maintenance of equipment in the form of standard operating procedures (SOPs) that should include also troubleshooting measures to be adopted for preventing equipment malfunction. In this sense, a copy of SOP should be readily available for the staff.[6]

Table 10.1: Parameters and verification frequency for the supervision of the laboratory equipment.

Equipment	Type of external measurement	Measurement frequency
Incubators	Carbon dioxide (CO_2) and T^a	Daily
Heating surfaces	Temperature	Daily
Heating blocks	Temperature	Daily
Freezers and refrigerators	Temperature	Daily
Automatic pipettes	Volume	Annual
Cryotanks	Temperature	Daily

Incubators

The incubator number is critical and should be based on the number of cycles and embryo culture duration. As a general rule, gametes and embryos should be conveniently distributed across incubators to minimize door openings, hence to maintain stable culture conditions.

- *Working incubators:* Adjusted to 35–37°C and 5–6% CO_2; to be used for the storage of bicarbonate-based media and as working incubators when handling gametes and embryos. The number will depend on the workload but it is advisable to have at least one in the IVF laboratory, one in the cryoroom and one in the andrology laboratory. There is a high variety of models available in the market, i.e. Penguin from Astec, Heracell from Thermo Fisher Scientific™, LabX from Sanyo, Cell Culture™ from ESCO, Galaxy from Eppendorf, etc.
- *Culture incubators:* Adjusted to 35–37°C and 5–6% CO_2 or those designed to work in hypoxia at 6%; to be used for the culture of gametes and embryos. Any of the previous mentioned could be used for this purpose but there are other incubators with different characteristics that could be included in this group. Those adjusted to low-oxygen culture conditions could be either because of the Tri-gas use (i.e. MINC from COOK) or the N_2 use (miriESCO from ESCO) (Figs. 10.1A to F). There is another group of culture incubators that include time-lapse technology: the possibility of recording the development of the gametes or embryos. Part of them are devices to be included in regular incubators, hence the culture conditions (hypoxia or normoxia) will depend on the "external" incubator (i.e. Primo Vision™ from Vitrolife or Eeva from Auxogyn). The other type includes independent incubators with in-built cameras in which the culture conditions are autonomously decided (i.e. EmbryoScope from Vitrolife or Geri from Genea Biomedx).

Heating Devices

Those should be installed to maintain the temperature of media and reproductive cells during handling (Figs. 10.2A to D).

- *Laboratory ovens:* Adjusted to 35–37°C without CO_2 for liquefaction of semen samples and warming of buffered media and mineral oil (this can be used in both the IVF and andrology laboratories) (i.e. Thermo Scientific™ Precision™ from Thermo Fisher Scientific or the High Temperature Laboratory Oven from Bio Technics India)
- *Block heaters or dry bath incubators with heating blocks:* Adjusted to 35–37°C; to be used during the oocytes pick up (OPU) to maintain the temperature of the follicular fluid before the oocyte cumulus complex screening. Usually those are present inside the operating theater (OT)

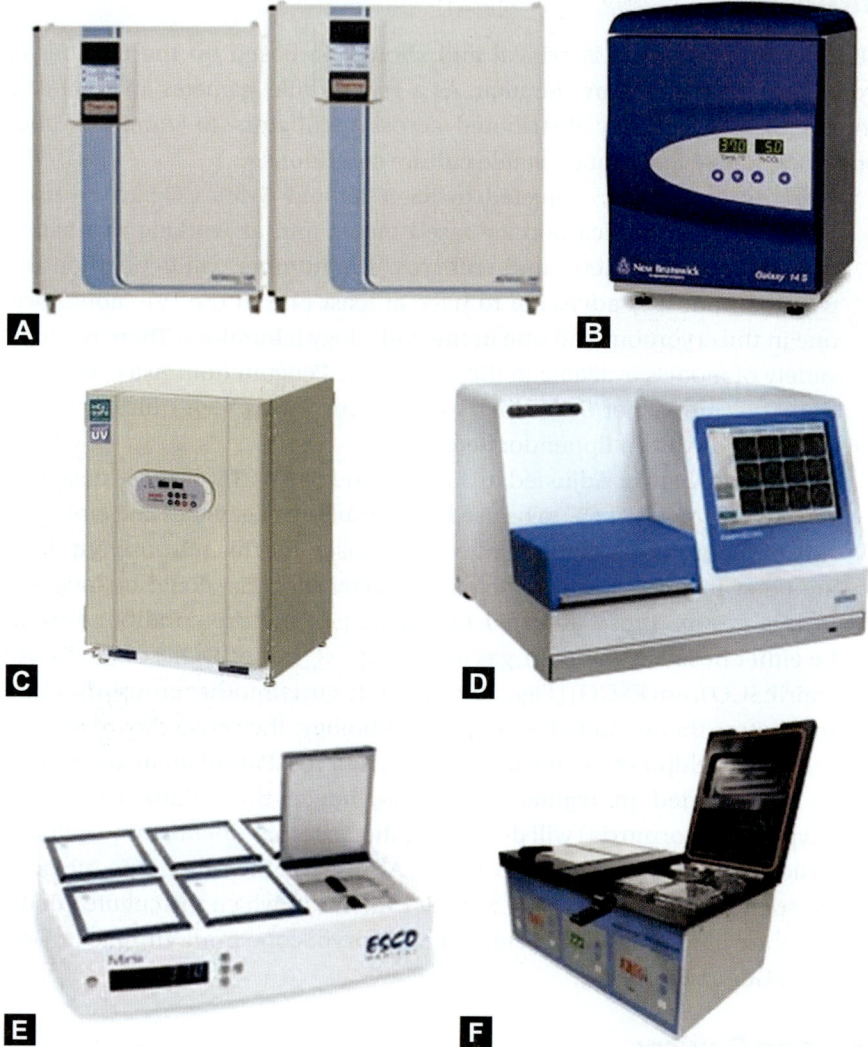

Figs. 10.1A to F: Different types of incubators used in an assisted reproductive technology (ART) laboratory. (A) Heracell from Thermo Fisher Scientific; (B) Galaxy from Eppendorf; (C) LabX from Sanyo; (D) EmbryoScope from Vitrolife; (E) MiriESCO from ESCO; and (F) MINC from COOK.

and in the pass box that ideally communicates it with the IVF laboratory (i.e. G73 Dry Bath Incubator from K-systems or the Tube Warmer from IVF Tech).

Gas Cylinders

Those should be located outside of the laboratory. There should be an automatic change-over system and sufficient cylinders stocked for immediate

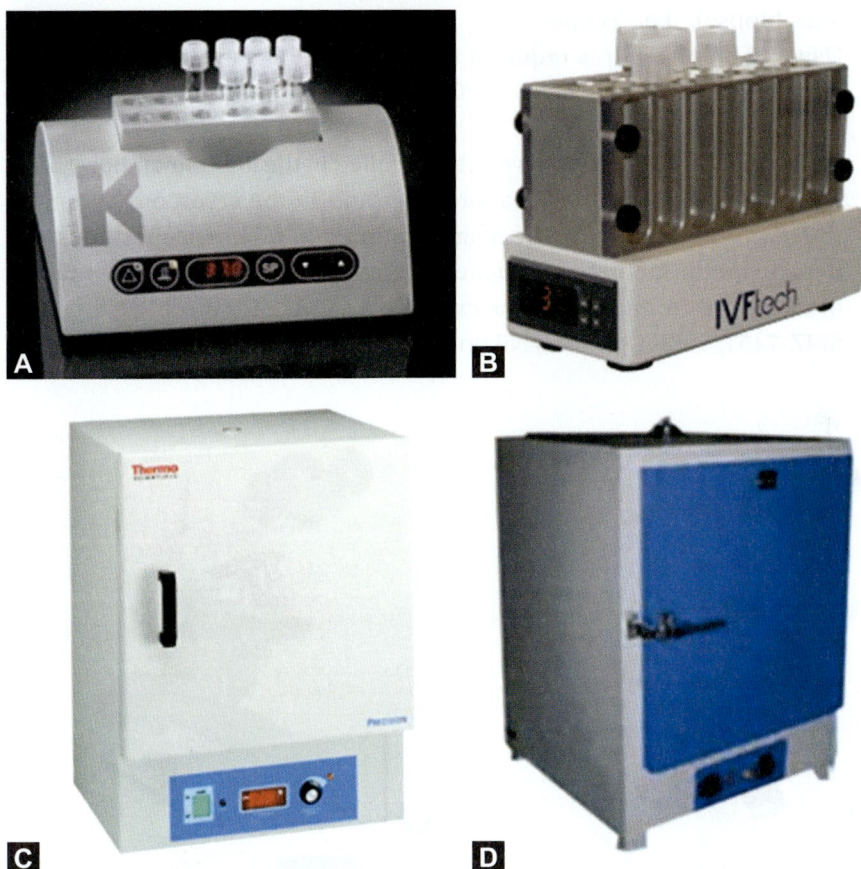

Figs. 10.2A to D: Different types of heating devices used in an assisted reproductive technology (ART) laboratory. (A) G73 Dry Bath Incubator from K-systems; (B) Tube Warmer from IVF Tech; (C) Thermo Scientific™ Precision™ from Thermo Fisher Scientific; and (D) High Temperature Laboratory Oven from Bio Technics India.

replacement. High-purity gas and inline HEPA and VOC filters are highly recommended.

Microscopes and Stereomicroscopes

- Binocular phase contrast microscope with 20x, 40x and 100x objectives and 10x eyepiece for the andrology laboratory (semen analysis: sperm count, motility and morphology). Oil immersion lens should be available, and if possible, also photography or video camera attached if training is desired, i.e. Olympus CX21 or Nikon Eclipse E200.
- Inverted microscope with 4x, 10x, 20x and 40x objectives and heating stage for the IVF laboratory (for oocyte and embryo assessment, microinjection

and biopsy), i.e. Eclipse Ti-U from Nikon or IX73 from Olympus (Figs. 10.3A to D). It is required to add a heating stage to maintain the temperature constant at 35–37°C (i.e. glass or metallic Tokai heating stage).

- *Stereomicroscopes:* These have to be installed in the laminar air flow (LAF) hoods of the IVF and PGD laboratories and in the cryoroom to handle the oocytes or embryos. The magnification and other specifications will depend on the laboratory designer discretion. There are different models available in the market as for example SZX10, SZ61 from Olympus or SMZ-745T, SMZ-1270 from Nikon.

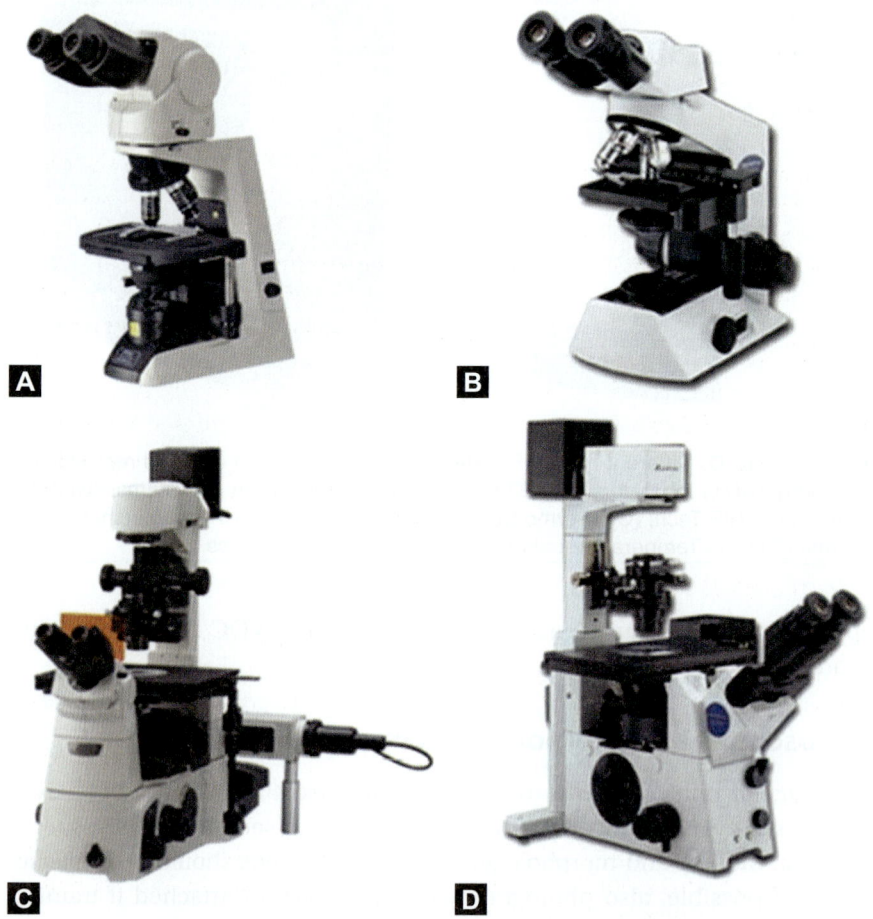

Figs. 10.3A to D: Different types of microscopes used in an assisted reproductive technology (ART) laboratory. (A) Nikon Eclipse E200; (B) Olympus CX21; (C) Eclipse Ti-U from Nikon; and (D) IX73 from Olympus.

Injection System

The injection system as to be installed in the inverted microscope and it is highly recommended placing the whole station over an antivibration table to provide stability during the microinjection or biopsy procedures. There are different models available in the market but mainly all consist into: Four-axis Hanging Joystick Micromanipulators, adaptor for the microscope (usually they are available for the main microscope brands), injectors (pneumatic/air or oil systems) and injection holders. The most common systems are from Narishige, Eppendorf, Research Instrument (RI), etc. (Fig. 10.4).

If PGD procedures are performed in the IVF laboratory, the micro-manipulation system will require the attachment of a laser for the embryo biopsy. Basically laser systems can be fixed or portable. There are different fixed systems, being the most commonly used Laser Shot or NaviLase from Octax, regarding portable laser probably the most commonly used is the one from Hamilton Thorne.

Laminar Air Flow Hoods

A laminar flow hood is recommended. The hood reduces contamination of the samples as well as offering protection to laboratory personnel. A laminar flow hood can be either a vertical or a horizontal flow. Vertical flow is less harmful to the laboratory workers as the airflow is not directly aimed at their faces. On the other hand, a horizontal flow is more effective in reducing contamination. In any case, they should include HEPA filters to provide a particle free work environment and should have a heated stage to maintain the temperature of the samples handled constant at 37°C. The only LAF hoods that do not need to be with heated stage are those destined to vitrification or thawing procedures, media preparation and tubing after embryo biopsy. The desired stereomicroscopes have to be built-in as under them will happen the manipulation of samples (Figs. 10.5A to C).

Fridges and Freezers

Laboratory refrigerators and freezers are generally used for storing culture and buffer media, and nonvolatile biological specimens with temperature ranges from +2°C to +15°C (in case of refrigerators) and from −10°C to −40°C (in case of freezers).

Nitrogen Tanks

There are several items related with the cryopreservation procedures that should be present in both the cryopreservation area of the IVF laboratory and the andrology laboratory.
- *Liquid nitrogen storage containers:* Specific tanks to storage the nitrogen in liquid phase for the vitrification procedures. There are different brands and sizes available (depending on the nitrogen volume to storage),

Micromanipulation station

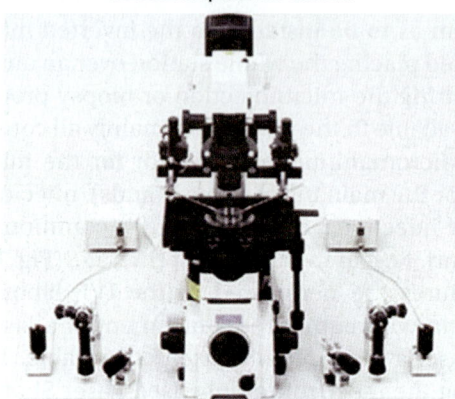

Microinjectors

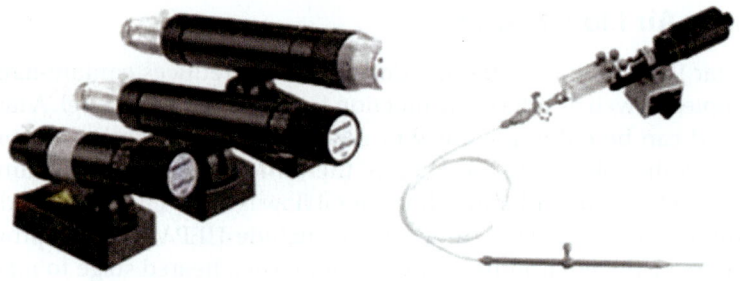

Micromanipulation system

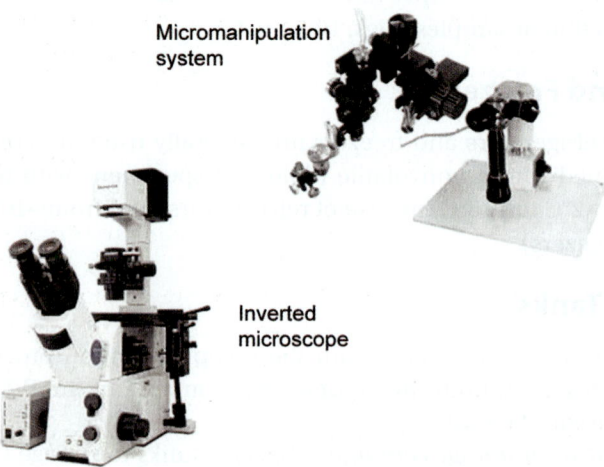

Inverted microscope

Fig. 10.4: Different components of a micromanipulation station.

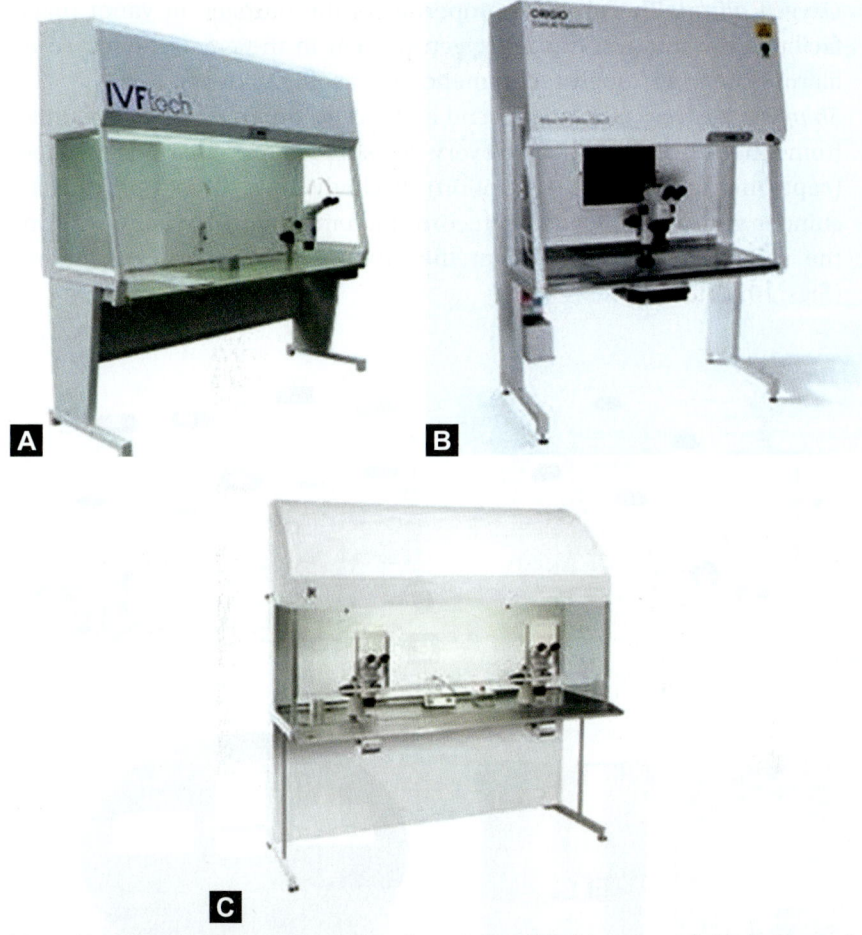

Figs. 10.5A to C: Different types of laminar air flow (LAF) hoods available in the market. (A) IVF Tech Sterile Cabinet, from IVF Tech; (B) Fortuna Clean Air from Origio; and (C) L125 IVF workstation from K-systems.

and can be complemented with semiautomatic or manual bombs and dispensers.

- *Frozen sample containers:* Specific tanks to storage the samples once frozen or vitrified. There are containers in which the samples are stored in LN and others (called dry containers) in which they are immersed in nitrogen in vapor phase. The choice should be based on each laboratory necessities, capacities and expected use. It is strongly advised to provide each tank with a nitrogen level or temperature sensor. The first one measures the level of nitrogen and the alarm is activated when the level decreases below a certain preset level; the temperature sensor detects the decrease of temperature below a certain preset level also so ultimately both ensure the triggering of the alarm when the samples are under risk.

- *Oxygen alarm:* The physical properties of the nitrogen in vapor phase facilitate the removal of the oxygen present in the environment, so an alarm system is strongly recommended to avoid accidents.
- *Shippers:* It is very frequent to send and receive frozen or vitrified samples from other clinics or banks, so every unit should have at least one shipper (vapor nitrogen is the best option). It is advisable also to provide the shipper with a data logger to record the temperature variations during the shipment and ensure that they have been properly maintained (Figs. 10.6A to E).

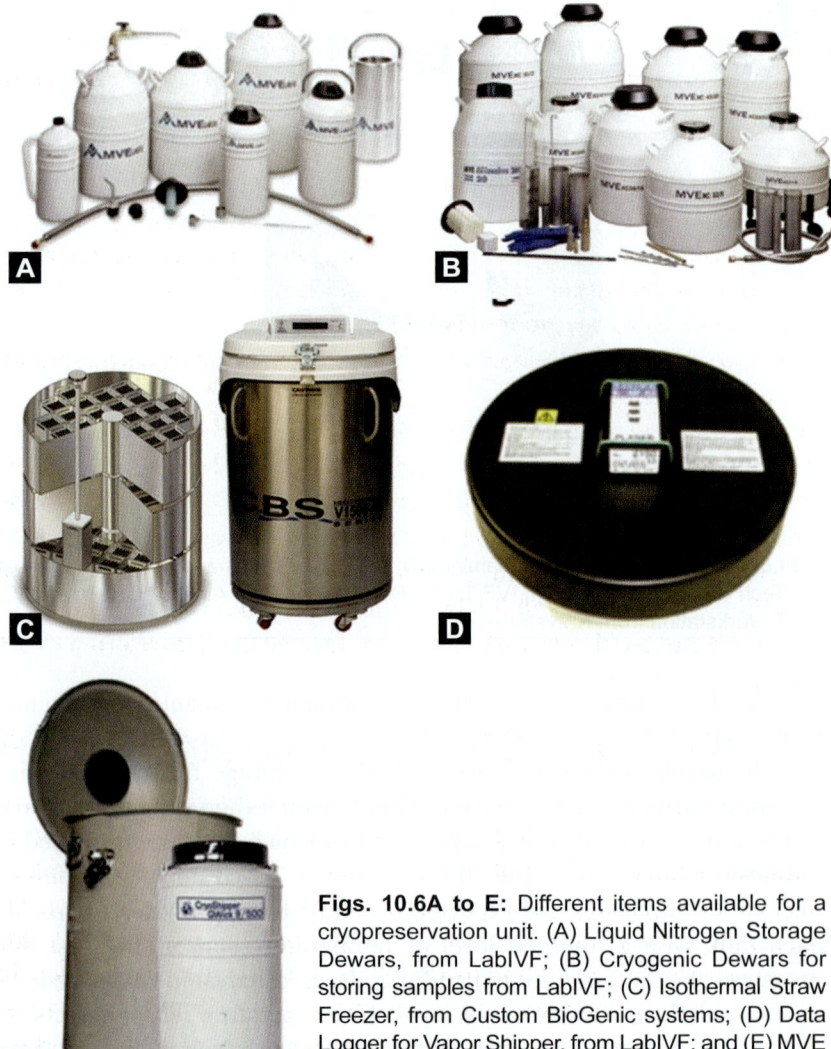

Figs. 10.6A to E: Different items available for a cryopreservation unit. (A) Liquid Nitrogen Storage Dewars, from LabIVF; (B) Cryogenic Dewars for storing samples from LabIVF; (C) Isothermal Straw Freezer, from Custom BioGenic systems; (D) Data Logger for Vapor Shipper, from LabIVF; and (E) MVE CryoShipper QWick, from LabIVF.

Small Items

- A bench centrifuge for sperm processing with a rotor (calibrated in g or in revolutions per minute) and a timer, to control the speed and time (andrology laboratory)
- Micropipettors 10–100 μL, 20–200 μL, 100–1,000 μL, automatic pipettor (andrology, and IVF laboratories, cryoroom and PGD units)
- Test tube racks to place the sample tubes (andrology, and IVF laboratories, cryoroom and PGD units)
- Sperm counting chamber, such as Neubauer or Mackler (andrology laboratory)
- Spirit burners (andrology and IVF laboratories)
- Laboratory counter, to make easier the counting of the semen samples moreover in laboratories with a large volume of work (andrology laboratory)
- Calculator
- Thermometers for both incubators or heater and fridges or freezer (andrology, and IVF laboratories, cryoroom and PGD units)
- *Timer:* It is used for control the time incubation of the sample, indicating the end of the processing. It is used also during the freezing or vitrification procedures (andrology laboratory and cryoroom)
- Protective gloves and glasses for the nitrogen related activities (cryoroom and andrology laboratory)
- Dustbins for the safe disposal of biological and laboratory materials; they can be recipients made of paperboard, plastic sharped containers or waste plastic bags, always with the international "biohazard" symbol. If possible, glassware should be omitted in the laboratory, otherwise the Pasteur pipettes and broken glassware should be discarded in special containers (andrology, and IVF laboratories, cryoroom and PGD units)
- Computer, preferably networked, to introduce all the date referred to the patient's sample.[4,5,7]

CONSUMABLES AND MEDIA

In the laboratory, all supplies and materials should be sterile single-use and disposable, and must be tested also by the supplier as being nontoxic to gametes and embryos. This aspect is fundamental to prevent contamination and makes the whole process as safe as possible minimizing the risks. If appropriate quality control testing for IVF purposes is not provided, this must be performed by the laboratory itself or by a designated company. In addition, packaging integrity and appropriate delivery conditions must be checked. Documentation of quality control testing must be supplied for any commercial media and this must correspond with the delivered batch.[3]

Most consumables and media have more than one manufacturer and model but the specific branch to be used depends on costs, preference of laboratory and medical personnel, location of the manufacturer, and the availability of after-sales service.

The essential consumables include tips, pipettes, round bottom test tubes, conical bottom tubes, culture dishes, injection dishes, injection, holding and biopsy pipettes, denudation tips, pH test paper, slides and coverslips, intrauterine insemination (IUI) catheters, embryo transfer (ET) catheters, OPU needles, BD syringes and semen containers; also stains and jars to stain the slides for morphology assessment. Specific disposables for vitrification or freezing procedures have to be considered also. Gloves to be used in the IVF unit should ideally be powder-free.

Respect to media, the best option for IVF laboratories is to purchase buffer solutions and media that are sterile and already cell culture tested. Today it is uncommon for each laboratory prepares their own media, as the commercial ones offer all the necessary guarantees and are optimized to the maximum. These are easily available, nontoxic, tested for quality control and have consistent performance. The commonly used media are simple balanced salt solutions or complex solutions supplemented with proteins, vitamins, glucose and antibiotics, but can be supplemented with two different types of buffer. It can be supplemented with 4-(2-hydroxyethyl)-1-piperazineethanesulfonic acid (HEPES) buffer (when exposed to atmosphere, it maintains the pH between 7.2 and 7.4, so these media do not require CO_2 incubation to maintain pH) or bicarbonate buffer (it requires a 5% CO_2 atmosphere to maintain the pH between 7.2 and 7.4).[5]

Cryopreservation requires a ready supply of LN and its own special supplies and media.

The size of the bottles and other packaging must be appropriate to minimize openings and time between first and last use.[3]

Appropriate refrigeration facilities must be available for storage of media and reagents. The correct temperature during their shipment to the clinic should be verified. Repeated shifts of temperature should be avoided while handling in the laboratory.[3]

An appropriate stock management system for media, oil and consumables, including the batch number, date of entry and expiration date should be available.[3] Each batch of culture media should be tested before use for osmolarity. Media pH testing should be performed following equilibration with CO_2 at concentrations used for assisted reproductive technology (ART) procedures. All lots of media and media components should be recorded and traceable to each patient procedure.[8]

Reagents, media and consumables should always be used prior to the manufacturer's expiry date.[3]

PERSONNEL MANAGEMENT

Personnel are one of the most important parts of an IVF laboratory. Staff resources shall be adequate to carry out all the procedures and functions in the laboratory according to the level of facility and the workload. The ESHRE recommends that clinics that perform up to 150 retrievals and/or cryopreservation cycles per year should have always a minimum number of two qualified clinical embryologists. This initial number will increase depending not only on the number of treatments, but also on the complexity of the procedures, techniques and tasks undertaken within the laboratory. Other duties such as administration, training, education, quality management and communication also need consideration.[3] The American Society for Reproductive Medicine (ASRM) coincides on the same ratios: always a minimum of two qualified clinical embryologists and increasing according to the number of cycles (Table 10.2).[8]

Appropriate human resources should provide an adequate climate to perform all laboratory tasks in a timely manner, to ensure patient safety and quality care. Sufficient qualified personnel should be available to provide backup for the laboratory staff.[3]

The hierarchical laboratory organization depends on staff size (larger facilities will need to delegate responsibilities to different levels). A person with officially recognized qualifications and expertise in clinical embryology and biological or medical sciences should direct the laboratory. According to the Guidelines for Good Clinical Laboratory Practices (GCLP) from the Indian Council of Medical Research (ICMR) each laboratory should designate a Head of the laboratory who should be overall incharge of the daily functioning of the laboratory including administration.[6] A quality manager should be designated for monitoring and maintaining of day-to-day quality management system (QMS). This laboratory manager shall have an organizational plan, personnel policies and job descriptions to define responsibility and authority of all personnel. Clinical embryologists represent the first line of participation in daily clinical practice. Their responsibilities include execution of SOPs, participation in daily practice, communication and

Number of cycles	Minimum number of embryologists
1–150	2
151–300	3
301–600	4
>600	1 additional embryologist per additional 200 cycles

Table 10.2: Recommended staff according to volume.

organization, contribution to laboratory clinical decisions and training of staff members and students.[3]

A program for technical training and updating of skills on a regular basis should be in place. Laboratory management should be committed for providing continuing professional development and training opportunities to staff. Action plan for improvement in the laboratory should be determined and revised according to the feedback received from previous trainings and experiences, as reflected in the International Organization for Standardization (ISO) 15189:2007 and document 112 of National Accreditation Board for Testing and Calibration Laboratories (NABL).[9]

Qualification level and experience required of the staff are also specified in the latter document.

The roles and responsibilities of the staff should be also clearly outlined, even more, policies defining the competency of each person to perform tasks such as using the computer system, access to patient data, enter and charge patient results or correct billing shall be established. However, all personnel shall maintain confidentiality of information and data regarding patients.

Laboratory should organize or conduct periodic staff evaluation, preferably, once a year, but the frequency and method of evaluation should be decided by the laboratory.

LABORATORY SAFETY AND INFECTION CONTROL

As a general rule, procedures and policies on laboratory safety must be available to all laboratory personnel and should be reviewed annually by the laboratory director. The following guidelines are recommended:

- All patient worksheets should have clear patient identifying information as well as laboratory accession numbers that uniquely identify the patient during related procedures. All disposable material used during the preparation of the sample should be properly labeled or identified
- Disposable, and nontoxic (nonpowdered) gloves should be worn when handling fresh or frozen semen samples or any material that has come in contact with them. Gloves should be removed and discarded when leaving the laboratory or handling the telephone. Gloves should never be reused
- Hands should be washed after removing gowns and gloves and immediately if they become contaminated with body fluids. All hand washing should be done with body fluids. All hand washing should be done with disinfectant soap and hot water or alcohol-based solutions
- A laboratory coat or appropriate gown should be worn in the laboratory and removed upon leaving the laboratory
- Safety glasses or goggles are suggested where appropriated

- Disposable laboratory supplies must be used whenever possible
- All discarded body fluid samples and disposable laboratory supplies should be disposed of properly in a container marked "biological hazard" and disposed of accordingly
- Protocols should be available for fire and electrical safety and internal and external disaster preparedness (including provisions for equipment backup in the event of equipment failure)
- Mechanical pipetting devices should be used for the manipulation of liquids in the laboratory. Mouth pipetting is never permitted
- Eating, drinking and smoking are not permitted in the laboratory
- Use of cosmetics should be minimized and perfumes should be avoided.

Infectious Agents

All ARTs involve handling of biological material, and pose a potential hazard of transmitting diseases to personnel and to other patient's biological material (cross-contamination).

- Vaccination of all personnel against hepatitis B or other viral diseases, for which vaccine is available, is recommended
- All patients must be screened for infectious diseases according to national and international regulations
- Staff must be informed when a viral-positive patient is to be treated and be aware of the risks of handling infected biological material
- Extraordinary precautions should be taken to avoid accidental wounds from sharp instruments contaminated with body fluids. Accident/incident/injuries record of laboratory personnel should be maintained and reported to the designated authority. The report should include description of the event, factors contributing to the event and information on first aid or other health care provided. This information can be analyzed periodically toward effectively controlling and preventing future events
- Contaminated laboratory equipment and/or work surfaces should be disinfected and sterilized after a spill.[8]
- To ensure adequate safety measures, the treatment of viral-positive patients should be only performed in IVF laboratories with dedicated areas and equipment. Alternatively, such patient treatments could be allocated to specific time slots provided processing of their biological is followed by a thorough disinfection of the allocated areas and equipment.

RECORD MAINTENANCE

Records may include but not limited to request forms, report results, staff training, quality control records, audit records, examination procedures, instruments printout, interlaboratory comparison or management reviews and SOPs.

The laboratory shall establish and implement policies and procedures for identification, indexing, access, storage and overall control of the registers. Records shall be legible and stored in a suitable environment to prevent damage, loss or unauthorized access but they should be retrievable in any moment.

The laboratory shall decide the retention time of records as per the national, regional and local regulations. However, NABL requires following minimum retention time for ensuring the quality service and patient care. The minimum period for retention of IUI related test reports issued shall be 1 year.[9]

QUALITY MANAGEMENT SYSTEM

Working in compliance with a QMS is mandatory and it is the mechanism to review the quality of all factors involved in laboratory functioning. It is recommended that a clinical embryologist is made responsible for quality management within the laboratory.

The requirements cover the organization, management personnel, equipment and materials, facilities or premises, documentation, records and quality review. This includes:

- Defining responsibilities and ensuring all personnel are qualified and competent
- Having validated, and written instructions for each process (SOP) in order to optimize outcomes, including management of adverse events. The laboratory director or designated supervisory personnel should review and update all procedures on at least an annual basis. Any changes must be approved, signed and dated by the laboratory director or by designated proxy
- Ensuring full traceability of cells and tissues, materials, equipment and personnel involved in specific laboratory activities, with records maintained accordingly
- Ensuring proper and periodic equipment maintenance, service and calibration. It should include aspects referred to equipment maintenance and calibration, validation and documentation of new protocols, vendor certification of media batch, safety laboratory procedures and record maintenance. Moreover, a written procedure manual must be readily available and followed by laboratory personnel
- Taking corrective action to keep procedures under conformity
- All relevant data concerning laboratory work must be recorded in a database that allows key performance indicator (KPI) extraction and statistical analysis. Corrections, either written or electronic, should be traceable. Data should include
- Morphological characteristics of gamete and embryos

- Detailed information of the procedures, including timing and staff involved
- All information needed to comply with the requirements of national and international data registries
- Every relevant communication with the patients should be recorded in the patient's files or in the informatics system
- Key performance indicators should be objective and relevant, regularly checked and discussed, and communicated to all staff. For each indicator incorporated, a threshold needs to be established for setting the critical level of quality laboratory performance. These markers may concern a wide variety of parameters such as technical aspects of the laboratory (e.g. temperature of working surfaces, percentage of CO_2 in incubators or pH in culture media) or clinical variables (e.g. concerning percentage of progressive mobile spermatozoa recovered per sample or gestational rates by group of analysis)
- In addition to laboratory and clinical performance, operator performance should be checked regularly to ensure competence, compliance and consistency, via direct observation of procedural skills (DOPSs) and/or individual KPIs. If necessary, retraining should be implemented
- Participation in internal quality control (IQC) and external quality assurance (EQA) programs, either commercial or in collaboration with other laboratories, is highly recommended. IQC records should be maintained and reviewed, including documentation of results and any corrective action
- An audit system, both internal and external, must be in place. An independent, competent auditor should verify compliance of all procedures with SOPs and requirements. Any findings, corrective actions and their effectiveness must be documented.[3,9]

CONCLUSION

The important components that make a laboratory great are the people, procedure, equipment and the laboratory design. All those aspects are fundamental to provide a service catalogued as excellent to fullfill patient's expectations.

REFERENCES

1. Pai RD. Pai's Textbook of Intrauterine Insemination. New Delhi: Jaypee Brothers Medical Publishers (P) Ltd; 2011. pp. 39-54.
2. Gianaroli L, Plachot M, van Kooij R, et al. ESHRE guidelines for good practice in IVF laboratories. Committee of the Special Interest Group on Embryology of the European Society of Human Reproduction and Embryology. Hum Reprod. 2000;15(10):2241-6.
3. De los Santos MJ, Apter S, Coticchio G, et al. Revised guidelines for good practice in IVF laboratories (2015). The ESHRE Guideline Group on Good Practice in IVF Labs. Hum Reprod. 2016;31(4):685-6.

4. Mahmud N, Malhotra N, Malhotra J. Manual on IUI. What, When and Why. New Delhi: Jaypee Brothers Medical Publishers (P) Ltd; 2013. pp. 12-23.
5. Mukherjee GG, Chakravarty BN. Intrauterine Insemination. New Delhi: Jaypee Brothers Medical Publishers (P) Ltd; 2012. pp. 62-75.
6. Indian Council of Medical Research (ICMR). Guidelines for Good Clinical Laboratory Practices (GCLP), 2008. [online] Available from www.icmr.nic.in/guidelines/GCLP.pdf. [Accessed March, 2017].
7. Mukherjee GG, Chakravarty BN. Intrauterine insemination. In: Shah R (Ed). Infertility Management Series. New Delhi: Jaypee Brothers Medical Publishers (P) Ltd; 2015. pp. 115-34.
8. Practice Committee of American Society for Reproductive Medicine, Practice Committee of Society for Assisted Reproductive Technology. Revised guidelines for human embryology and andrology laboratories. Fertil Steril. 2008;90 (5 Suppl):S45-59.
9. National Accreditation Board for Testing and Calibration Laboratories (NABL). Specific Criteria for Accreditation of Medical Laboratories., 2012 [online] Available from www.nabl-india.org/nabl/file_download.php?filename=201210 170522-NABL-112-doc.pdf. [Accessed March, 2017].

Chapter 11

Future Perspectives: Developing Gametes from Stem Cells

José V Medrano, Carlos Simón

INTRODUCTION

Regenerative medicine is an emerging multidisciplinary field that comprises knowledge from cellular biology, developmental biology, genetics, molecular biology and tissue engineering, aiming to the study of stem cells and their potential clinical application to regenerate tissues and organs.

Among the multiple translational applications of regenerative medicine, the study of stem cells for their use in reproductive medicine has achieved significant progress in the last years. In particular, the use of animal models for the study of germ cell development, together with a significant improvement of current knowledge of human germ cell biology, recently achieved thanks to the access to early human embryos for research purposes, has allowed an important step forward in the possibility of obtaining human functional gametes from different cell sources that convert this promise in a reality that is closer than ever (Flowchart 11.1).

Here, we will discuss the different approaches and applications that regenerative medicine is currently developing in order to offer a solution to infertile patients aiming to have genetically matched children.

PLURIPOTENT STEM CELLS (ESCs AND IPSCs) AS A SOURCE OF HUMAN FUNCTIONAL GAMETES

The potential use of mouse embryonic stem cells (mESCs) as a source of gametes was first reported in 2003 when some oocyte-like structures able to achieve parthenogenetic activation and form pseudoblastocysts were spontaneously formed upon culture of mESCs without feeders nor leukemia inhibitory factor (LIF).[1] Upon this first probe of concept, a variety of strategies have been reported to achieve the formation of both male and female gametes from mESCs and induced pluripotent stem cells (iPSCs) with disparaging results.[2-7]

However, the real functionality of these *in vitro* generated gametes was not demonstrated until very recently when a Japanese group achieved for the first time the generation of viable offspring from sperm and oocytes

Flowchart 1: Schematic diagram of the circuitry of different approaches that regenerative medicine offers for the development of gametes.

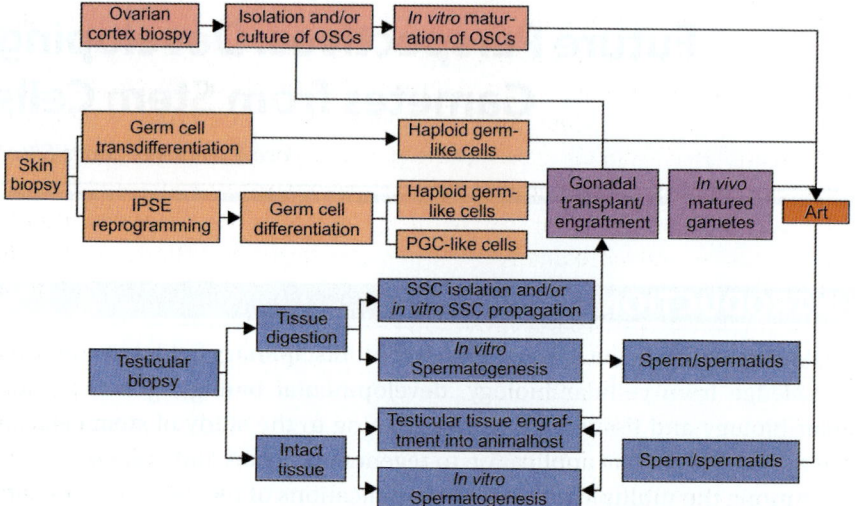

(ART: Assisted reproductive technology; iPSC: Induced pluripotent stem cell; OSCs: Ovarian stem cells; PGC: Primordial germ cell; SSC: Spermatogonial stem cell).

derived from mESCs and iPSCs.[8,9] In their experiments, authors based in the unique potential of epiblastic cells to give rise to primordial germ cells (PGCs) in response to bone morphogenetic proteins 4 (BMPs4) and BMP8b secreted from the adjacent extraembryonic ectoderm (ExE) at embryonic day 6.25 (E6.25) *in vivo*.[10,11] Based on this, they designed an *in vitro* induction protocol to induce naive mESCs and iPSCs cultured in 2i + LIF conditions into epiblast-like cells (EpiLCs) resembling their *in vivo* counterparts by treating them with activin A and basic fibroblast growth factor (bFGF). Subsequently, in a second induction step, EpiLCs were exposed to LIF, stem cell factor (SCF), epidermal growth factor (EGF) and BMP4 or 8b to trigger the acquisition of a PGC-like cell (PGCLC). Resulting PGCLCs showed a phenotype resembling *in vivo* mouse PGCs, including the expression of key PGC markers, but also signs of epigenetic reprogramming including genome-wide demethylation, loss of H3K9me2 and gain of H3K27me3, as their *in vivo* counterparts. Moreover, PGCLCs were able to differentiate either into sperm or germinal vesicle oocytes when transplanted into the mouse testicular lumen or under the ovarian bursa in reconstituted mouse ovaries that produced healthy and fertile offspring upon intracytoplasmic sperm injection (ICSI). These works were complemented by a third report of the same group showing that the ectopic expression of the key transcription factors downstream of BMP signaling Prdm1, Prdm14 and Tfap2c over preinduced mouse EpiLCs resulted also in a PGCLC phenotype that formed sperm and gave rise to healthy offspring after transplantation into mouse testes.[12] In summary, these three complementary reports demonstrated for the first time the possibility to create functional gametes from pluripotent cells. At the same time, they described the regulatory signaling network of mouse PGC specification, where Prdm1, Prdm14 and AP2γ together constitute a transcriptional network necessary to enable the repression of somatic genes by Prdm1 and Prdm14 blocking of Hox enhancers, the expression of pluri-potency and PGC-specific genes (executed mainly by Prdm14 and AP2γ) and the induction of epigenetic reprogramming by Prdm14 and Prdm1 repression of the de novo deoxyribonucleic acid (DNA) methyltrans-ferase Dnmt3b and its cofactor Uhrf1; at the same time Prdm14 recruits 10–11 topoisomerases TET1 and TET2 to activate active hydroxylation of 5-methylcytosines and induce methylation marks erasure.

Following this approach, an interesting report has recently demonstrated the BMP independent function of Nanog as a master regulator of PGCLC specification from EpiLCs *in vitro*.[13] In this study, ectopic expression of Nanog over EpiLCs resulted in the activation of Prdm1 and Prdm14 as well as the acquisition of a PGCLC phenotype *in vitro*. Thus, this new study high-lighted the plasticity of PGC specification with the context-dependent role of a pluripotency-related transcription factor, such as Nanog, acting as a member of the core pluripotency network in mESCs and iPSCs, but inducing PGCLC formation in EpiLCs.

Although there exist several reports on differentiation of human pluri-potent stem cells into germ cells using different approaches,[14-21] the success of the reports described earlier in the mouse model inspired another recent works that adopted a very similar approach on human ESCs (hESCs) and iPSCs, demonstrating its reliability.[22-24] With slight differences in the cocktails employed to induce a mesodermic epiblast state from hESCs and human iPSCs (hiPSCs), in all three studies authors achieved the formation of a human PGCLC (hPGCLC) phenotype upon exposure of preinduced cells to BMPs, LIF, SCF and EGF. With similar conclusions, these works highlighted the mesodermic origin of hPGCLCs based on the need of creating a meso-dermic epiblast phenotype expressing T (Brachyury) for their efficient derivation. Also, resulting human PGCLCs from all three studies displayed several differences compared to the ones obtained in mouse, such as null activation of SOX2, a delayed expression of PRDM14 and an upregulation of SOX17 and GATA4. Results from one of the studies also concluded that in contrast with mouse PGC specification, SOX17 might play an essential role in human germ line specification by acting upstream and synergistically with BLIMP1 or PRDM1 as the master regulators of PGC specification, at the same time that BLIMP or PRDM1 acts as a repressor of the somatic program in human PGCLCs.[22] However, compared with mouse studies were PGCLCs were matured into functional gametes by transplanting them into mouse gonadal hosts, further maturation of human PGCLCs obtained *in vitro* was not investigated.

Related to the need of an animal host to achieve the complete maturation of human PGCLCs, it has recently been reported a new mouse study that based in the same approach has overcome this need and achieved the formation of functional gametes totally *in vitro*.[25] In this report, authors also followed the two-step induction of PGCLCs from EpiLCs. However, instead of transplanting them into a mouse gonad recipient, they used testicular somatic cells from KITW or KITW-V mice lacking germ cells to coculture with PGCLCs. After 2 weeks of PGCLC or testicular cells coculture with follicle-stimulating hormone (FSH), testosterone and bovine pituitary extract, around 14% of PGCLCs matured into spermatid-like haploid cells that were able to generate healthy offspring upon ICSI. This new achievement has supposed a new landmark since avoids totally the need of an animal host to generate gametes from pluripotent cells, offering an exceptional tool for the study of germ cell development and paves the way to its translation to humans.

Compared to the current knowledge of murine germ cell development, data regarding this process in humans has been scarce and based in classical histological studies.[26] However, the use of *in vitro* models of human germ cell derivation from pluripotent cells, together with very recent reports focused on the study of the germ cells development in early human embryos from a molecular point of view have supposed a new landmark.[27-29] Thanks to these last reports, now we have a better knowledge of the transcriptomic and epigenetic dynamics of human germ cells and indeed, the recent discovery of some evolutionary young transposable elements such as SINE-variable number of tandem repeats-Alu elements (SVAs) to resist epigenetic reprogramming of germ cell development *in vivo* opens new lines of study of the possibility of epigenetic inheritance with hPGCLCs obtained *in vitro*.[27]

MILLION-DOLLAR QUESTION: ARE THERE STEM CELLS IN THE HUMAN OVARY?

It is generally accepted that follicular regeneration occurs in most non-vertebrate animals[30] and in some vertebrates.[31] However, one of the central dogmas in reproductive medicine is that female mammals are born with a finite number of germ cells (follicular reserve) that decreases along individual's lifespan until become completely depleted at the start of menopause.[32] However, this view was questioned few years ago when John Tilly's group at Harvard University postulated the existence of ovarian stem cells in postnatal mammalian ovaries.[33] After counting the amount of atretic follicles in mouse ovaries, Tilly's group hypothesized that the ovarian reserve should become depleted at a much faster rate than what actually occurs, suggesting the presence of some kind of germinal stem cells within mammalian ovaries that replace atretic follicles by neofolliculogenesis. In order to test this hypothesis, ovarian fragments from wild-type mice were transplanted into the ovarian bursal cavity of transgenic green fluorescent protein (GFP) mice, resulting in the appearance of newly formed chimeric follicles with GFP positive oocytes surrounded by non-GFP expressing granulosa cells.[33] This first report on neofolliculogenesis caused great criticism since many argued against the methods employed to calculate follicle atresia and the ovarian graft results.[34,35]

In response to these criticisms, only 1 year later, based on the observation that stage-specific embryonic antigen-1 (SSEA-1) positive cells isolated from either disassociated mouse ovaries or bone marrow shared the expression of early germ line markers, Tilly's group suggested the bone marrow as the putative source of germ stem cells for adult neofolliculogenesis in mammals.[36] Supporting this idea, transplantations of both bone marrow and peripheral blood from GFP transgenic mice into chemotherapy-ablated wild-type females resulted in the formation of new chimeric follicles with GFP-positive oocytes.

In response to the intense discussion derived to these reports,[37] a new study comprising parabiosis experiments in which the circulatory systems of wild-type and GFP transgenic female mice were joined for up to 6 months demonstrated the presence of some GFP-positive granulosa cells associated with ovulated oocytes in wild-type mice, but no evidence of GFP-positive oocytes derived from GFP donors in wild-type females. In contrast to Tilly's results, transplantation of bone marrow from a GFP donor into wild-type females treated with cyclophosphamide or busulfan also failed to demonstrate the presence of oocyte chimerism, suggesting that the recovery of ovulation in chemically sterilized mice could be explained by incomplete depletion of endogenous follicles by the alquilant drugs, whereas the presence of some GFP-positive cells within the granulosa cell layer could be a consequence of the infiltration of white cells from the GFP donor.

After the publication of several reports supporting[38-42] or arguing against[43-45] the neofolliculogenesis hypothesis in mammalian ovaries, a new report in 2009[46] established germ stem cell lines *in vitro* from mouse vasa homolog (Mvh)-positive cells isolated from mouse ovaries. *In vitro* cultured Mvh cells expressed pluripotency-associated markers as well as early germ cell markers. Since Mvh is a ribonucleic acid (RNA) helicase that localizes in the cytoplasm of all germ cells, the use of an antibody for Mvh to isolate germ cells based on its surface membrane localization generated scepticism about these results.

More recently, Tilly's group published a new report in 2012 describing a similar approach to isolate Mvh or VASA germ cells from both mouse and human ovaries and establish germ cell line cultures *in vitro*.[47] Additionally, this report also demonstrated the spontaneous formation of oocyte-like cells (OLCs) able to complete meiosis in ovarian germ cell cultures. As a functional assay, *in vitro* cultures were labeled with GFP and either transplanted into mouse ovaries or cocultured with disassociated adult human cortical tissues and transplanted into immunosuppressed mice, resulting in the formation of GFP-positive oocytes that were able to form healthy embryos upon ICSI fertilization in the case of mouse oocytes. However, another recent report from a consortium of independent groups replicating the same experimental approach did not support the presence of VASA positive cells in the human ovary.[48]

With the exciting controversy upon the existence of neofolliculogenesis in the mammalian ovaries, some authors proposed an ovarian cell dedifferentiation process that, under specific *in vitro* conditions or stress may produce cells with certain potential to develop into germ-like cells in the same way as previously described for other cell types,[49-52] as one possible explanation for the existence of germinal stem cells in mammalian ovaries. Related to this hypothesis, some authors have even postulated a possible relationship between the existence of stem cells in the ovarian surface epithelium (OSE) and the origin of ovarian cancer of epithelial cells.[53] Alternatively, others also propose the presence of very small embryonic-like (VSEL) stem cells resident in the ovaries which have the potential to differentiate into both germ and somatic cells.[54]

Besides the great interests on demonstrating the existence of germ stem cells in the mammalian ovary that may lead to neofolliculogenesis and thus the design of strategies to restore the fertility of infertile women without follicular reserve, as can be the case of patients suffering premature follicular reserve depletion due to cancer treatments, their existence is not fully supported and further research is needed in order to solve this scientific debate. Nevertheless, with independence of the existence of stem cells in the ovary, other methods for fertility preservation, such as oocyte or embryo vitrification currently offered to this kind of patients is a worldwide employed technique with excellent results. Alternatively, in prepubertal patients or patients without possibility of obtaining oocytes before the initiation of their oncological treatment, ovarian cortex cryopreservation for its reimplantation after the disease has been overpassed is an experimental technique that has already probed its efficiency to restore fertility of oncological patients.[55]

SPERMATOGONIAL STEM CELLS: TAKING ADVANTAGE OF PLASTICITY OF SPERMATOGENESIS FOR FERTILITY PRESERVATION

Spermatogonial stem cells (SSCs) are the resident stem cells in the mammalian testes and the origin of the process of spermatogenesis during adulthood. The SSC pool is comprised by a subset of spermatogonia attached to the basal layer of the seminiferous tubules.[56] SSCs were first described in 1994 by Brinster's laboratory using a murine germ cell transplant model, and were defined as "the spermatogonial subpopulation of spermatogenic stem cells with the ability to colonize the seminiferous epithelium and fully reconstitute spermatogenesis".[57,58]

Due to their ability to potentially restore full spermatogenesis, there is great interest in the study and use of SSCs as a tool for fertility restoration. Specifically, patients unable to generate sperm such as prepubertal boys in risk of acquired permanent azoospermia due to the gonadotoxic effect of oncologic treatments can be potential beneficiaries from biotechnology derived of the study of SSCs.[59] Indeed, having in mind the use of SSCs to restore spermatogenesis, based in the Oncofertility Consortium of Northwestern University database, there are currently more than 120 health centers around the world offering the cryopreservation of testicular biopsies to prepubertal oncological patients in risk of permanent azoospermia as a consequence of their oncologic treatment.[60-65]

Among the strategies designed to restore spermatogenesis in azoospermic patients, the SSC transplantation (SSCT) is probably the most interesting.[66,67] Described for the first time by Brinster's laboratory in mice, transplantation of testicular cell suspensions containing spermatogonial cells into the germ cell depleted seminiferous lumen of mice results in its colonization and fully restoration of spermatogenesis, producing sperm able to give rise to healthy offspring.[57,58] Moreover, this technique has been applied to other animal models including nonhuman primates with successful results.[68] However, despite these encouraging results, there are three main issues to solve before the use of SSCT in humans. First, since transplantation of human SSCs (hSSCs) into germ cell depleted mouse testes results in colonization of the seminiferous epithelium, but fails to restore spermatogenesis because of phylogenetic discrepancies,[69] there is a need for appropriate models for spermatogenic restoration in humans beyond the technical trials performed in human cadaveric testes.[70] Second, the lack of appropriate markers to isolate SSCs has hampered their study, leaving their ability to colonize mouse testes is the best approach to identify them. By using this approach as a read out, several surface markers, such as GFRA1,[71] CD9,[72] fibroblast growth factor receptor 3 (FGFR3),[73,74] epithelial cell adhesion molecule (EpCAM),[75] integrin alpha 6 (ITGA6)[75-77] and THY-1,[76] as well as intracellular markers, such as PLZF, Sal-like protein 4 (SALL4), UTF1 and UCHL1[76] have been identified as putative hSSCs markers. The isolation of pure SSC populations is not only necessary for their study, but also as a technique to prevent the transplantation of malignant cells back into the testes of cancer survivors.[75] Finally, due to the limited size of testicular biopsies, *in vitro* propagation to increase the number of SSCs to transplant is a necessary step prior to perform SSCT in humans. However, although long-term *in vitro* propagation of mouse SSCs was first reported in 2003,[77] *in vitro* propagation of hSSCs[78,79] has been difficult to replicate.[80-83]

An alternative promising strategy to restore spermatogenesis is the testicular tissue grafting.[84] This approach consists of the engraftment of small pieces of immature (prepubertal) testicular tissue under the skin of immunosuppressed mice previously castrated in order to prevent the feedback inhibition of gonadotropins by their own testes. In this way, the host animals serve as bioreactors that activate spermatogenesis of engrafted tissue after few weeks, producing sperm that can be retrieved for ICSI and production of healthy offspring. As happened with the SSCT, this technique has also demonstrated its feasibility in other donor species, using always mice as hosts,[85,86] as well as slight improvement of results by modifying the engraftment in the scrotum[60] or even in intratesticular orthotopic grafts.[87] However, xenografts from other species with higher than average daily sperm production such as pig, goat and human donors show limited survival of the engrafted tissues and fibrosis probably due to insufficient vascularization causing ischemia.[60,61,85,88,89] Thus although data suggests that grafts from immature tissue show better resistance to ischemia due to the quiescent nature of tissue, so far human grafts designed to preserve spermatogenesis have not been able to develop beyond the spermatocyte stage,[61] highlighting once again that probably the mice are not the most appropriate hosts for human testicular grafts. Thus, despite its success in other animal models, this approach still needs further research to prevent ischemia of engrafted tissue as well as improvements to the technique to support full maturation of sperm cells before an eventual possible clinical application to produce functional human sperm in azoospermic patients.

In vitro spermatogenesis is a third approach that has gained interest in the last years as a possible source of sperm from SSCs. Despite the achievement of a recent report describing the production of haploid human spermatids able to fertilize mouse oocytes from SSCs obtained from cryptorchid patients and treated with SCF and retinoic acid (RA),[90] due to the three-dimensional (3D) structure of the spermatogenesis with several maturation stages of germ cells tightly dependent of sertoli cells regulation, most efficient strategies to achieve the production of sperm from mouse SSCs comprise 3D cocultures of both somatic and immature germ cells.[91] In a similar way to these 3D models of *in vitro* spermatogenesis, in 2011 a Japanese group obtained for the first time sperm able to be used in ICSI in a model of mouse 3D testis tissue culture.[92,93] In their work, authors used immature testicular pieces from newborn mice carrying GFP gene expression under the control of the postmeiotic markers Gsg2 (haspin) and acrosin, and were placed them in a liquid-gas interphase onto agarose rafts soaked in a medium containing knockout serum replacement and were placed at 34°C to mimic *in vivo* testicular conditions. After around 3 weeks, GFP spermatids and sperm were retrieved and used for ICSI, giving rise to healthy offspring. Although this technique has been reproduced in further reports,[94,95] no data regarding the feasibility of this technique with human tissue has been reported so far. However, the use of cytocompatible scaffolds from decellularized human testicular tissue may be an interesting approach to test the potential of hSSCs to mature *in vitro*.[96]

With an experience of more than 15 years of cryopreserving immature testicular biopsies from prepubertal patients, it seems a matter of time that the first reports on fertility restoration in azoospermic men appear.[97] However, even the success of different techniques of spermatogenesis restoration in animal models, as described earlier, there are still important issues to solve before the application of SSCs as a clinical cell therapy in the next years, making this possibility still an experimental procedure that should be offered only to patients with a high-risk of acquired azoospermia as the unique via to preserve their fertility.

ANSWER OF REGENERATIVE MEDICINE TO REPRODUCTIVE NEEDS: THE PROMISE MAY NOT BE SO FAR TO BE ACCOMPLISHED

Apart from the important advances of regenerative medicine about the potential use of stem cells as a source of functional gametes for human reproduction, their study itself has provided key insights for the better understanding of gamete-related diseases, as well as the design of new strategies to help patients affected by them.

Based in the expression of germ cell markers such as DAZL in hESCs, suggesting that this pluripotent stem cell stage could be formed by a heterogeneous population in which some cells may be primed toward a germ cell fate,[14] further investigation on the role of evolutionary conserved germ cell RNA-binding proteins such as the DAZL family[17,18] or VASA[21] suggested their role in the initiation of meiosis of *in vitro* differentiated germ cells from hESCs upon their exogenous expression. In the same line, another report demonstrated that DAZL may function in limiting pluripotency as well as differentiation to control apoptosis in PGCs through a robust interactive network. If this network is broken or DAZL expression is lost, the consequence is teratoma formation.[98] Moreover, by the employment of xenotransplantation of *in vitro* derived human germ cell-like cells into seminiferous tubules of immunosuppressed mice, one study demonstrated that ectopic expression of VASA in hiPSCs improved their colonization efficiency, highlighting the role that VASA plays in controlling the pluripotency state in a combined *in vitro* or *in vivo* model.[99] In the same line, recent reports have also designed a potential cell therapy for azoospermic men with microdeletions of the Y chromosome (AZFα), demonstrating the decreased ability of iPSCs derived from this kind of patients to colonize the seminiferous tubules of mice, and how the complementation via ectopic expression of DDX3Y can be a potential genetic therapy to rescue their ability to colonize this niche and form germ cell-like cells *in vivo*.[100,101] This same approach has also been used recently to demonstrate that germ cell-like cells can be formed *in vivo* independently of X chromosomes genetic profile.[102] In this case, hiPSCs from infertile Turner syndrome patients (46, XO) were derived and xenotransplanted into mice testes, resulting in proper colonization and demonstrating that the presence of a second X chromosome is not required for human germ cell formation, although is necessary for their maintenance until adulthood.

Finally, a recent study performed by our group opened a new interesting strategy for the obtention of human gametes by direct reprogramming of somatic cells.[103] Based in the success of direct transdifferentiation of somatic cells into other somatic cell fates,[104-108] human male somatic cells were directly transdifferentiated into a meiotic germ cell-like phenotype by the ectopic expression of PRDM1, PRDM14, LIN28A, DAZL, VASA and SYCP3 *in vitro*. Induced germ cell-like cells were able to colonize the seminiferous tubules of germ cell depleted mouse testes, showed their ability to form haploid cells and evidences of epigenetic reprograming toward an oocyte-like expected epigenetic profile. Despite the low efficiency of the germ cell-like transdifferentiation, it can represent a step forward to the creation of human functional gametes and serve as an *in vitro* model to test the role of critical key factors in human germ cell development.

CONCLUSION

The study of germ cells is critical for our society not only because of their potential use in human reproduction but because they have the extremely important task of transmitting genetic and epigenetic information to the next generation. In summary, all the advances discussed earlier represent significant improvements to our current knowledge of germ cell biology. Those may have important implications in reproductive medicine from the point of view of the future clinical use of the *in vitro* obtained gametes, but also for the information that they provide about germ cell biology for the design of new strategies to offer to infertile patients. Ultimately, with the proper ethical precautions, the combination of the study of germ cells with the new molecular techniques of gene editing can even be the next scientific landmark for the eradication of genetic diseases, as demonstrated by some preliminary reports.[109-111]

Taking together, for the first time in recent history it seems that the promise of regenerative medicine as a tool for treating all kind of diseases, including reproductive diseases, may not be so far to be accomplished.

ACKNOWLEDGMENT

This work was supported by a private donation of the Villarreal CF to Hospital Universitario y Politécnico La Fe intended to promote the scientific research on fertility preservation in child with cancer.

AUTHOR CONTRIBUTIONS

José V Medrano and Carlos Simón conceived this work and José V Medrano wrote the manuscript.

REFERENCES

1. Hübner K, Fuhrmann G, Christenson LK, et al. Derivation of oocytes from mouse embryonic stem cells. Science. 2003;300(5623):1251-6.
2. Toyooka Y, Tsunekawa N, Akasu R, et al. Embryonic stem cells can form germ cells in vitro. Proc Natl Acad Sci U S A. 2003;100(20):11457-62.
3. Geijsen N, Horoschak M, Kim K, et al. Derivation of embryonic germ cells and male gametes from embryonic stem cells. Nature. 2004;427(6970):148-54.
4. Novak I, Lightfoot DA, Wang H, et al. Mouse embryonic stem cells form follicle-like ovarian structures but do not progress through meiosis. Stem Cells. 2006;24(8):1931-6.
5. West JA, Viswanathan SR, Yabuuchi A, et al. A role for Lin28 in primordial germ-cell development and germ-cell malignancy. Nature. 2009;460(7257):909-13.
6. Nicholas CR, Haston KM, Grewall AK, et al. Transplantation directs oocyte maturation from embryonic stem cells and provides a therapeutic strategy for female infertility. Hum Mol Genet. 2009;18(22):4376-89.
7. Hayashi K, Surani MA. Self-renewing epiblast stem cells exhibit continual delineation of germ cells with epigenetic reprogramming in vitro. Development. 2009;136(21):3549-56.
8. Hayashi K, Ohta H, Kurimoto K, et al. Reconstitution of the mouse germ cell specification pathway in culture by pluripotent stem cells. Cell. 2011;146(4): 519-32.
9. Hayashi K, Ogushi S, Kurimoto K, et al. Offspring from oocytes derived from in vitro primordial germ cell-like cells in mice. Science. 2012;338(6109):971-5.
10. Okamura D, Hayashi K, Matsui Y. Mouse epiblasts change responsiveness to BMP4 signal required for PGC formation through functions of extraembryonic ectoderm. Mol Reprod Dev. 2005;70(1):20-9.
11. Günesdogan U, Magnúsdóttir E, Surani MA. Primoridal germ cell specification: a context-dependent cellular differentiation event. Philos Trans R Soc Lond B Biol Sci. 2014;369(1657).
12. Nakaki F, Hayashi K, Ohta H, et al. Induction of mouse germ-cell fate by transcription factors in vitro. Nature. 2013;501(7466):222-6.
13. Murakami K, Günesdogan U, Zylicz JJ, et al. NANOG alone induces germ cells in primed epiblast in vitro by activation of enhancers. Nature. 2016;529(7586): 403-7.
14. Clark AT, Bodnar MS, Fox M, et al. Spontaneous differentiation of germ cells from human embryonic stem cells in vitro. Hum Mol Genet. 2004;13(7):727-39.
15. Kee K, Gonsalves JM, Clark AT, et al. Bone morphogenetic proteins induce germ cell differentiation from human embryonic stem cells. Stem Cells Dev. 2006;15 (6):831-7.

16. Tilgner K, Atkinson SP, Golebiewska A, et al. Isolation of primordial germ cells from differentiating human embryonic stem cells. Stem Cells. 2008;26(12): 3075-85.
17. Kee K, Angeles VT, Flores M, et al. Human DAZL, DAZ and BOULE genes modulate primordial germ-cell and haploid gamete formation. Nature. 2009;462 (7270):222-5.
18. Panula S, Medrano JV, Kee K, et al. Human germ cell differentiation from fetal- and adult-derived induced pluripotent stem cells. Hum Mol Genet. 2011;20 (4):752-62.
19. Park TS, Galic Z, Conway AE, et al. Derivation of primordial germ cells from human embryonic and induced pluripotent stem cells is significantly improved by coculture with human fetal gonadal cells. Stem Cells. 2009;27(4):783-95.
20. Easley CA, Phillips BT, McGuire MM, et al. Direct differentiation of human pluripotent stem cells into haploid spermatogenic cells. Cell Rep. 2012;2(3):440-6.
21. Medrano JV, Ramathal C, Nguyen HN, et al. Divergent RNA-binding proteins, DAZL and VASA, induce meiotic progression in human germ cells derived in vitro. Stem Cells. 2012;30(3):441-51.
22. Irie N, Weinberger L, Tang WW, et al. SOX17 is a critical specifier of human primordial germ cell fate. Cell. 2015;160(1-2):253-68.
23. Sasaki K, Yokobayashi S, Nakamura T, et al. Robust In Vitro Induction of Human Germ Cell Fate from Pluripotent Stem Cells. Cell Stem Cell. 2015;17(2):178-94.
24. Sugawa F, Araúzo-Bravo MJ, Yoon J, et al. Human primordial germ cell commitment in vitro associates with a unique PRDM14 expression profile. EMBO J. 2015;34(8):1009-24.
25. Zhou Q, Wang M, Yuan Y, et al. Complete Meiosis from Embryonic Stem Cell-Derived Germ Cells In Vitro. Cell Stem Cell. 2016;18(3):330-40.
26. Napalkov P, Felici DM, Chu LK, et al. Incidence of catheter-related complications in patients with central venous or hemodialysis catheters: a health care claims database analysis. BMC Cardiovasc Disord. 2013;13:86.
27. Tang WW, Dietmann S, Irie N, et al. A Unique Gene Regulatory Network Resets the Human Germline Epigenome for Development. Cell. 2015;161(6): 1453-67.
28. Gkountela S, Zhang KX, Shafiq TA, et al. DNA Demethylation Dynamics in the Human Prenatal Germline. Cell. 2015;161(6):1425-36.
29. Guo F, Yan L, Guo H, et al. The Transcriptome and DNA Methylome Landscapes of Human Primordial Germ Cells. Cell. 2015;161(6):1437-52.
30. Lin H. The stem-cell niche theory: lessons from flies. Nat Rev Genet. 2002;3 (12):931-40.
31. Nakamura S, Kobayashi K, Nishimura T, et al. Identification of germline stem cells in the ovary of the teleost medaka. Science. 2010;328(5985):1561-3.
32. Green SH, Zuckerman S. The number of oocytes in the mature rhesus monkey (Macaca mulatta). J Endocrinol. 1951;7(2):194-202.
33. Johnson J, Canning J, Kaneko T, et al. Germline stem cells and follicular renewal in the postnatal mammalian ovary. Nature. 2004;428(6979):145-50.
34. Gosden RG. Germline stem cells in the postnatal ovary: is the ovary more like a testis? Hum Reprod Update. 2004;10(3):193-5.
35. Bristol-Gould SK, Kreeger PK, Selkirk CG, et al. Fate of the initial follicle pool: empirical and mathematical evidence supporting its sufficiency for adult fertility. Dev Biol. 2006;298(1):149-54.
36. Johnson J, Bagley J, Skaznik-Wikiel M, et al. Oocyte generation in adult mammalian ovaries by putative germ cells in bone marrow and peripheral blood. Cell. 2005;122(2):303-15.

37. Eggan K, Jurga S, Gosden R, et al. Ovulated oocytes in adult mice derive from non-circulating germ cells. Nature. 2006;441(7097):1109-14.

38. Lee HJ, Selesniemi K, Niikura Y, et al. Bone marrow transplantation generates immature oocytes and rescues long-term fertility in a preclinical mouse model of chemotherapy-induced premature ovarian failure. J Clin Oncol. 2007;25 (22):3198-204.

39. Bukovsky A, Caudle MR, Svetlikova M, et al. Origin of germ cells and formation of new primary follicles in adult human ovaries. Reprod Biol Endocrinol. 2004;2:20.

40. Bukovsky A, Svetlikova M, Caudle MR. Oogenesis in cultures derived from adult human ovaries. Reprod Biol Endocrinol. 2005;3:17.

41. Virant-Klun I, Zech N, Rozman P, et al. Putative stem cells with an embryonic character isolated from the ovarian surface epithelium of women with no naturally present follicles and oocytes. Differentiation. 2008;76(8):843-56.

42. Szotek PP, Chang HL, Brennand K, et al. Normal ovarian surface epithelial label-retaining cells exhibit stem/progenitor cell characteristics. Proc Natl Acad Sci U S A. 2008;105(34):12469-73.

43. Liu Y, Wu C, Lyu Q, et al. Germline stem cells and neo-oogenesis in the adult human ovary. Dev Biol. 2007;306(1):112-20.

44. Begum S, Papaioannou VE, Gosden RG. The oocyte population is not renewed in transplanted or irradiated adult ovaries. Hum Reprod. 2008;23(10):2326-30.

45. Veitia RA, Gluckman E, Fellous M, et al. Recovery of female fertility after chemotherapy, irradiation, and bone marrow allograft: further evidence against massive oocyte regeneration by bone marrow-derived germline stem cells. Stem Cells. 2007;25(5):1334-5.

46. Zou K, Yuan Z, Yang Z, et al. Production of offspring from a germline stem cell line derived from neonatal ovaries. Nat Cell Biol. 2009;11(5):631-6.

47. White YA, Woods DC, Takai Y, et al. Oocyte formation by mitotically active germ cells purified from ovaries of reproductive-age women. Nat Med. 2012;18(3): 413-21.

48. Zhang H, Panula S, Petropoulos S, et al. Adult human and mouse ovaries lack DDX4-expressing functional oogonial stem cells. Nat Med. 2015;21(10):1116-8.

49. Lei L, Spradling AC. Female mice lack adult germ-line stem cells but sustain oogenesis using stable primordial follicles. Proc Natl Acad Sci U S A. 2013;110 (21):8585-90.

50. Wei S, Zan L, Hausman GJ, et al. Dedifferentiated adipocyte-derived progeny cells (DFAT cells): Potential stem cells of adipose tissue. Adipocyte. 2013;2 (3):122-7.

51. Herreros-Villanueva M, Zhang JS, Koenig A, et al. SOX2 promotes dedifferentiation and imparts stem cell-like features to pancreatic cancer cells. Oncogenesis. 2013;2:e61.

52. Lee ST, Gong SP, Yum KE, et al. Transformation of somatic cells into stem cell-like cells under a stromal niche. FASEB J. 2013;27(7):2644-56.

53. Bowen NJ, Walker LD, Matyunina LV, et al. Gene expression profiling supports the hypothesis that human ovarian surface epithelia are multipotent and capable of serving as ovarian cancer initiating cells. BMC Med Genomics. 2009; 2:71.

54. Bhartiya D, Unni S, Parte S, et al. Very small embryonic-like stem cells: implications in reproductive biology. Biomed Res Int. 2013;2013:682326.

55. Donnez J, Dolmans MM, Pellicer A, et al. Restoration of ovarian activity and pregnancy after transplantation of cryopreserved ovarian tissue: a review of 60 cases of reimplantation. Fertil Steril. 2013;99(6):1503-13.

56. de Rooij DG. The spermatogonial stem cell niche. Microsc Res Tech. 2009;72 (8):580-5.
57. Brinster RL, Avarbock MR. Germline transmission of donor haplotype following spermatogonial transplantation. Proc Natl Acad Sci U S A. 1994;91(24):11303-7.
58. Brinster RL, Zimmermann JW. Spermatogenesis following male germ-cell transplantation. Proc Natl Acad Sci U S A. 1994;91(24):11298-302.
59. Geens M, Goossens E, De Block G, et al. Autologous spermatogonial stem cell transplantation in man: current obstacles for a future clinical application. Hum Reprod Update. 2008;14(2):121-30.
60. Wyns C, Curaba M, Martinez-Madrid B, et al. Spermatogonial survival after cryopreservation and short-term orthotopic immature human cryptorchid testicular tissue grafting to immunodeficient mice. Hum Reprod. 2007;22 (6):1603-11.
61. Wyns C, Van Langendonckt A, Wese FX, et al. Long-term spermatogonial survival in cryopreserved and xenografted immature human testicular tissue. Hum Reprod. 2008;23(11):2402-14.
62. Baert Y, Van Saen D, Haentjens P, et al. What is the best cryopreservation protocol for human testicular tissue banking? Hum Reprod. 2013;28(7):1816-26.
63. Goossens E, Van Saen D, Tournaye H. Spermatogonial stem cell preservation and transplantation: from research to clinic. Hum Reprod. 2013;28(4):897-907.
64. Poels J, Van Langendonckt A, Many MC, et al. Vitrification preserves proliferation capacity in human spermatogonia. Hum Reprod. 2013;28(3):578-89.
65. Gassei K, Orwig KE. Experimental methods to preserve male fertility and treat male factor infertility. Fertil Steril. 2016;105(2):256-66.
66. Medrano JV, Martinez-Arroyo AM, Sukhwani M, et al. Germ cell transplantation into mouse testes procedure. Fertil Steril. 2014;102(4):e11-2.
67. Ogawa T, Aréchaga JM, Avarbock MR, et al. Transplantation of testis germinal cells into mouse seminiferous tubules. Int J Dev Biol. 1997;41(1):111-22.
68. Hermann BP, Sukhwani M, Winkler F, et al. Spermatogonial stem cell transplantation into rhesus testes regenerates spermatogenesis producing functional sperm. Cell Stem Cell. 2012;11(5):715-26.
69. Nagano M, Patrizio P, Brinster RL. Long-term survival of human spermatogonial stem cells in mouse testes. Fertil Steril. 2002;78(6):1225-33.
70. Faes K, Tournaye H, Goethals L, et al. Testicular cell transplantation into the human testes. Fertil Steril. 2013;100(4):981-8.
71. von Schönfeldt V, Wistuba J, Schlatt S. Notch-1, c-kit and GFRalpha-1 are developmentally regulated markers for premeiotic germ cells. Cytogenet Genome Res. 2004;105(2-4):235-9.
72. Kanatsu-Shinohara M, Toyokuni S, Shinohara T. CD9 is a surface marker on mouse and rat male germline stem cells. Biol Reprod. 2004;70(1):70-5.
73. von Kopylow K, Schulze W, Salzbrunn A, et al. Isolation and gene expression analysis of single potential human spermatogonial stem cells. Mol Hum Reprod. 2016;22(4):229-39.
74. von Kopylow K, Staege H, Schulze W, et al. Fibroblast growth factor receptor 3 is highly expressed in rarely dividing human type A spermatogonia. Histochem Cell Biol. 2012;138(5):759-72.
75. Dovey SL, Valli H, Hermann BP, et al. Eliminating malignant contamination from therapeutic human spermatogonial stem cells. J Clin Invest. 2013;123(4): 1833-43.
76. Valli H, Sukhwani M, Dovey SL, et al. Fluorescence- and magnetic-activated cell sorting strategies to isolate and enrich human spermatogonial stem cells. Fertil Steril. 2014;102(2):566-80.e7.

77. Kanatsu-Shinohara M, Ogonuki N, Inoue K, et al. Long-term proliferation in culture and germline transmission of mouse male germline stem cells. Biol Reprod. 2003;69(2):612-6.

78. Sadri-Ardekani H, Mizrak SC, van Daalen SK, et al. Propagation of human spermatogonial stem cells in vitro. JAMA. 2009;302(19):2127-34.

79. Sadri-Ardekani H, Akhondi MA, van der Veen F, et al. In vitro propagation of human prepubertal spermatogonial stem cells. JAMA. 2011;305(23):2416-8.

80. Chikhovskaya JV, Jonker MJ, Meissner A, et al. Human testis-derived embryonic stem cell-like cells are not pluripotent, but possess potential of mesenchymal progenitors. Hum Reprod. 2012;27(1):210-21.

81. Chikhovskaya JV, van Daalen SK, Korver CM, et al. Mesenchymal origin of multipotent human testis-derived stem cells in human testicular cell cultures. Mol Hum Reprod. 2014;20(2):155-67.

82. Eildermann K, Gromoll J, Behr R. Misleading and reliable markers to differentiate between primate testis-derived multipotent stromal cells and spermatogonia in culture. Hum Reprod. 2012;27(6):1754-67.

83. Baert Y, Braye A, Struijk RB, et al. Cryopreservation of testicular tissue before long-term testicular cell culture does not alter in vitro cell dynamics. Fertil Steril. 2015;104(5):1244-52.e1-4.

84. Honaramooz A, Snedaker A, Boiani M, et al. Sperm from neonatal mammalian testes grafted in mice. Nature. 2002;418(6899):778-81.

85. Arregui L, Rathi R, Zeng W, et al. Xenografting of adult mammalian testis tissue. Anim Reprod Sci. 2008;106(1-2):65-76.

86. Shinohara T, Inoue K, Ogonuki N, et al. Birth of offspring following transplantation of cryopreserved immature testicular pieces and in-vitro microinsemination. Hum Reprod. 2002;17(12):3039-45.

87. Van Saen D, Goossens E, Bourgain C, et al. Meiotic activity in orthotopic xenografts derived from human postpubertal testicular tissue. Hum Reprod. 2011; 26(2):282-93.

88. Geens M, De Block G, Goossens E, et al. Spermatogonial survival after grafting human testicular tissue to immunodeficient mice. Hum Reprod. 2006;21(2): 390-6.

89. Schlatt S, Honaramooz A, Ehmcke J, et al. Limited survival of adult human testicular tissue as ectopic xenograft. Hum Reprod. 2006;21(2):384-9.

90. Yang S, Ping P, Ma M, et al. Generation of haploid spermatids with fertilization and development capacity from human spermatogonial stem cells of cryptorchid patients. Stem Cell Reports. 2014;3(4):663-75.

91. Stukenborg JB, Wistuba J, Luetjens CM, et al. Coculture of spermatogonia with somatic cells in a novel three-dimensional soft-agar-culture-system. J Androl. 2008;29(3):312-29.

92. Sato T, Katagiri K, Gohbara A, et al. In vitro production of functional sperm in cultured neonatal mouse testes. Nature. 2011;471(7339):504-7.

93. Sato T, Katagiri K, Kubota Y, et al. In vitro sperm production from mouse spermatogonial stem cell lines using an organ culture method. Nat Protoc. 2013;8 (11):2098-104.

94. Sato T, Yokonishi T, Komeya M, et al. Testis tissue explantation cures spermatogenic failure in c-Kit ligand mutant mice. Proc Natl Acad Sci U S A. 2012;109 (42):16934-8.

95. Yokonishi T, Sato T, Komeya M, et al. Offspring production with sperm grown in vitro from cryopreserved testis tissues. Nat Commun. 2014;5:4320.

96. Baert Y, Stukenborg JB, Landreh M, et al. Derivation and characterization of a cytocompatible scaffold from human testis. Hum Reprod. 2015;30(2):256-67.

97. Picton HM, Wyns C, Anderson RA, et al. A European perspective on testicular tissue cryopreservation for fertility preservation in prepubertal and adolescent boys. Hum Reprod. 2015;30(11):2463-75.

98. Chen HH, Welling M, Bloch DB, et al. DAZL limits pluripotency, differentiation, and apoptosis in developing primordial germ cells. Stem Cell Reports. 2014;3(5):892-904.

99. Durruthy Durruthy J, Ramathal C, Sukhwani M, et al. Fate of induced pluripotent stem cells following transplantation to murine seminiferous tubules. Hum Mol Genet. 2014;23(12):3071-84.

100. Ramathal C, Angulo B, Sukhwani M, et al. DDX3Y gene rescue of a Y chromosome AZFa deletion restores germ cell formation and transcriptional programs. Sci Rep. 2015;5:15041.

101. Ramathal C, Durruthy-Durruthy J, Sukhwani M, et al. Fate of iPSCs derived from azoospermic and fertile men following xenotransplantation to murine seminiferous tubules. Cell Rep. 2014;7(4):1284-97.

102. Dominguez AA, Chiang HR, Sukhwani M,et al. Human germ cell formation in xenotransplants of induced pluripotent stem cells carrying X chromosome aneuploidies. Sci Rep. 2014;4:6432.

103. Medrano JV, Martinez-Arroyo AM, Miguez JM, et al. Human somatic cells subjected to genetic induction with six germ line-related factors display meiotic germ cell-like features. Sci Rep. 2016;6:24956.

104. Kim J, Efe JA, Zhu S, et al. Direct reprogramming of mouse fibroblasts to neural progenitors. Proc Natl Acad Sci U S A. 2011;108(19):7838-43.

105. Vierbuchen T, Ostermeier A, Pang ZP, et al. Direct conversion of fibroblasts to functional neurons by defined factors. Nature. 2010;463(7284):1035-41.

106. Szabo E, Rampalli S, Risueño RM, et al. Direct conversion of human fibroblasts to multilineage blood progenitors. Nature. 2010;468(7323):521-6.

107. Ieda M, Fu JD, Delgado-Olguin P, et al. Direct reprogramming of fibroblasts into functional cardiomyocytes by defined factors. Cell. 2010;142(3):375-86.

108. Buganim Y, Itskovich E, Hu YC, et al. Direct reprogramming of fibroblasts into embryonic Sertoli-like cells by defined factors. Cell Stem Cell. 2012;11(3):373-86.

109. Chapman KM, Medrano GA, Jaichander P, et al. Targeted Germline Modifications in Rats Using CRISPR/Cas9 and Spermatogonial Stem Cells. Cell Rep. 2015;10(11):1828-35.

110. Sato T, Sakuma T, Yokonishi T, et al. Genome Editing in Mouse Spermatogonial Stem Cell Lines Using TALEN and Double-Nicking CRISPR/Cas9. Stem Cell Reports. 2015;5(1):75-82.

111. Vassena R, Heindryckx B, Peco R, et al. Genome engineering through CRISPR/Cas9 technology in the human germline and pluripotent stem cells. Hum Reprod Update. 2016;22(4):411-9.

Index

Page numbers followed by *f* refer to figure and *t* refer to table.